SOUL MEDICINE

RETURNING THE SPIRIT
TO HEALING

Helen Graham

Newleaf

Newleaf

an imprint of
Gill & Macmillan Ltd
Hume Avenue
Park West
Dublin 12

with associated companies throughout the world
www.gillmacmillan.ie
© Helen Graham 2001
0 7171 2999 3

Index compiled by
Susan Williams
Design and print origination by
O'K Graphic Design, Dublin

Printed by ColourBooks Ltd, Dublin

A catalogue record is available for this book from the British Library.

1 3 5 4 2

For Janet

CONTENTS

Integration + Common ?
Why the book is good - for me.

INTRODUCTION

J anet is a friend of my sister Anne. Anne and her family had been invited to spend part of their summer holiday with Janet and her husband Dominic at their cottage in France. These plans were suspended when Janet suddenly and dramatically became ill. Within days of developing a persistent headache and symptoms independently diagnosed by three general medical practitioners as those of 'flu, she was in a coma in a hospital intensive care unit (ICU). Baffled doctors could only surmise that Janet's brain had been attacked by an unspecified virus. They told Dominic that the prognosis was very poor. This was confirmed when a few days later Dominic was told that Janet had no hope of recovery. She was severely neurologically impaired demonstrating no signs of mental function and in the absence of more specific treatment for her condition the decision was made that she would be moved to a general ward where, given her physical state, and without intensive care she was expected to succumb quickly to infection. If Janet were to survive she would remain in a persistent vegetative state — an irreversible coma.

Dominic was distraught. He refused to accept that Janet was beyond hope and pestered the doctors to keep treating her in the intensive care unit — to no avail. Before Janet was due to be moved from the ICU, Dominic and his daughters were sitting at her bedside when he noticed her eyeballs move under her eyelids. The nurses assured him that this was a reflex action. Yet, it seemed to Dominic that Janet was following the family conversation. When he tested this by asking Janet to look first in one direction and then in the other he felt she responded accordingly. Moreover, when Dominic took Janet's hand she responded by lightly squeezing it. Some days later when settled on the ward, Janet spoke, and when she did so it was to answer a question that had been preoccupying her daughters. Everyone else was speechless.

So too was my sister when she visited Janet in hospital shortly after she was allowed to receive visitors. Janet insisted that she had been 'with' Anne one night during her illness, a night Anne recollected all too vividly. She had been so upset to learn of Janet's apparently hopeless condition that she had been unable to sleep and had spent a very disturbed and disturbing night thinking about her and a mutual friend who was dying. Without having been told, Janet knew of the friend's subsequent death and details of the funeral my sister had attended while Janet lay technically 'dead' in a hospital sixty miles away. Janet also knew that one of her daughters was pregnant, although her daughter was still unaware of this at the time, and that she would give birth to a daughter, which subsequently she did.

Although just about able to speak, Janet was otherwise effectively paralysed as a result of almost total muscular collapse throughout her body. She required intensive physiotherapy to restore movement to her wasted limbs. It was two months before she could feed herself and six months before she could walk, having had to completely re-learn this skill. Eventually, though, she was able to return to work.

It was some time before Janet was able to visit the staff of the ICU to thank them for their efforts on her behalf. They were shocked to find that Janet, who had been comatose throughout her stay in the unit, recognised nursing staff she had not 'seen' before, and recalled personal details about them that she had learned while there. One nurse was astonished when Janet commented on her hairstyle, which was now different from when she had attended to Janet. It was clear that Janet had seen and heard a good deal of what was occurring around her when she was lying in coma, including comments made directly to her by medical staff and family members and conversations between medical staff. Her doctors confessed that her case had shaken them considerably.

It has taken time for everybody concerned with Janet's illness and recovery to come to terms with what occurred. No one, least of all her doctors, can explain what happened or why. Dominic and his daughters have been too relieved and delighted to delve into the whys and wherefores. They have Janet with them. That, and her continued health and well-being are all that matter. They also have a new family member, the granddaughter whose existence Janet knew of before it was medically confirmed, and with whom Janet feels a particularly special bond.

Janet eluded death at the eleventh hour, although technically she was considered to have severe neurological impairment for some time beforehand. Her experience, while remarkable, is by no means unique. Such cases often highlight tremendous advances in medical technology, particularly in relation to methods of life saving and support. Inevitably, however, they also draw attention to the shortcomings of contemporary Western medicine with its materialistic emphasis on the body. Janet's illness and recovery challenge almost every principle of orthodox scientific medicine. Her case highlights the limitations of contemporary medicine, and raises questions about human life and nature that Western medicine generally chooses to ignore.

Janet's case also challenges contemporary Western psychology. It raises questions that are simply not addressed, as yet unresolved and unanswered questions about mind and consciousness and their relationship to the body.

The questions raised by Janet's experience are as old as mankind itself. Ultimately they are concerns about human nature, life and death. Throughout history, and until relatively recently, attempts to consider these questions have focused upon the soul, in particular its importance in relation to health and illness and the dangers in ignoring it, and so traditional approaches to healing throughout history and all over the world have tended to address the person in body, mind and soul or spirit. Yet in present day orthodox medicine and psychology the soul is completely ignored. So why then do we still speak of the soul in this age of science? As physician Larry Dossey answers the question he poses:

> The main reason is that something vital has been left out of almost all modern efforts to understand our mental life — something that counts as a first principle, without which everything is bound to be incomplete and off base.[1]

He points out that virtually every modern explanation of mind assumes it can be found in a certain place in time or space:

> The spatial place to which the mind has traditionally been fixed is the brain of an individual person; the temporal place to which it is assigned is the present moment and a single lifetime. Thus, a mind is consigned and isolated to an individual person. And, what is worse, it is thus doomed to oblivion, for with the death of the brain it must also die.[2]

These local assumptions underlie almost all the scholarly Western attempts to describe the human mind, but Dossey believes that trying to *locate* the mind, to try to fix it in time and space, is a flaw in this approach. He tells us there is good evidence that mind cannot be localised; that it displays its non-local character in millions of ways, showing that it is free in space and time, that it bridges consciousness between persons, and does not die. He supports his claims with scientific evidence and observations drawn from his many years as a doctor.

Janet's experience is fully consistent with, and reinforcing of, these claims. It points to a non-local aspect of mind that can transcend the body, can travel in time — in her case into the future — and in space, that has valid and accurate knowledge and information unobtainable by her ordinary senses. Dossey indicates that this non-local aspect of mind closely resembles what has traditionally been described as the soul — a timeless, spaceless and immortal aspect of the person — and that 'recovering the non-local nature of mind, then, is essentially recovery of the soul'.[3] This, he suggests, redirects 'the imperatives of medicine' away from its 'sole' concern with the body.

Certainly, Janet's case highlights the need for a truly psychological medicine which literally (from the Greek words *psyche*, 'soul', and *logos*, 'study' or 'knowledge'; and the Latin *medicina*, the art of healing) means applying knowledge of the soul in the art of healing. As such, psychological medicine is not an alternative to or substitute for orthodox Western medicine but provides a more inclusive context for it, embracing and integrating body, mind and spirit. It is my hope that this book, which examines the scope and nature of such an endeavour, may help Janet come to terms with her experience; and that her experience may persuade others to recognise the vital importance to medicine of healing the soul.

The problems in achieving the latter goal cannot be underestimated. At the present time the concept of soul has no status at all within medicine or psychology and the term is virtually absent from the literature of both disciplines. More surprisingly, it is also not found in contemporary theological literature and is not even listed in the index of a major encyclopaedia of religion published in the 1990s.[4] While 'soul' as a prefix is common in everyday language (soul searching, soul sickness, soul destroying, soulless, soulful, soul mate, soul food, soul music and so on) and 'soul' frequently appears in titles of books, journal and newspaper articles, it is rarely defined. In popular usage its meaning is taken for granted. So much so that those wishing to understand the term, let alone study it, and apply the findings in the attainment and maintenance of health or the treatment of illness, have a difficult task on their hands.

The aim of this book is to make this task easier. It presents a digest of information concerning the soul as it has been understood historically and cross-culturally since the earliest times. The book examines the ways in which this knowledge has traditionally been applied within medicine and how it is currently supported by contemporary scientific thinking and research. It also discusses the implications of new understanding of the soul for psychology and medicine of the future.

The book takes as its starting point the fact that belief in the existence of the soul is common to all cultures and that the beliefs themselves are remarkably similar throughout the world. Within Western culture the idea of the soul as a vehicle for personal existence — as the life force or principle — is continuous from antiquity to the present day and until the seventeenth century Western psychology consisted essentially of a variety of doctrines concerning the soul.

Chapter One traces Western thinking about the soul and its psychology (literally, the 'study of the soul') from its origins in the mystically inspired ancient wisdom of early civilisations through to the scientific wisdom of the twentieth century. It examines the shift away from animism — the belief that everything has a soul — to a rationalism that brings the concept of soul and, indeed, its very existence, into question. Consideration is also given to the impact of the emergence of rational thinking in Western civilisation, Western religions and the scientific revolutions of the seventeenth and twentieth centuries.

Chapter Two indicates how the history of medicine in the Western world until the nineteenth century largely consisted of the application of knowledge concerning the soul to healing. The chapter identifies some of the influences that have led to the widespread belief in the West that medicine has little or nothing to do with the soul and looks at the contemporary scientific challenges to this view.

Chapter Three shows how Eastern psychologies, which originate in similar sources of wisdom to the psychology of the West, retain the soul as their central focus, yet are fully consistent with contemporary

Western scientific thinking about the universe.

Chapter Four shows how the traditional spiritual concerns of the psychologies of the East are reflected in Eastern healing practices, notably in Ayurveda and Tibetan, Chinese, Japanese and Sufi medicine, and how these practices embody principles that are increasingly admitted within orthodox Western medicine.

Chapter Five examines the implications of the loss of soul in the twentieth century for Western psychotherapy, traditionally and literally, 'the cure of the soul'. It traces the shift from soul to self and back to soul in psychodynamic psychology, humanistic psychology and transpersonal psychology.

Chapter Six presents arguments and evidence that allow for the readmission of the soul as a legitimate subject of concern and investigation within contemporary Western science. It examines the key principles of twentieth century physics and their implications for medicine and psychology. It also examines growing scientific evidence for human energy fields and the overlap between these discoveries and the long-standing, universal ideas about the soul.

Chapter Seven discusses the implications for medicine and psychology of a scientific redefinition of the soul, arguing the need in the twenty-first century for psychological medicine that treats the whole person, body, mind and soul. It examines the implications of models of medicine for the therapeutic relationship and assesses the nature and outcomes of effective therapeutic relationships.

Chapter Eight examines the nature of diagnosis in psychological medicine and how this relates to the scientific principles established in the twentieth century and traditional approaches to divining the soul.

Chapter Nine examines the applications of psychological medicine in treatment, considering the therapeutic uses of colour; light and sound; other subtle energy medicines such as homeopathy and flower essences; touch; 'imaginative' approaches involving the application of mental imagery and the arts; and the involvement of animals as therapeutic agents.

The postscript describes in more detail the experiences of Janet, and concludes by arguing the case for a literal psychological medicine — healing the soul — as the medicine of the twenty-first century, the medicine of the new millennium.

1

STUDENTS OF THE SOUL

The mystical origins of psychology

L.S. Hearnshaw begins his scholarly survey of the development of psychology[1] from the dawn of civilisation to the present day with Francis Bacon's claim (1609) that 'the most ancient times are buried in oblivion and silence.' He indicates that while this is certainly true of humans' earliest speculations and beliefs concerning their own nature, the obscurity is not quite so dense as it was in Bacon's time. Some information about human prehistory has emerged from archaeological excavations. Anthropological studies of still primitive and isolated peoples have also made possible tentative reconstructions of prehistoric man and his mode of life, and from these sources a primeval psychology can be gleaned. Prehistoric art shows that early humans were conscious of the world around them and, by the time they had begun to bury their dead with provision for an afterlife, they were tacitly postulating a part of themselves that survived death. Hearnshaw indicates that primitive psychology is grounded in these experiences, and that anthropological evidence provides a glimpse of it.

He suggests that as soon as humans became actively conscious they must inevitably have searched for meanings in order to explain the mysterious and uncertain world they occupied. They did so by postulating a soul, a tenuously physical substance such as breath or spirit, possessed of all natural phenomena and the universe itself; an immaterial force that animates the entire universe. Accordingly, all things have souls, not merely humans. This belief, which in the nineteenth century became known as **animism** (after the Latin word *anima*, meaning soul), is a universal feature of primitive thought, suggesting that it must be based in some common human experience. The pioneering English anthropologist Sir Edwin Tylor (1832–1917), who coined the term, believed that animism probably originated in dreaming which suggests existence independent of the physical body.

Ancient wisdom

Certainly it might be supposed that for early humans the world was shrouded in mystery and that without modern-day understanding of mundane phenomena the world was a magical and awesome place. However, there are indications in ancient mythology and in various teachings passed down through history that early humans were inherently attuned to nature, instinctively and collectively understood its fundamental forces and lived in accordance with them. Such wisdom was not a function of intellect or reasoning but rather of an intuitive grasp of the truth of things, a seeing into them, or insight. This instinctive aspect of the ancient mind appears to have been a feature of pre-literate cultures. Human nature was part of a whole. Hence, 'there was no need for the search for unity and meaning before human beings became self-conscious, when humans (just as other animals still seem to be) were at one with their universe.'[2] This ancient wisdom has largely, although not totally, been lost by mankind during the course of intellectual evolution, as the parts of the brain specialised for language and related functions evolved and eclipsed those parts of the brain specialised for non-verbal intuitive processes. Consequently it is very difficult for people today to understand the ancients or the world in which they belonged.

Nevertheless, the ancient wisdom, although fragmented and obscured, has never fully disappeared but has been passed down in various, mostly secret, traditions. 'It runs like an underground river emerging now and then into the light of day, then disappearing again beneath the surface.'[3] Within the West it has surfaced in a number of orders and fraternities, such as the Order of the Golden Dawn, the Order of the Temple, the Albigenses, the Brethren of the Golden and Rosy Cross, the Illuminati, Magnetists, Theosophists and Kabbalists. Furthermore, primitive thought survives in occultism, spiritualism, witchcraft, esotericism and many cults of the contemporary world and is far from dead.

All of these traditions share the aim of realising the truth of the world through the development of insight and intuition. They assert that certain learned ways of perceiving confine human awareness to what is immediately apparent. Yet a far greater, hidden, or occult, reality exists beyond normal awareness and ordinary comprehension. This is an infinite, ever-changing, expanding, indivisible and ultimately indescribable universe of harmonious relationships and interrelationships of which man is part. Those individuals with insight into the true nature of the universe and its mysteries are variously referred to as visionaries, seers, clairvoyants, or mystics.

> In the true mystic there is an extension of normal consciousness, a release of latent powers and a widening of vision, so that aspects of truth unplumbed by the rational intellect are revealed to him. Both in feeling and thought he apprehends an immanence of the temporal in the eternal and the eternal in the temporal ... Though he may not be able to describe it in words, though he may not be able logically to demonstrate its validity, to the mystic his experience is fully and absolutely valid and is surrounded by complete certainty. He has been 'there', he has 'seen', he 'knows'.[4]

Accordingly, throughout history and all parts of the world, **mysticism** is characterised by certain beliefs. These include the concept of a timeless reality beyond and utterly different to the world of ordinary appearance, a reality which, though interwoven with the external world of material phenomena, is not of it. Knowledge of this reality and awareness of the unity and indivisibility of all phenomena come by revelation, sudden insight or intuition 'certain beyond the possibility of doubt'.[5] Mysticism is not a doctrine or learned dogma, but a personal experience, an inner knowing or conviction.

Mysticism appears to underpin the beliefs of early man and to be prior to, and the root of all, religious traditions. It is evident in the thinking of the Australian Aborigines, who are among the best documented of the primitive peoples studied by anthropologists. They had been almost totally isolated for tens of thousands of years and were still living in a Stone Age culture at the end of the eighteenth century when Australia was colonised by Western Europeans. The Aborigines' ancient ways of life disappeared only gradually as Europeans spread across the continent and the first anthropologists were able to study them while their culture remained intact.

The soul in pre-literate cultures

The whole structure of life for Aborigines was underpinned by an elaborate system of mythical ideas and beliefs. These expressed the essential unity of man and nature, the earth and all creatures, and the solidarity of the present with the ancestral beings of the 'eternal dreamtime', or *alcheringa*, a Golden Age of the past. The dreamtime permeated all aspects of Aboriginal life, gave it meaning and a deeply felt spiritual character. The core of each person, his or her true nature or soul, belonged to this pre-existing realm of spirits, descending from and returning to the spirit world after death, as did all the diverse forms assumed by persons and objects. The spirit world was not divorced from the natural world and material bodies as these were impregnated with spiritual qualities and everything was sacred and linked. As it integrated the world, living in harmony with the dreamtime was essential. Hence Aboriginal lore proclaimed that 'he who loses his dreamtime is lost.' So, it would seem, in the primitive 'there is existent and permeating on earth, in the air and on the water, in all the diverse forms assumed by persons and objects, one and the same essential reality; both one and multiple, both material and spiritual.'[6]

From the all-pervading dreamtime of the Aborigines, animism developed in three directions. In the supernatural sphere a host of gods, demons and other spiritual beings proliferated. In the world of nature, animal, plant and object souls accounted for the ways in which natural objects and living things function and behave. In the human domain spiritual powers explained the vicissitudes of man's experience and the fluctuations of his behaviour and destiny. During the long primeval period of humanity the rate of change by historical standards was slow and systems of belief were static. Hence beliefs and practices comparable to those of the Aborigines probably prevailed for many millennia in prehistoric times, almost certainly as far back as the earliest burials. Signs of elaboration are found only in the much more advanced cultures of the Neolithic period, such as the Maori of New Zealand.

The Maori believed that humans inherit a sacred spark of divine nature. This *ira atua* represents true vitality and is the source of physical and moral well-being. It has to be protected because once defiled the links between the individual and the ruling forces of the world are broken and he or she is helpless. This unity of man and nature, physical and spiritual worlds, individuals and their fellows is all-important.

The Maori also believed that, like all other things, living and non-living, humans possess a life principle (*mauri*) that cannot leave the body and ceases to exist at death. This is distinct from the soul, or *wairua*, a tenuous material substance which is not located in any particular body organ, departs the body at death and during dreaming sleep, and after death becomes a refined, immaterial immortal spirit. The Maoris believed that the soul is visible to persons possessing second sight. This belief supports the view that early humans did not *postulate* the existence of the soul, as claimed by Hearnshaw, but perceived it directly. That is, their beliefs about the soul were not arrived at by reasoning but through experience.

> Apparently, there is something fundamental to human experience that usually requires such a label. Such evidence does not establish the ontological status of the soul, but it does point to something being signified.[7]

Extensive research on tribal societies points to a similar conclusion. Not only are ideas about the soul similar throughout the world, but belief in the soul and ideas about its nature and function have also been repeatedly confirmed and strengthened by the actual living experience of people in all cultures and epochs. 'The belief in a soul is therefore not a tradition but a living reality.'[8]

Historical and ethnological studies reveal beliefs about the soul common to all primitive cultures. The soul is the life principle, the prerequisite of consciousness, the source of health and strength, and can exist independently of the body, which lives only by virtue of the soul, is of secondary importance and completely dependent on it. Unlike the body, the soul is immortal and imperishable. In most cultures it is identified with breath because it signifies life. Therefore life, soul and breath and all equivalent. In Egyptian, Greek, Hindu, Semitic, Aryan and Slavonic languages and gypsy dialects, words for soul originated in words for breath. The soul is present throughout the body or certain parts of it but can leave through all bodily orifices, and may do so in the shape of a bee, butterfly or bird. This occurs in dreaming sleep, and in states of shock, fear, emotional disturbance, or unconsciousness, during childbirth, in illness, fits and trance, some time before the actual moment of death, and at death when it departs to a spirit world. It may travel to the spirit world before death and bring back evidence of this on wakening. When no soul is present the body is unconscious or as if dead. Aborigines refer to someone insensible or unconscious as *wilyamarraba*: without soul. In this state the body continues to function in a purely mechanical manner, but is incapable of generating wakefulness. Comprehension declines and the body collapses. It is exhausted, weary and feels cold. Sneezing may indicate the return of the soul into the body.[9] However, the soul can also leave the body during sneezing, which is why, even in the modern day, it is common to bless someone who sneezes.

Indigenous peoples believe that disease is caused by loss of the soul. In North American Indians sickness is accounted for by a person's soul being unsettled or detached from the body. Algonquin Indians account for recovery from coma by saying that the soul has travelled to the banks of the River of Death but has been driven back to reanimate the body.

In most animistic thinking it is taken for granted that souls set free from their earthly bodies are recognised by a likeness to them that is retained either on earth or in the world beyond. Irrespective of whether the individual is considered to have one soul or several, each is conceived as a 'body' or vehicle for various different functions such as physical being, feelings and thought. Most commonly the soul is conceived as a second body, consisting of more or less subtle matter — a double or *doppelgänger* — extending outside the body.[10] This 'soul body' is generally described as a subtle vapour, smoke or shadow. It is perceptible by clairvoyants or seers, and by ordinary people during dreams when it goes wandering, or occasionally as the ghost of a deceased person. In some tribal societies ordinary people in coma are thought to be able to perceive the soul. Others believe that it is particularly easy to see it during illness. The idea of present objective figures and the identification with the shadow or breath has led to the treatment of souls as substantial material entities, and explicit statements of the substance of the soul are found in many races.[11]

It is widely believed that just as souls have visible forms they also have voices. They speak in a low murmur or whisper (a ghost of a voice), typically during dreams or visions.[12] Moreover, the primitive knows how to converse with the soul; 'it is vocal within him because it is not simply he himself and his consciousness ... it is something objective, self-subsistent, and living its own life.'[13]

The primitive therefore experiences the soul as the source of life, the prime mover; 'he does not imagine that he directs it, but feels himself dependent on it in every respect.'[14] To the primitive the soul is a ghost-like presence that has objective reality, and so always has both earthly and ghostly qualities. The soul is life itself.

From the evidence available there seems to be little doubt that the concept of soul is the oldest, most original and most firmly based idea about human existence and the most enduring.

> The notion of the existence of a life principle beyond the body is central to all tribal cultures. They, in turn, form the first link in a long chain of cultures, all of which subscribe to that one idea. True, each society has added its own specific adornments and intellectual colourings and has adapted the philosophy of the soul to the mythology and lifestyle of its culture, but the idea of the existence of an animatory principle behind our corporeal world has been preserved throughout history, nourished again and again by Man's spontaneous experiences.
>
> There is hardly any need to produce specific examples for the existence of this leading theme in the history of mankind. The fact that the primary and most universal factor of human existence is the idea of a life-giving energy that is independent of the body and directs or guides each individual speaks for itself. Our material existence is only a reflection of our immaterial soul, just as a shadow has no existence of its own but is dependent on the presence of a solid body. The existence of a soul and its postmortal connection with our lives is the ground of all traditional spiritual philosophy.[15]

Certainly, the soul is a key feature of what is referred to as the world's 'perennial philosophy'. This has been defined as 'the metaphysics that recognises a divine Reality substantial to the world of things and lives and minds; the psychology that finds in the soul something similar to, or even identical with divine Reality; the ethic that places man's final end in the knowledge of the immanent and transcendent Ground of all Being.'[16] It asserts that human beings are from or grounded in the One Self, estranged from or unaware of their origin, and can return, not by learning something new, but by remembering their true identity.

Yet in his classic history of psychology,[17] G.S. Brett denied that speculations about the supernatural soul have made any significant contributions to Western psychology. Hearnshaw disputes this claim. While accepting that there is little psychology in the modern sense in the mythically expressed ideas of ancient cultures, he argues that 'they constituted the common matrix from which systematic psychology developed.'[18] The philosopher Karl Popper also considered primitive and prehistoric humans to have provided significant psychological insights that were the starting point of more systematic psychology. As such they were important.

> But even more important was the tacit recognition in these primitive forms of animism of the soul as an active agent, a principle of movement and feeling — a recognition that the visible body was not self-sufficient, but that there was something within man which accounted for his experiences and behaviour, and which bound him in sympathy, not only with his fellow beings but with nature and the supernatural. These insights have not always been accepted. Indeed they have frequently in recent times been rejected by psychologists. Nevertheless they have played, and continue to play, a far from insignificant part in the shaping of psychology.[19]

Moreover, there may also be an essential and important core of truth in the outlook of primeval peoples; a lost unity that humans in their intellectual strivings have sought to restore.[20]

The soul in ancient civilisations
However, no significant advances in thinking occurred even in the more complex civilisations of the Middle East from 10,000 BC onwards. The Coffin Texts give the clearest identification of the soul with nature,[21] personified as Osiris, but ancient Egyptians recognised a number of souls and regarded the body as one of a series. The

Egyptian *ka* represented the human spirit or life force, equivalent with breath. It was the ethereal projection of eternal being. The *ba*, or soul, seated in the heart, corresponded with the individual's own spirit and as such was remarkably similar to the Maori soul or *wairua*. It was symbolised as a human-headed bird and was thought to survive death, when it would leave the body and later reunite with it in the afterlife. In the meantime it was able to haunt the scenes of the person's life. 'The *ba* is thus the spiritual principle which could appear independently of its physical support and act on its own account, as the representative, as it were, of its owner ... the itinerant soul of a living being, capable of physical action.'[22] The heart was left in place after death, although other bodily organs were removed. Hence the immortal element still preserved a link with this world through the body, and depended on the food and other offerings left at the tomb for its continued sustenance in the next world. The soul was therefore central to the Egyptian cult of the dead.

Death preoccupied the ancient Egyptians. It was regarded as an initiation through which humans have to pass in order to attain eternity, so the art of dying was of the greatest importance. The complex funeral rites of the ancient Egyptians were intended to provide the eternal soul with a body to inhabit so that it would be recognisable in the afterlife. Primarily, however, the death rites were to assist the soul in coming forth from this life into another life. Guidance on this sacred art of dying was given in *The Coming Forth from Day*, or *Egyptian Book of the Dead*, which was chanted to the dying and dead person, and its text inscribed on the inner walls of his or her tomb. The future of the soul in the afterlife depended critically upon the outcome of the Day of Judgement, when Osiris, the god of the underworld, and forty-two other divinities assessed the dead person. The deceased affirmed the purity of his or her soul by reciting the 'negative confession', a declaration that no serious offences had been committed during life. The heart of the deceased, the seat of the soul representing emotions and intellect, was then weighed against a feather, the symbol of truth and justice, by Anubis the jackal-headed god, while the soul looked on, awaiting the outcome. If the heart and feather balanced equally the deceased was declared free of sin, and could pass into the blessed afterlife. If the scales did not balance and the deceased was found guilty of having sinned and deemed

unworthy of passing into eternity, his or her heart was thrown to a
fearsome creature to be devoured.

The soul in the Old Testament

The Hebrews also provided an archaic account of man, and the soul
is frequently mentioned in the books of the Old Testament. The word
for soul, *nephesh*, like the Arabic *nafs*, is related to that for breath.
Breathing is the mark of life and so the term refers to living beings.
The first reference to the soul is when God, customarily spoken of as
Spirit or *ruah*, which also means breath or wind, breathes 'the breath
of life' into man at the creation. By the breath of God man becomes a
living soul.[23] Hence spirit animates the soul, and so man possesses
spirit. 'Soul' and 'spirit' are generally used interchangeably, so the case
for a strict separation between them cannot be made solely on the
basis of Scripture. However, in the biblical tradition the soul is clearly
described in angelic images. The mythic tradition of the fall of angels
can be understood as a description of how the soul, from realms of
pure energy, or spirit, incarnates and descends into the material
paradox of human life.[24]

The *nephesh* or soul is comparable to a life force and is identified
with blood, which is why the Israelites were forbidden to imbibe
blood[25–7] and why, when a person dies, the *nephesh* leaves the body.[28]
However, the Hebrew soul was more than a vital force permeating the
organism: human beings do not *have* a soul, they *are* soul. They are a
unity with no division between body and soul or the living and the
dead. This unity of the person is the focus of the Old Testament.

The *nephesh* is able to know[29] and to remember[30] and it also
'appears to refer to one's intra-personal dynamics, including all that
makes up personality'.[31] Inasmuch as it thinks, feels and is the source
of activity, it is synonymous with inner human nature.

The soul in Judaism

In the Old Testament the soul is much more than a vital force
permeating the organism. It is the seat of affective experience and an
expression of man's oneness with God. The Talmud, the main
authoritative compilation of ancient Jewish law and tradition (from
talmuah, literally, instruction), rests entirely on biblical foundations.
Central to it are the ideas of the Bible concerning a transcendent God

and the Torah — the whole body of Jewish sacred writings and oral traditions — as the embodiment of his moral demands. The Talmud speaks of the pre-existence of the soul and states that before birth the soul knew the entire Torah, forgetting it only at the moment of birth.[32] The hidden teachings of the Talmud, or *Kabbalah*, said to have originated with the angels and to have been passed on by great figures of biblical times, concern the return of the individual soul to God. The Torah constitutes the law and order of the universe, the blueprint of creation. It is often referred to as light through which a person is able to 'see' reality. Just as it is the structure of the universe, so it is the structure of consciousness.[33] The hidden God has neither qualities nor attributes but is symbolised as a flame, whose latent powers manifest as light. The spiritual seeker thus seeks union with the light, or enlightenment, and when his soul achieves this union 'he no longer needs to study Torah, for he has become Torah.'[34]

Biblical religion stands in marked contrast to mysticism and pantheism, largely because of the different relationship between God and the world. In mysticism God is not a sovereign will ruling the universe but a hidden source from which all emanates or an inner life force that pulsates through the universe. In mysticism there is no personal communion between God and man but a union with the Godhead: what is envisaged is an essential identity of the self with the divine life of the universe, or as a merging of the soul in the mysterious divine ground of being. The living relationship between persons is replaced by the extinction of personal individuality that is felt to be the main barrier separating the person from God. The transcendence of God as personal creator is foreign to mysticism and pantheism because according to the latter the world is not subject to a sovereign divine will. In mysticism the God is the principle underlying the suprasensual world. These ancient magical and mythical elements were purged in Talmudic Judaism. This development was inevitable because mythology and magic are possible only where gods in their actions and passions are conceived as natural forces. In biblical religion nature is of God's creation and hence an opposition between man and nature. A rejection of metaphysics is in accordance with a religiosity that promotes man's mastery of nature.

In the Talmud there is a dualism between body and soul which are regarded as being in sharp contrast. 'Because of his soul, which is destined for eternal life, man belongs to the superior world of the Spirit; in his body, he belongs to the earth. Thanks to his soul, he resembles the angels; thanks to his body, a beast.'[35] The relationship of the soul to the body is compared to that of God and the world. To the soul the Talmud attributes pre-existence and human higher powers of moral reasoning and moral consciousness; to the body lower passions. However, it is not a battle between body and soul. The body is not the ground of evil and the moral task of humans doesn't lie in separating soul from body. The warfare between good and evil occurs within the soul. This is where good and evil impulses face each other. They represent two directions of the human will and the individual must choose between them. 'The body and the senses should be subordinate and subservient to the soul; they are not, of themselves, enemies of its heavenly destiny.'[36]

The Celtic soul

The Celts, an Indo-European people who inhabited much of Europe, including Britain, Gaul and Spain, identified the soul with both spirit and breath. The panceltic word for soul, *anamon*, is closely related etymologically to the word for harmony and represents 'the fullness of the individual's potential as a spiritual being'.[37] The immortality of the soul was one of the basic doctrines of Druids, an ancient order of pre-Christian priests who gain their name from the Celtic *dru-wid-es* (similar to the Old Irish word for 'wizard' or 'sorceror') meaning 'clear seeing', or clairvoyant. The Celts believed that after death the soul continued to exist in the Beyond in much the same way as it had on earth.

The soul in ancient Greece

Similar ideas existed in early European civilisation. Though commonly identified with life-giving substances such as blood or, more usually, breath, in Greek mythology *psyche*, or *psukhe* from which the term is derived, had many meanings. In its widest sense it referred to life in general. More specifically, however, it was the principle of life or life force. The term was used in such a way as to suggest that it was felt as something objective and was not merely an abstraction treated metaphorically.[38] In this archaic period of Greek thought the soul or psyche was believed to leave the body in the form of a butterfly (*psyche* also means butterfly in Greek), withdrawing when a person faints and departing the body at death. Until the eighth century BC 'psyche' was always used in its original sense of life but thereafter it also came to denote that which exists after life has ceased: 'life in death'. Homer (*circa* 800 BC) used the term 'psyche' to refer to the life that is lost at death and which survives afterwards as a wraith — the individual's spirit, joined in life to the body, separated from it at death, and surviving after death in Hades, the abode of departed souls. By the sixth century BC 'psyche' had come to mean 'a something of man which leaves the body at death',[39] a separable soul. Even so, in the fifth century BC 'psyche' still retained its quality of objective existence.

After Homer, use of the term 'psyche' was extended to embrace new aspects of psychological life and the character of the individual. Progressively it was used as a psychological agent and came to be seen as the source of sexual desire, emotion, non-rational knowledge and courage and as an inner self. It began to designate the comprehensive personal soul; the immortal and divine part of man; the self as a centre of being; the seat of rational intelligence and moral choice; and that which is not body but is related to the body as master is to slave.[40] Indeed, as the meaning of 'psyche' shifted from life to soul, its opposite term *soma*, which had meant corpse or deadness, came to mean body, and this introduced a fundamental dualism or separation between soul and body that was to have far-reaching significance. More and more 'psyche' came to mean the conscious mind 'trapped' in the body.

Distinctions were made between the intellectual functions of the soul (*nous*) and its emotions, which were generally located in the middle parts of the body. These distinctions between functions and their locations were imprecise and variable, as was the terminology used to describe them. Similar vague conceptions also occurred in Egyptian, Babylonian, Jewish, Celtic, Slavic, Germanic and other Indo-European cultures.

Within Greek literature until the fourth century BC the soul was variously seen as breath, air, incarcerated angels and ectoplasmic wraiths, and the body was viewed as a tomb or prison. Over the same period the use of the term 'psyche' in philosophical texts was very much more varied. It was conceived as breath by Heraclitus and

Xenophon; air by Diogenes and Pythagoras; water by Hippo; fire or heat by Parmenides, Heraclitus, Democritus and Leucippus; blood by Critias; number by Hippasus; flux by Heraclitus; that which imparts movement to living things by Democritus; the moving principle by Anaxagorus and Thales; mind by Democritus; the proportion of bodily parts by Empedocles; a mixture of elements by Empedocles, Plato and Zeno; a harmony of its constituents by Pythagoras; mortal by Democritus; and immortal by Alcmaeon and Heraclitus. Despite their differences, almost all thinkers distinguished three attributes of the soul: movement, sensation and incorporeality.

However, the changing meaning of 'psyche' cannot properly be traced only through a sequence of ideas attributed to philosophers. Two different and important contexts for the psyche — rationalism and Pythagorean mysticism — merged almost invisibly in the fifth century BC, and as a result the soul acquired comprehensive powers.

The emergence of rationalism

Until the sixth century BC, thinking in ancient Greece was clearly rooted in mysticism and the conviction that 'true being, the world in which the soul can find itself at home, must *somehow* be other than "all this",'[41] that is, the superficial world of appearances. The aim of the ancient Greeks was *physis* (the word from which the term 'physics' derives), the attempt to perceive the essential nature or soul of all things. All knowledge, or *scientia*, concerned understanding the meaning and purpose of natural phenomena and living in accordance with the natural order. Two ideas were of central importance: the concepts of harmony and measure.

Maintaining a sense of proportion or 'right measure' was vital because all things were considered to have measure. This was viewed not as an overt feature of phenomena but as a deeper hidden harmony that was deemed to lie in the ratio of its inner proportions to one another and the whole. To understand this ratio, and so have the measure of a thing, was a form of insight into its essential nature or harmony: its soul.

This concept of the soul cannot be attributed to any one person, but Hearnshaw identifies Heraclitus (*circa* 535–475 BC) as the father of modern Western psychology. He viewed the essential nature or underlying *physis* of everything as continual and cyclic change, which he represented as 'fire'. This was not imagined as a visible flame or glow but as a kind of invisible vapour or exhalation, the least corporeal of substances[42] and was identified with the soul. Like a flame it may appear steady and unchanging but it is constantly renewing itself by the destruction of fuel and giving of heat, light and smoke. It represents the basic truth of the universe, apparent or formal stability coupled with continuous change of material.[43] For Heraclitus, therefore, the soul is the exhalation that composes all other things. It is the intelligent governing principle of the universe within each person, its living and divine 'stuff'. Heraclitus therefore proclaimed, 'I search myself, for truth lies within.'

Unquestionably, however, the sixth century BC was a turning point in Western history. It was a period when 'rational thought was emerging from the mythological dream world'[44] and the mystic vision of the ancients began to become obscure and lost to Western civilisation. Heraclitus' emphasis on the importance of inner wisdom or intuition was no longer fashionable and had been overtaken by belief in external truth. This was largely because of the influence of Pythagoras (*circa* 580–500 BC) 'whose influence on the human race was probably greater than any single man before or after him'.[45]

Ironically, Pythagorean philosophy is the perfect embodiment of the mystical view of the universe. Pythagoras was a mystic and his philosophy reflects ideas and specific details that have their origins in earlier religious doctrines of the surviving soul; many of his ideas originate in magic. Consistent with this thinking, Pythagoras viewed the world as a form of divine power or Soul that was the cause of physical motion. His universe was a living, breathing creature and human beings gained their life from breathing. Essentially they are immortal because they retain a fragment or spark of the divine, cut off and imprisoned in a perishable body. Knowledge of this higher nature gives them an aim in life — to cultivate the soul, shake off the body and rejoin the universal soul of which each individual soul is in essence a part. Pythagoras believed in *metempsychosis* — the transmigration of the soul, and reincarnation.

> So long as the soul was to stay on the wheel of transmigration — to enter a new human or animal body after death — so long was it still impure. By living the best and highest life it might

ultimately shake off the body altogether, escape from the wheel of rebirth and attain the final bliss of losing itself in the universal, eternal and divine soul to which its own nature belong.[46]

The re-emergence of these older modes of thought was a feature of the sixth-century religious revival known as **Orphism** whose doctrines interpenetrate the whole mystical tradition of Greek philosophy. Orphism, which probably reached Greece from Eastern sources, laid stress on the unity of life, on the double nature of man and the inferiority of body to soul. Pythagoras provided powerful arguments to support these mystical ideas. He revealed a supersensible world of mathematical relations that could not be reduced to matter. The life principle of the world, he argued, was a system of numbers. Harmony was a property of numbers and underlay both the beauty of art and the health of the body and soul. The soul is a state of arrangement of numbers, a harmony of its own parts. The Eleatic philosophers, Parmenides and Zeno, who followed, proved that the fabric of reality would not be broken into units, that only the 'One', the indivisible whole, could exist in the full and proper sense of the term.

In the course of these controversies the seeds of what later became known as psychology were sown. Gradually the concept of the soul was crystallised and clarified. Its functions were defined and its differences from body distinguished. The broad outlines of psychology as we know it today were sketched. Hence, it has been argued that 'in a very real sense the Greeks discovered the human mind.'[47]

However, Pythagoras' discovery that the pitch of a note depends on the length of the string that produces it, and that concordant intervals in the scale are produced by numerical ratios (2:1 octave; 3:2 fifth; 4:3 fourth and so on) reduced the ancient concept of harmony to mathematics and quality to quantity. As such, it was the first step towards the quantification of human experience and hence the beginning of science in the modern sense.

Pythagorean mathematics were to prove the greatest single influence on Western thought because mathematics are the chief source of belief in external and exact truth and an intelligible world. The exactness of geometry, which is not matched in the real world, suggests that all exact reasoning applies to ideal as opposed to sensible objects, and when taken further, it leads to the belief that the objects of thought are more real than those of sense perception. Contrary to mysticism, Pythagorean mathematics elevated the status of intellect and reduced that of the senses, intuition and feeling. The early followers of Pythagoras were aware that the symbols of mythology and mathematics expressed different aspects of the same reality. Nevertheless, before long the concept of measure lost its mystical significance. It became routinised and habitual as it began to be learned mathematically by formula, rather than acquired intuitively through the development of insight. Ratio came to be conceptualised as that point on a line that divides it into segments in such a way that the smaller is to the larger as the larger is to the whole. This measure or ratio, known as the Golden Mean or Section, came to be imposed by rule, that is, an objective fact or absolute truth about reality rather than some intuitive feeling about the inner essence of a thing. Thereafter, measure came to denote mainly a process of comparison with some external standard. As such it was handed down by the Greeks via the Romans to all Western civilisation. The only sense in which its original meaning is retained is in the notion of 'getting the measure' of a person, thing or situation.

Consequently Western civilisation came to view knowledge as essentially linear — as meaning objective 'out there' fact or objective reality — and such facts as constituting the only valid knowledge of the world. This idea had enormous implications for all subsequent thinking. From this same concept the West derives its notion of time — the idea of a linear sequence from the past, through the present to the future. Such a concept carries with it the idea of progress: given enough time man will discover and discern all possible truth.

From the concepts of measure or ratio Western science also derives its emphasis on measurement, standardisation, rationality and reason, all of which involve dissection and analysis. Gradually Western civilisation came to believe in an orderly linear universe that in time could be explored rationally, that is, through reason, the possession of which set man above and apart from the rest of creation. Nevertheless, the Greeks acknowledged two valid forms of reason: *ratio*, or discursive reason, by its nature analytic and reductionist; and *intellectus*, which was more akin to intuition in being holistic and integrative. It was viewed as a higher faculty of mind than ratio, capable of bringing man to a more profound knowledge than could be gained by reason. Intuition thus held an acknowledged status in Greek thought, but wherever the mystic tradition was filtered through the sieve of Greek culture the enduring emphasis on reason and rationality remained.[48] Hence the Greeks made a profound and lasting contribution to the development of Western thought, and reductionism with its implicit dissection and analysis has come to characterise Western thinking and science.

Dissection is first evident in Greek thought in the fifth century BC when Parmenides of Elea opposed Heraclitus, who, in the mystical tradition, had asserted that man should have knowledge of the whole of things. By contrast, Parmenides proposed a clear distinction between spirit and matter — a substance made of passive, dead particles moving in a void. The smallest individual units of matter were termed atoms, from the Greek word *atom* meaning indivisible. Hence Parminides' theory became known as **atomism**. The movement of atoms was unexplained but assumed to be spiritual in origin.

The followers of Parmenides initially assumed a divine unifying principle standing above all gods and men, but this devolved into a personal God who stood above and directed the world. God was external to or other than man and, as such, was a fact or truth — the Ultimate Fact or Truth — and the very embodiment of Western thought. Indeed, the philosopher Bertrand Russell[49] pointed out that were it not for the Greek concept of an external world revealed only to the intellect not to the senses, the notion of God as it is known in the West might not have existed. In mysticism 'god' is the ground in which all things have their being and live; it is immanent in the soul of all things and can be realised by looking inwards. However, the concept of an external supernatural God, on which Western religion is based, created a gulf between man and the Divine. Accordingly human nature was no longer seen as part of a whole and infused with God-nature, but as separate and distinct.

> Religion's supreme function is to destroy the dream-harmony of Man, Universe and God, to isolate man from the other elements of the dream stage of his mythical and primitive consciousness. For in its classical form, religion signifies the creation of a vast

abyss, conceived as absolute, between God, the infinite and transcendental Being and Man, the finite creature.[50]

By the end of the classical period in Greek history when Greek civilisation was in its ascendancy, several developments in thinking had occurred that were to have profound implications for subsequent Western thought. Eventually they eclipsed the instinctive wisdom of early man.

However, it was several centuries before they did so. In the latter half of the fifth century BC another significant shift in thinking occurred when man rather than the universe became the focus of enquiry. The concept of measure came to be of particular importance to human affairs because, as Protagoras (*circa* 485–411 BC) observed, by nature of his perception and insight, man is the measure of all things. Accordingly, man was seen as the most significant subject of enquiry, and the main focus of study was his soul, essence or psyche.

The Socratic soul
Until this time the soul had been conceived in many different ways and as possessing many different faculties. It was generally viewed as the vital principle of living things and as containing an element that produces knowledge. Nowhere had it been affirmed that the soul is the whole person or total self. The concept of the soul as the self is attributable to Socrates (469–399 BC) whose teachings are known only through the writings of his devoted pupil Plato. He used 'soul' and the 'whole person' as interchangeable terms. His 'soul' is the total self of which the body is an integral part and, as such, represented a concept previously unvoiced by the Greeks. Thus, with Socrates the ancient Greek injunction to 'know thyself' becomes an injunction to know one's soul.[51] For Socrates, knowing about the body is knowing about one's possessions, but not about oneself. He considered care of the soul man's most important task and curing the soul the indispensable preliminary to any curing of the body. However, while the core of his teaching lays stress on care of the soul, it sheds little light on its nature.

Socrates defined death as the separation of the soul from the body and the state of being dead as that in which the body and soul exist separately. He claimed that souls can be separated from bodies but they cannot be destroyed. As such, the soul is an independent substance with powers of cognition and, though the soul guides the body and has it under its charge, the exercise of its cognitive powers is likely to be hindered by 'bodily sensation'.[52] So, although Socrates was not responsible for the concept of the soul as it later became accepted, he acted as a catalyst, preparing the way for his devotee, Plato.

The Platonic concept of soul

Plato (428–347 BC) profoundly influenced thinking about the soul, which was central to his view of human nature, and so made a significant contribution to psychology. He claimed that 'the Soul, since it is immortal and has been born many times, and has seen all things both here and in the other world, has learned everything that there is.' He often used 'soul' and 'self' synonymously and appeared to view them as one and the same. However, in his writings Plato uses 'soul' in several distinguishable senses with the result that the nature of the self is ambiguous and the body–soul relationship is expressed in different ways. While soul is seen as the true self or person, as a cognitive principle and a principle of moral activity, sometimes its moral characteristics and at other times its cognitive characteristics are emphasised. At times the soul appears to include the body as an integral part of itself; at others the body is excluded from the concept of the soul; elsewhere it is a possession or instrument of the soul but enjoys a 'special relationship' with it that other possessions do not. In two of his dialogues, partition of the soul is suggested, as is its continued conscious active existence after separation from the body. Over against this general view is the picture of the soul as a counter-person, a duplicate or inner person possessed of cognitive faculties imprisoned in the body as in a tomb.[53] The soul is rational and substantial; it pre-exists and is immortal. It is an invisible, noetic substance that is the direct and physical cause of human existence. It is not a homogenous entity but a complex of elements, notably reason and impulse, the balance or imbalance of which will characterise it as morally good or bad. Virtue is health of the soul, which is equivalent with balance, harmony and order between its different constituent elements. Parallel harmony and order in the body is equivalent with health.

The relationship between the soul and body advanced by Plato is one of extreme dualism. The soul has the body in its charge. It is the dominant partner, and can be seen as the true self without reference to the body. The body is at best a nuisance and at worst an evil that hinders the soul from gaining truth and intelligence, so a person must spend their lifetime purifying the soul from it. The soul can oppose the feelings and inclinations of the body. Yet in the *Republic* conflict in a person is within the soul not between soul and body. Such conflict within the soul is the source of illness or disease.

As to the nature of the soul, Plato considered it to be dynamic activity or movement — *energeia*. More specifically it was self-motion. According to his definition, the soul is 'that which moves itself'. It is a first principle and, since it does not come into being, it is immortal and imperishable. According to Plato, any body that has an external source of motion is soulless but a body deriving its motion from a source within itself is animated or ensouled. The material universe qualifies as ensouled because he conceived it as a living creature possessing intelligence. Hence soul pervades the universe. Plato identified the movement of the soul with the spatial movement of heavenly bodies; in his writing (*Phaedo*), added to the notion of soul as life principle or life carrier, is the idea of the soul as some sort of spatialistic fluid in the body rather like ectoplasm.

In Plato's thinking the universe is a prototype of man, and so primordial being is reflected within him. The soul is the real man trapped within the body, which is the image of the soul: a complex, hierarchically ordered entity intermingled with the body, but totally different from it. At its lowest level it is simply the principle of life without perception, memory or desire. The next level, the 'mortal', contains passions, affections and sensations. These lower appetites and lusts are distinguished from higher, or spirited, emotions. Finally, there is the rational, intelligent, 'immortal' part of the soul, akin to the divine. The soul therefore has three kinds of function: rationality; will and resolution; and desire. Plato located the will in the chest and the rational faculty in the head, as far removed as possible from the lower impulses.

There can be little doubt as to the strong mystical character of Plato's thinking. It was his view that human beings see not the true nature of reality, but its pale image or shadow. They live in a false reality, alienated from the truth of themselves and all things. Perfect reality is an ideal archetype and within it are forms that are the original blueprint or archetype of the physical world.

The realm of forms is the highest reality, the eternal world of ideas or the divine mind, and only the soul, the divine within each person, can see things as they really are. Only by 'the rising of the soul into the world of the mind' can a person acquire true knowledge. Plato suggested that true knowledge is remembering what the soul once knew, the wisdom it possessed long before it became embodied. Therefore, in his thinking the soul's origin is prior to that of the mundane order; it is not subject to the process of decay and is connected intrinsically with the eternal world of ideas. The body may perish but the soul continues to exist. Accordingly there are two kinds of existence, visible and invisible: the former constantly changing and the latter pure, everlasting, immortal and unchanging. Plato thus distinguished the realm of ideas from the world of experience.

However, ultimate knowledge is not attained or discovered, but comes upon or is revealed to the soul. Accordingly, in Plato's thinking the purpose of philosophy and of life is to pursue true knowledge, to become aware or awakened rather than asleep to the true nature of reality. The first step towards awakening, or perceiving and connecting with this realm of ideas — the Higher Reality — is by looking inward, achieving insight and clear vision.

Plato considered the ideal attitude to life as the renunciation of all that pertains to bodily wants and desires and aspiration towards the spiritual purity of an other-worldly life of the soul. The effects of such striving were reflected in sexual morality, education, philosophy and everyday living and so, under the influence of Plato, the health of the soul became the ideal of Greek culture. It was the role of politics to attend to the soul, and medicine to attend to the body.

In elaborating on the nature and functions of the soul in his various writings, Plato 'illuminated the entire field of psychology'.[54] He outlined the nature of motivation and emotion, addressed the problem of knowledge and highlighted the importance of mental health, with which he was much preoccupied. He constantly reverted to this topic because he considered care of the immortal soul to be the primary task of man.

Aristotle's view of the soul

Plato established an academy that endured for nine hundred years after his death. His most distinguished student was Aristotle (384–322 BC), and his was the most influential and enduring system of psychology ever put forward. His stated aim at the beginning of his treatise on the soul, *De Anima*, was to investigate and ascertain the essential nature of the soul. Although profoundly influenced by Plato, as his thought developed Aristotle showed an increasing aversion to the mystical aspects of his master's teachings, and concern for the accumulation of empirically established facts. His study of the soul was therefore based more on biology than metaphysics.

Aristotle's view of the soul is as the principle of all living things, the vital force that directs life. He located the seat of the soul in the heart and emphasised its physiological primacy within the human body. Nevertheless, he was convinced that the soul was a transcendent principle, a 'quintessence' — in effect, all reality — and so ultimately could not be wholly explained in empirical terms. He did not consider the soul and body as two substances, but as two aspects of all living things, neither of which could exist without the other. He emphasised the psychophysical entity of the living being, and explained the relationship between the soul and the body as that between matter and form. Just as matter cannot be conceived apart from a particular form, and as the form cannot exist simply as form, so the soul and the body can be apprehended only together, by virtue of each other. Moreover, as living matter is always in process of motion and growth, in living creatures form is more a principle of perfection, a life plan or design that becomes increasingly evident as it unfolds. Accordingly, the soul is the form or archetype of the natural body endowed with the capacity of life. It is the perfect realisation of the material body and its inherent potentialities, or *entelechy*, the actualised condition that represents the fundamental design of such a body. From the outset this body is other and more than an inert object. It is an organic and organised body and the function of the soul is to utilise the body and give it purposive direction.

Because for Aristotle psychology was an extension of biology, vital and mental processes were regarded as lying in a common dimension. The psychologist therefore needed to consider the soul, not only of man but also animals and plants, because 'nature proceeds little by little from things lifeless to animal life in such a way that it is impossible to determine the exact line of demarcation.'[55] Man is part of a series that includes all living creatures. He therefore takes his place in the scale of living creatures and does not enjoy exceptional status. Aristotle considered the soul to manifest at three principle levels: the nutritive, found principally in plants and lower life forms, and concerned mainly with nutrition and reproduction; the sensitive, found in animals proper with sensory-motor capacities and corresponding desires; and the rational, found only in man. Thus for Aristotle the soul is the means by which feeling and learning occur.

He believed that qualities of mind — the intellectual capacity to learn, reason and analyse — were present in all animals but that different creatures display more or less of each of these qualities, and animals and humans differ only in the degree to which they possess certain mental abilities. Both have emotions, but human emotions are more complex; both learn, remember, solve problems and benefit from experience, but humans are more able in each of these. Animals and humans therefore differ only qualitatively in the degree to which their mental abilities are expressed, rather than quantitatively in the nature of those mental processes. However, according to Aristotle the soul of man is the highest form of soul attributable to beings in this world by virtue of the reflective faculty peculiar to man. He proposed a hierarchy based on the powers of the soul possessed by each being. Each order possesses all the powers of the order below it and also those powers peculiar to it. This was the origin of what in the Middle Ages became known as the 'great chain of being' composed of countless links. This notion, portraying everything as belonging to one unified and complete chain extending from man to the smallest particles of inanimate matter, was subsequently embellished by Christian thinking:

> The picture of the Chain of Being is of God at the apex of the universe, suffusing the whole, purely spirit: at the base is matter — the most primitive matter that can exist, rocks, earth, the most simplest forms of the universe — these are purely matter and not spirit. In between is the hierarchy of all living things. Mankind is midway between the depth of matter and the heights of spirituality. Below the human race come all animal forms in

descending order of complexity to simplicity. Above mankind are the angels and other spiritual beings.[56]

This metaphor was accepted as the basis of reality in the universe throughout the medieval and renaissance periods in Western civilisation until the early nineteenth century. Only in the twentieth century was this ancient paradigm lost sight of.

Having defined the nature of the soul, Aristotle also analysed its properties and powers. In so doing he gave psychology an identity and a basic conceptual framework, and can be considered the founding father of systematic psychology. In due course his psychology became highly influential in the West. It had no serious rivals for nearly four hundred years and even after its displacement by newer psychologies continued to exert an influence.

Cicero's soul

Aristotle's death in 322 BC marked the end of an era in that he was the last of the ancient masters of all knowledge. After him developments in the study of the soul shifted to Rome. The writings of the Roman orator and statesman Cicero (106–43 BC) represent a landmark in the history of psychology because through them he transmitted Greek ideas to the West, where Latin was the common medium of communication.

Cicero wrote at length about the soul, which he conceived as an immortal, spiritually self-moving principle possessing powers, particularly memory, creativity, active attention and wisdom. For him, the soul is in part physical or mortal in that it is embodied, but it also has higher immortal aspects. Much of his writing concerned psychotherapy and the treatment of pain, distress and various mental disorders. He insisted that diseases of the mind are more numerous and pernicious than those of the body and should be treated as medical matters. He distinguished insanity, mental deficiency and mental deterioration, claiming that they arose psychologically in emotions such as anger and fear, and that, accordingly, they should be treated psychologically. These disorders, he claimed, could be deadly and could also destroy the soul. Other disorders were largely the result of attitudes of mind and disregard of reason. Hence all disorders are within the individual's control and aspects of judgement and are voluntary. His remedy for such disorders was impregnability against life's afflictions. This required 'outstanding intelligence', truth-seeking and philosophical study. It was not a view that found wide support. It led instead to disillusionment with philosophy as a source of guidance on all-important questions relating to the soul. The common people turned instead to Christianity and oriental religions for answers to their questions, and some of the intelligentsia looked back to mysticism.

Plotinus' mystical vision of the soul

One of the latter was the last great philosophical figure of the pagan era, Plotinus (AD 205–70). A strong mystical element and the influence of Platonic thought are evident in his ideas, although his psychology was in many ways original. He was the principle founder of what became known as **neoplatonism**, which is essentially a philosophy of divine unfolding. Neoplatonic thought rests on the assumption of an ordered cosmological reality crowned not by an intellectual principle but by the 'One', an ineffable, timeless, non-local reality, prior to all form, motion and permanency. This ultimate One is the ground of all existence, unifying all apparently diverse life forms. It is the life of the cosmos, making the world a living and blessed thing. Derived from this divine unity there emerged pure intelligence from which the world soul and individual souls derive. Hence in Plotinus' thinking there is a trinity. At the top is the One, or God principle, from which Spirit, the intellectual principle is derived, and finally soul, which is the source of all living things. Soul suffuses all nature, so the apparent diversity of life forms an overall unity.

The individual soul emanates from and communicates with the soul of all. Within it are three levels: one that 'always resides on high'; another that is 'conversant with sensibles', concerned with the maintenance of bodily functions; and another that exists between the two.

> The soul is many things, linked to the realm of sense by what is lowest in us, linked to the intelligible realm by what is highest. For each of us is an intelligible cosmos. By what is intellective, we are permanently in the higher realm; by our lower part we are prisoners of sense.[57]

At the base of the hierarchy is matter. Each of these levels is derived dynamically from the one above it and ultimately from the 'One', and each is concerned with a reverse upward striving towards assimilation with higher levels. 'As life comes more into form, as it moves further down the "chain of being", it is more diversified, more in conflict, more fragmented. The individual soul can, if it so wishes, ascend to become more united again through purification and simplification.'[58]

For Plotinus, therefore, the soul is a superior principle. It is not material, nor is it the perfection of the body, which is merely an instrument of the soul. It is separate from the body, produces the body and inspires all life. He insisted that 'We are not bodies, but souls resident in bodies.'[59] Although the human soul is of divine origin it is imprisoned in material clothing. As a result it is tainted, gross and dark. It is the individual's duty to cleanse the soul of its bodily form so that it might return to God. Despite being resident in a material body, the soul can purify itself even in this life and liberate itself from the senses and all earthly concerns because by its very nature it is unbounded. 'It is as great as it wishes to be.'[60]

The soul also integrates and coordinates. It is a unity that subsists with invariable sameness in the subject and in essence. Nevertheless, although a unity it functions at various levels and with a variety of powers or faculties. Important among these is awareness of the inner world and of personal identity. Plotinus considered that because of the integrative function of the soul it is necessarily a centre from which the senses extend, and which has what might be considered an overview of the whole situation. The soul's power of perception is therefore not directed to the object of sensation but to the impression it creates in the living being. Hence, for the first time in history, psychology, the study of the soul, became the science of consciousness, conceived by Plotinus as self-consciousness. It recognised for the first time in Greek psychology a distinction between the inner and the outer world and the concept of individual personality. However, Plotinus' views were ultimately mystical, not scientific. He held that the purified soul can, by a mode of intuitive knowledge superior to that of reason, achieve perception of the One and reunification with it, and he considered this ecstatic mystical vision to be the ultimate goal in life.

> As the soul ascends to the One it enters more deeply into itself.
> To find the One is to find itself.[61]

The worst sin is isolation from and ignorance of the unity of the creative source.

Plotinus' thinking brings to an end the period of history of early Greek thought that can be seen to originate in a mystical vision of unity, to progress through abstract analysis and the shattering of the primordial feeling of oneness bonding nature and man, and to conclude in a mystical reunification. In the process, the concept of soul was crystallised and clarified, its functions were defined and its differences from the body distinguished. Hence the broad outlines of psychology as we know it today were sketched. 'The way was paved for the philosophical and scientific reflection on the nature of the psyche and the subject matter of psychology began to get focus and organisation.'[62] From being the breath or principle of life and a diffuse presence in the universe, the soul took over the properties of mind and the emotions, formerly considered separate. Man was distinguished from other animals by the additional power of reason. Soul became distinguished from the body, but whether it was itself substantial or immaterial remained unresolved, and the basic functions of the soul came to be regarded as movement and sensation. At this level the soul was a vehicle for sensory-motor activities. At its lowest level the soul was simply the breath or principle of life, but 'in its highest reaches the soul seemed to have an affinity with the reason that ordered the universe.'[63] It was an aspect of universal intelligence, rather than merely the source and centre of human life: it was a transcendent principle and part of the divine. As such the soul was immortal. Plutarch writing 'on the soul', in the first century AD claimed that at the point of death it has the same experience as those who are initiated into great mysteries.

The Christian soul

The views of Plotinus mark the end of early Greek pagan psychology and the beginning of a new era. Though not himself a Christian, his thinking influenced his Christian successors and, with its development during the first centuries AD, neoplatonism in turn became influenced by Christianity. In the third century AD, Porphyry, a disciple of Plotinus, became its principal exponent and advocated asceticism as necessary for the salvation of the soul. Neoplatonism was not a religion but a philosophical movement. Nor was it an abandonment of Greek rationalism but an adaptation of Greek thought to inner experience. However, in the sixth century AD neoplatonism was denounced as a heretical movement by orthodox Christianity. Nevertheless, it continued as an underground movement for many centuries.

The teachings of Plotinus influenced Christianity because they gave St. Augustine (AD 354–430) 'a sight of the invisible things above' shortly before his conversion, and he transmitted them to the medieval world. By so doing Augustine can be considered an important psychologist who added new dimensions to the understanding of the soul.

Augustine believed that the nature of God and the mysteries of the world could be revealed by an analysis of the human mind. Accordingly the most important truths were revealed by looking inwards. Psychology was therefore the main key to reality. Consciousness of self was immediate and beyond all doubt and quite different from the mediate knowledge of things and so the immediacy of conscious experience was the starting point of all knowledge. Of particular importance to Augustine was the relationship between soul and body. He insisted that man is not just a body or a soul but a being made up of both. Together they comprise 'man'. However, while the soul is not the whole man, it is the better part and the body its inferior. He viewed the soul as immaterial and incorporeal, made by God out of nothing. It is thus a spiritual entity and, though not extended in space, it somehow resides in the body and can act upon it, without itself being acted on in turn. Every movement of the soul affects the body to some degree. It is therefore dynamic and forceful but not measurable. As ideally the soul rules the body, the will is more important than the soul's other faculties, reason and memory, as it drives the rest of the soul and the body.

For Augustine, the soul, though not in space, is in time. It measures time, so immediate human experience is temporal — a concept that came to be known as the 'stream of consciousness'. However, in Augustine's view, man's destiny is eternal and the progress of his soul involves an integration and transcendence of time.

Augustine's descriptions of the stream of consciousness and of its depths were unlike anything that had preceded him and were his main contribution to psychology.

His views on the soul also influenced Christian theology. This dominated Western thinking between AD 400–1450, in particular psychology whose subject matter was intimately connected with that of religion. The value and importance of the soul was central to Christian teaching: 'For what shall it profit a man, if he shall gain the whole world and lose his own soul.'[64] Accordingly every soul had to be saved.

The soul in the New Testament

The Old Testament scriptures were not translated into Greek until several hundred years after the death of Aristotle. In the Greek-language version of the Old Testament, known as the *Septuagint*, the Hebrew term *nephesh* was usually translated with 'psyche'. However, by the time Christianity was founded Roman culture had been dominant for some time and Latin had superseded Greek as the scholarly language in Europe and the Latin *anima* was now used to refer to the soul. Nevertheless, the authors of the New Testament used 'psyche' as it had been used in the Septuagint to refer to inner human nature. It is referred to 101 times, mostly in the synoptic gospels,[65] and generally resonates with early Greek thought, but 'psyche' is also used in a distinctly religious sense as a human's connectedness to God. This psyche or soul is not destroyed by biological death and continues to exist in an afterlife unless destroyed eternally by God[66] until reunited with the body at the final resurrection. The New Testament implies that souls have conscious extra-bodily existence after death prior to resurrection.[67, 68] So, although similar, the New Testament and Greek uses of the term 'psyche' are not identical, but both essentially view the soul as life and the invisible, inner dynamics of the person. At times, therefore, the soul is used, along with the body, to represent the whole person, and at times it is distinguished from the body as that which cannot ultimately be affected by physical death. The soul and body are different entities that, taken together, form a unity — the whole person — and so in its most comprehensive sense the New Testament soul stands for the entire person, the human being as a 'living soul'.[69] Implicitly, then, the actions or characteristics of the soul are those of the whole person.

The soul in the Dark Ages

It took three hundred years before the Roman world converted to Christianity when it became the dominant religion of the Roman Empire and its founder was elevated from the status of a master of ancient knowledge to that of a God who embodied the character of the Roman Empire. In the process, Christianity was transformed from a humanistic tradition based on Christ's teaching that 'the Kingdom of God is within you' to a religion in which God is viewed as the ultimate, external, supreme power and authority to which man is subjugated. All practices that emphasised the development of human powers and potentials were systematically eradicated in Western culture, and all bodies of knowledge were framed within the context of its dominant religion, with the result that sources of occult knowledge and mysticism were eclipsed. Nevertheless, pagan heresies were never fully eliminated and pagan ideas and practices continued to survive 'underground' throughout the centuries. However, in the dark ages following the final collapse of the Roman Empire in AD 476 and until around AD 1000, concern was with salvation or saving the soul rather than understanding it, and preserving surviving knowledge rather than adding to it.

The knowledge of the ancient world that survived was conserved in the Eastern Roman Empire, the Moslem civilisation of the Middle East, and in the monasteries of Europe where early Christian monks devoted themselves to compiling elaborate digests. One of these was *De Anima*, written by Cassiodorus (*circa* 490–585), which provided a summary of classical and Christian views about the soul. However, much of the ancient wisdom had been lost and nothing was added to psychology. It was only after the First Crusade in 1097 and the occupation of Constantinople in 1204 that Arabic and Greek knowledge became accessible.

In the second half of the twelfth century, mystical ideas that had lain dormant within Judaism for many centuries were reawakened as the *Zohar*, the classic medieval text on the Kabbalah, based on ancient teachings, became known throughout Europe. Arabic translations of the works of Aristotle and the commentaries of Arabic scholars such as Avicenna were also influential and during the twelfth and thirteenth centuries European universities provided a home for the learning revival and — in the course of some centuries — a home for psychology. In Europe, *psyche* and *anima* were generally replaced by the German word *Seele* and the English word 'soul'. Both these terms derive from the Gothic *saiwala* and the Old German *Saiwalo* signifying a moving, life force and are connected to the Greek *aiolos* which means mobile, coloured and iridescent. As such the words are true to the senses conveyed by the Greek and Latin terms *psyche* and *anima* in earlier philosophy and literature. Indeed, the culture of the universities was initially literary rather than scientific. Ancient texts, the philosophical discourses and writings of Plato and Aristotle, treatises on medicine by Galen, legal works by Justinian and the scriptures and contributions of the Church Fathers not only constituted the substance and verbal analysis of what is known as **scholasticism** but also debated its methodology.

The soul in the Middle Ages

Two of the great figures of scholasticism had a long-lasting impact on psychology: the theologian Thomas Aquinas (1225–74) and John Duns Scotus (1265–1308). Aquinas followed Aristotle in regarding the soul as the incorporeal form of the body and as unique to each individual. It is not part of a universal soul, and in spite of its diverse functions, it is a unity: 'In man the sensitive soul, the intellectual soul and the nutritive soul are numerically one soul.'[70] Of the faculties which he distinguished within this unity, Aquinas considered intellect the most noble. It is incapable of functioning independently of the senses, which supply the basic data of all knowledge. Sensory processes are, however, insufficient by themselves to produce knowledge; the intellect must always be actively involved. Hence there is inevitably a subjective aspect to knowledge. It is not merely objective. The converse is equally true. Thus the soul cannot know itself by its essence but by its acts, and can only be known by subtle enquiry. Aquinas also taught the biblical view that the rational soul exists apart from the body after death and is reunited with it at the final resurrection.

The emphasis on intellect as the highest faculty of the soul during this period meant that soul came to be equated with it. Unlike Aquinas, Duns Scotus maintained that the individual, in principle at least, has direct and immediate knowledge of his own mind. He also believed that the faculties of the soul, such as intellect and will, though distinguishable conceptually, are inseparable aspects of one reality. For him, the will was central and supreme because as an initiator it is free, whereas intellect is always bound or determined by the intelligible object. As the soul is free it is the origin of moral values. As a consequence of his thinking, ethical problems came within the remit of psychology for the first time. The changes of moral feelings and attitudes ushered in by Christianity subsequently changed the intellectual climate of psychology and society, and personality, rather than intellect alone, became the distinguishing feature of man.

During the Middle Ages a synthesis occurred in which biblical and ancient Greek thinking about the soul were interwoven. Augustine's ideas about the structure of the soul and its distinction from the body were largely shared by Aquinas, but his interest in the soul was more expressly religious. Aquinas focused on the universal nature of the soul among all people regardless of their relationship with God. His conceptual separation of the soul from its religious context brought about a partial secularisation of the soul that was subsequently taken much further.[71]

In the 300 years following the death of Aquinas in 1274 radical transformations in outlook, ideas and society produced novel conceptions of human nature out of which new psychologies emerged. Ironically, however, the 'soul' had almost disappeared from them.

Soul destroyers

By combining the scientific world-view of antiquity, first systematised by Aristotle, with Christian ethics, Thomas Aquinas had established the scientific framework that remained largely unquestioned and unaltered until the Middle Ages. Science was rooted in a view of the universe that rested on the authority of the Church. Man was seen as the centre of God's creation, and earth as the centre of the heavens. The pursuit of reason was maintained and progress in knowledge was rapid. The aim of science was wisdom, understanding the natural order and living in accordance with it, and this was tantamount to accepting man's powerlessness in the face of God. Ultimate knowledge and knowing too much constituted sin and consequently all visionary mystical movements were suspect. Therefore during the Middle Ages the Cathars, Albigenses, Bogomils, Freemasons, Rosicrucians and Kabbalists were intensely persecuted by the Church.

However, during the sixteenth century the orthodoxy of the Church was called into question when Copernicus (1473–1543) challenged the biblical notion of the earth as the centre of the heavens by suggesting that the planets circle the sun. This effectively removed the earth from its geometrical pre-eminence and made it difficult to attribute to man the cosmic significance assigned to him in Christian theology. The discovery of the laws of planetary motion by Kepler (1571–1630) created a new astronomy that further challenged the old view of the universe which was finally discredited when Galileo (1564–1642) demonstrated that the earth revolves around the sun.

The seventeenth-century soul

Although at the beginning of the seventeenth century scientists generally still believed in the transcendent God, the belief in an immanent God present in all things had largely disappeared. Until this time the aim of science had been to understand and live in harmony with nature. This altered entirely when Francis Bacon (1561–1626) introduced the idea that man was something apart from nature and could use science to gain mastery over 'her'. This view was essentially anti-theological in that it encouraged man to sequester powers formerly attributed to God. Bacon asserted that Nature must be 'bound into service' and made a 'slave', 'put in constraint' and 'moulded' by the mechanical arts, for by this time the idea of the universe as machine-like had emerged. In 1605 Kepler had stated his aim as 'to show that the celestial machine is to be likened not to a divine organism but to a clockwork'.[72] This created a schism between the physical and spiritual realms and brought about bitter conflict between science and the Church that continued throughout the seventeenth century.

> It was a strange century, this seventeenth century, which begot our modern epoch … it was the century that created modern science; but the minds of the individuals who created this science were all solidly planted in the mind of God.[73]

Philosophers of the period were obliged to reconstruct psychology.

Thomas Hobbes (1588–1679) made the first attempt to assimilate psychology to the models of the physical sciences. He was the first theorist to grasp the implications of the mechanical world-view of Galilean science[74] and to apply it uncompromisingly to explain human nature; as such he can be considered the father of reductionist, mechanistic psychology. He regarded the universe as a material continuum. As there was nothing other than matter, the concept of incorporeal substance or soul was entirely meaningless. He reduced everything to bodies in motion and attempted to explain human nature and society in terms of the general principles of mechanics. However, his psychology had serious limitations because, although his philosophy was derived from science, he was not truly a scientist and his knowledge of physics and mathematics was limited. 'Nevertheless, Hobbes' psychological manifesto was enormously important as initiating a line of thought which has persisted to our time ... In the last resort man was simply a machine to be explained wholly in naturalistic terms.'[75] Whereas formerly nature had been seen as organic and alive now 'mechanism took over from the magical tradition the conception of the manipulation of matter but divested it of life and vitality.'[76]

The influence of René Descartes (1596–1650) was greater than that of Hobbes, but is considered 'more malign'. 'He directed psychology along a cul-de-sac from which it took more than two and a half centuries to extricate itself.'[77] Descartes believed that the new knowledge of the era required philosophy to begin again from first principles. He chose to doubt everything in his search for certainty and concluded on this basis that he existed, as did God. In this sense he kept God and the soul at the centre of his thinking but his concept of soul was very different from that of previous scholars. 'The soul of Descartes is still a Christian soul; though the lineaments may sometimes be faint, they are still there. But it is a Christian soul that has undergone another crucifixion: this time on the cross of mathematical physics.'[78]

Certainly, within Descartes' philosophy lay the 'seeds of death for the soul'.[79] He distinguished soul and body from each other as 'spiritual' and 'material' respectively and equated mind with soul. Soul is thus a thinking, conscious substance rather than the 'form' of the body or the principle of life and, as such, has no resemblance to the substance of the body, which is quite different. However, although he regarded body and soul as different substances that could in principle exist one without the other, he suggested that body and soul form a unity: a self-subsistent whole, one substance; and that it is God who unites the soul to the body-mechanism. Taken individually soul and body are distinct and complete substances but, seen within their relationship to the whole human being, they are incomplete substances. Descartes considered the relationship between body and soul essential, for without a soul a man would not be a man. 'It is surprising that a thinker widely celebrated as the propagandist for a dualistic view of body and soul should lay so much stress on the cohesion between the two.'[80] Nevertheless, Descartes' philosophy effectively tore psychology apart.

Descartes conceived of the soul as situated in the human body rather like a captain in a ship. His picture of the soul and body has been characterised as a doctrine of 'the ghost in the machine'.[81] A consequence of distinguishing and separating soul from body — in Descartes' terms 'thinking substance' and 'extended substance' — is that the human body can be treated separately 'as a complex, vitalised piece of machinery'[82] which is inanimate. In contrast, the soul is characterised, not by extension and divisibility but by cogitation, that is, in a broad sense, as mental activity — will, understanding, doubt and imagination. Hence, although 'inside' the ship, the captain observes as an outsider that, for example, his ship has sprung a leak.[83]

> There were fateful consequences for both physics and psychology in these theories of Descartes. Physics became emancipated from all occult and animistic influences, and the mechanical, mathematical viewpoint received a total vindication. Psychology, on the other hand, became split in two; there was the realm of pure consciousness, thought and will, totally divorced from corporeality and matter; and there was the mysterious area consisting of sensation, movement and emotion, where mind and body interacted. Man alone possessed consciousness and thought; all lower animals were merely machines ... These doctrines of Descartes in effect placed large, and perhaps the most important, areas of psychology beyond the reach of science, as he conceived it; for Descartes believed

that science was necessarily quantitative and mathematical. Mind, on the contrary, in its essential nature could only be known intuitively, and, being indivisible, could not be analysed by the methods of science.[84]

This dualistic philosophy of Descartes shattered the psychosomatic unity of the Aristotelian model and burdened psychology with the impossible problems of mind–body interaction. Consciousness, which was identified with thinking, became the subject matter of psychological enquiry and the foundations were laid for the self to be defined by its mental functioning. The identification of mind with consciousness ruled out the possibility of unconscious mental processes. So, the human mind was divorced not only from its deeper nature and physiological substructure but also from the rest of the animal kingdom.

Aristotle's views that humans and animals differ only quantitatively in the degree to which their mental abilities express themselves, rather than qualitatively in the nature of those mental processes, was established by St. Thomas Aquinas in the thirteenth century as a formal doctrine of the Church. For some scholars in the Christian Church accepting that animals possessed qualities then regarded as aspects of the soul was tantamount to conceding that they were candidates for an afterlife, including heaven. 'A heaven occupied by such a collection of souls would fill to overflowing, and such an afterlife would not hold out adequate promise of a blissful existence to keep the congregation on the straight and narrow path of virtue during their earthly years.'[85] Existence of the animal soul raised a whole series of ethical problems, such as whether animals should be killed for food, denied free will by being forced into servitude or granted access to the church and baptism. Descartes' thinking provided a solution to these vexed questions. He wholeheartedly adopted the position that animals are simply machines, bodies without souls. For the sake of consistency, thinkers of the period also denied animals other aspects of mind. Thus, 'in order to prevent a population crisis in heaven and a philosophical problem on earth',[86] the possibility that animals had intelligence, emotions, consciousness and other aspects of mind was rejected. Given that there was no comparability between man and 'brutes', psychology lost the biological basis with which it had been endowed by Aristotle and became encapsulated in consciousness. Yet in spite of these enormous drawbacks, Descartes' ideas largely shaped the development of psychology for the next three centuries.

Descartes' views also determined the nature and development of science for the next three centuries and still exert a significant influence today. Indeed Descartes enunciated clearly 'something of which our whole culture is the living expression: the duality of the spiritual and the material'.[87] The split between mind and body he introduced enabled scientists to treat matter as inert and completely distinct from themselves and led to the belief that the world could be described objectively in terms of material objects that exist independently of human observers. As a result, objectivity became the ideal of science.

Descartes conceived of the material world of objects as assembled like a huge machine or cosmic clock which was operated by impersonal mechanical laws that could be explained in terms of the arrangement and movement of its parts and described using simple mathematics. His world-view was not only mechanistic and materialist but also analytic and reductionist in that he considered complex wholes to be understandable in terms of their constituent parts. He extended this mechanistic model to living organisms, likening animals to clocks composed of wheels, cogs and springs. Subsequently he extended this analogy to man, claiming that all the functions he attributed to this machine occurred naturally like the movements of a clock.

Descartes' ideas were opposed by Spinoza (1632–77), whose views were rooted in mysticism. He considered absurd the idea of two totally disparate substances that could interact. He regarded mind and body, which he referred to respectively as substance thinking and substance extended, as one and the same substance: two aspects of a single underlying reality. Accordingly all mental processes had physical correlates, and all material entities were correspondingly material. Therefore everything is animate, though in different degrees. In Spinoza's system all phenomena are merely 'modes' of the one ultimate reality, God or Nature, which could be viewed either as thought or extension, mind or matter. So, just as the body is a dependent part of the infinite natural world, the mind is part of the infinite intellect of God. His theory implied that the order and connection of ideas is the same as the order and connection of things, that memories possess a physical basis and that ideas are associated with physical correspondences.

Spinoza's views were largely ignored in his lifetime. This was partly because he wrote in Latin at a time when it was being replaced by vernacular languages, and his style of writing was dense and difficult. More significantly, Spinoza's ideas offended both Christians and Jews because his concept of God did not conform to the Western view of a personal and transcendental deity but was more akin to Eastern ideas, and he was denounced as an atheist. However, after his death, psychologists, most notably Sigmund Freud, were influenced by his double-aspect doctrine, and only now, in the light of contemporary scientific theories and discoveries, can their subtleties be appreciated for what they were — far ahead of their time.

> Reformulated in modern terminology, in which extension becomes energy, and thought becomes information, it seems increasingly attractive, and is, in fact, attuned to various recent developments in physics.[88]

Nevertheless, judged by the scientific thinking of his time, Spinoza's views were bizarre and unacceptable.

Although none of these thinkers of the seventeenth century used the term psychology they had laid the foundations for the scientific study of mind. 'In so doing, they shattered the intimate relationship between soul and body and the unity taken for granted in the older doctrines. All this represented a real impoverishment of the psychology which had come down through scholasticism from the ancient world.'[89] Nevertheless, this older psychology was never lost. It was studied in universities, albeit as philosophy, and some of its terminology was retained in the newer psychologies. Christianity also still exerted an influence. The existence of the soul, and the distinction between soul and body, in the sense of the mental and material aspects of man, was largely unquestioned.

Philosophy was concerned more with the highly problematic relationship between body and soul. Throughout history the soul had been defined in various ways and the soul–body relationship described accordingly. The particular soul in question therefore makes a profound difference. As soon as either body or soul is considered separately from the other they appear to have nothing in common. In contrast to the body the soul is invisible, formless, colourless, has no spatial extension, is indivisible and immaterial. So to speak of the soul as 'in' the body is to give it a spatial dimension it does not possess. Yet this idea of the soul being 'in' the body runs throughout the history of philosophy. Aristotle, Plato and Descartes considered the soul present in all parts of the body.

However, denigration of the body as in Plato's view of it as a prison, and Descartes' machine-like conception had 'negative implications for the prospect of the soul'.[90] While these conceptions of the body may be seen to exalt the soul in some way, from another perspective they also undermine it by taking 'from the soul the one setting in which it can plausibly be seen to exist'.[91] To the reasonable, materialistic thinker, if the soul cannot be 'inside' the body, some other means of connection is needed, for without any connection these two worlds can never meet, and man, as such, becomes an impossibility.

Plotinus had suggested that the soul is spoken of as 'in' the body because it is not generally seen, and he claimed that if it could be seen as it interpenetrates every part of the body it would appear that the body is an accessory. He claimed that the soul is not in the body but 'irradiates' it. This mystic vision is implicit in the idea that the body emanates from the soul, and in the ancient notion that the soul exists outside of the body as a *doppelgänger* or double. Either way, 'The soul is a presence that makes the body what it is. Nevertheless the *how* of this remains an open question.'[92] It was a question Descartes was unable to answer. He identified the pineal gland, a unitary structure situated in the mid-brain, as the point of interface between body and soul, and attempted to describe how the soul acts on the body, and vice versa, by way of it. But he explained the unity between body and soul as brought about by God. It was a question the highly influential seventeenth-century philosopher John Locke (1632–1704) did not attempt to answer. He affirmed Christian teaching on the soul, but did not try to explain its nature or relationship with the body, and tried instead to describe its mental structure and development.

The ancient idea that the psyche 'builds' itself a body was simply not part of the spirit of the age. In the new age of scientific materialism it was tantamount to heresy and thus unthinkable.

The soul in the eighteenth century

The eighteenth century proved to be a period of great significance in the development of Western psychology, not least because at this time 'psychology' was first identified as a scientific discipline. It was considered the age of enlightenment, the name given to a philosophical movement that stressed the importance of reason, and in which the psychological tradition established in ancient Greece reached its peak, only to decline rapidly thereafter. The philosophers of the enlightenment were students of the soul who spoke not in the name of any revelation or mystical insight but with the authority of reason about the unfolding of the human soul. They asserted that happiness could only be realised when inner freedom is achieved and argued for the abolition of those conditions of existence that required the maintenance of illusion and ignorance. However, within a very short period of time the tradition in which psychology was the study of the soul was abandoned and 'reason as the means of discovering the truth and penetrating the surface to the essence of phenomena ... relinquished for intellect as a mere instrument to manipulate things and men.'[93]

The thinking of Isaac Newton (1642–1727) dominated the latter part of the century. He formulated the mathematical laws or mechanics that were thought to operate the cosmic machine and to give rise to all the changes observable in the physical world. In the Newtonian universe all physical phenomena occurred in the three-dimensional space of classical Euclidian geometry. This is an absolute space, independent of the material object it contains, always at rest, immovable, constant and unchangeable. All changes in the physical world were described by Newton in terms of a separate dimension called time, which is also absolute, unconnected with the material world, and flows uniformly in linear sequence from the past, through the present, to the future. These notions of space and time were to become so deeply rooted in the minds of Western philosophers and scientists that they were taken as unquestionable properties of nature.

Within this absolute space and absolute time moved particles that Newton conceived as small indestructible objects, like tiny billiard balls or grains of sand, of which matter was made. Such a view was similar to that of the Greek atomists. The main difference was that Newton provided a precise description of the force acting between these particles, which he termed gravity. He saw this as rigidly connected with the bodies it acted on and as acting instantaneously over distance. The particles and the forces between them were both viewed as having been created and set in motion by God at the beginning of time. All physical events were thus reduced in Newtonian mechanics to the motion of material points in space caused by their mutual attraction. In order to express the effect of this force on mass points in precise mathematical terms, Newton developed differential calculus, and the resulting equations of motion form the basis of classical mechanics. The success of the latter in explaining the motion of the moon and the planets encouraged the clockwork view of the universe and inspired the invention of mechanisms that imitated these realities. Laplace (1749–1827) subsequently went further than Descartes or Newton in assuming that similar mechanical laws governed all things, including human beings.

Consequently, the scientific view of the universe was mechanistic, reductionist and deterministic. Everything occurring in the cosmic machine was considered to have a definite cause and to give rise to a definite effect, so that the future of any part could be predicted if its state at any time was known in sufficient detail.

In the Newtonian scheme the idea of God's intervention and influence on the universe was all but lost. 'Classical physics transmuted the living cosmos of Greek and medieval times, a cosmos filled with purpose and intelligence and driven by the love of God for the benefit of man, into a dead, clockwork machine.'[94] Matter was seen as the source from which universal forces originated, and the very existence of God, the creator of the cosmic machine, was progressively brought into question.

As the religious basis of knowledge was progressively eroded throughout the eighteenth century, the soul became a less tenable concept. The philosopher David Hume (1711–76) lacked Christian convictions and discarded Christian beliefs about the soul. He adhered to the traditional doctrine of the 'great chain of being', the idea of a hierarchically ordered universe of insensible gradations between animate and inanimate, and he also acknowledged mind and body as two different spheres of reality. The body comprehends physical substance, providing knowledge of the external world by way of sensation, and the mind comprehends spiritual substance, providing knowledge of the inner world of the mind by way of reflection. However, Hume recognised that 'spiritual substance' lacks precise content and so cannot form the basis of awareness of personal identity. Hume therefore argued that the existence of a substantial mind, self or soul can not be posited. What is called the self is simply a collection of perceptions retained from experience. He insisted that in the beginning the mind is empty of content, 'void of all characters, without any ideas'[95] and the only source of knowledge is experience. Hence learning is all-important in forming the mind. Hume, in his fundamental assumption that all knowledge comes from experience, had established the empiricist tradition in psychology, and under his influence the mind now became the focus of psychology.

Empiricists agreed with Hume that the concept of a substantial soul is false. 'They were encouraged in this by the influence of positivism, the assumption that all knowledge must be rooted in sensory experience and accessible to the methods of natural science. From such a standpoint the idea of a soul was truly nonsense.'[96] With the loss of the idea of soul as substance the 'death' of the soul in psychology became inevitable.

Immanuel Kant (1724–1804) was the first person to devise a psychology without a soul. He acknowledged that the idea of soul is not meaningless, that it is necessary to posit some transcendent unifying principle in the self, and he termed this the transcendental ego. However, he maintained that this ego could not be studied by empirical psychology. He insisted that human knowledge is confined to the phenomenal world and cannot penetrate beyond the phenomenal veil to its antithesis, the 'noumenal' world of 'things in themselves'. Hence he believed that the real nature of an ego that transcends phenomenal experience can never be known and used the term 'psychology' to refer to a phenomenal description of mind as it appears to individuals. In so doing, Kant legitimised knowledge within the world of experience but at the same time ruled out metaphysical knowledge of ultimate reality and the nature of the soul.[97] Effectively he had excluded the soul from psychology, but at the same time he held that it was impossible to establish psychology as a science, which he equated with quantification, because inner experience cannot be quantified. Unsurprisingly, therefore, Kant has been regarded by some as 'a disaster for psychology',[98] especially as he was extremely influential.

Loss of the soul in the nineteenth century

Johann Herbart (1776–1841) subsequently went further than Kant, declaring that the soul has no capacity nor faculty whatever either to receive or to produce anything. This was not a view shared by Gustav Fechner (1801–87) who opposed materialists of his day by arguing for the existence of a universal soul. He believed that all living things have souls, including plants. Indeed he wrote a book on the plant soul. He held that mind and body are the inner and outer aspects of one underlying reality and he set out to establish this experimentally and mathematically by establishing a constant and lawful relation between them. He found measurable relationships between the physical world and human sensory experience that he called *psychophysics*. Fechner thus initiated quantitative methods in psychology and what had formerly been an essentially philosophical discipline became quantitative and experimental.

Subsequently the first self-proclaimed psychologist Wilhelm Wundt (1832–1920) used Fechner's methods without his metaphysical speculations concerning the soul. He used the term 'psychology' to refer to measurable examination of elements of consciousness and so is commonly acknowledged as the founder of modern psychology, that is, psychology without a soul. Psychology was moving with the times.

> Most of those who followed Wundt into the field of modern psychology were more influenced by the positivism then current and were content to study the mind using only natural science methods. Some ... applied such methods to the study of higher mental phenomena like thinking and memory, something to which Wundt was opposed. However, virtually all early, modern continental psychologists were persuaded that the soul could not be the focus of psychological study.[99]

Until the nineteenth century it was still generally accepted that man and nature were linked in an almighty purpose and that the world was not 'soulless'. Then Charles Darwin explained man's evolution in scientific, materialistic, non-divine terms. In what has been claimed to be one of the most significant statements of the modern world[100] Darwin described the change from the spiritual to the mundane view of reality. 'Formerly I was led by feelings ... to the firm conviction of the existence of God, and of the immortality of the soul ... But now the grandest scenes would not cause any such convictions and feelings to rise in my mind. It may be truly said that I am like a man who has become colour blind.'[101]

As nineteenth-century science made belief in the creator increasingly difficult, the Divine gradually disappeared from the scientific world-view. The philosopher Nietzsche (1844–1900) could justifiably declare God 'dead' in the sense that traditional meanings and values had been negated and physical science had become the ultimate authority in Western culture: it had become 'God'. The new dogma, **logical positivism**, had at its core the argument that any principle that cannot be verified by empirical, observational means is utterly devoid of meaning. Anything that could not be seen with the eyes or touched with the hands was doubted. Effectively this relegated all non-empirical aspects of science and philosophy, such as metaphysics and theology, to the realm of emotion or belief. This left psychology with a dilemma because adopting scientific method and the total objectivity it implies precludes from study human experience, sensation, feelings and consciousness, all properties of the soul. If it was to be seen as a science, as a valid and respectable body of knowledge, psychology had to abandon both its methods and its traditional subject matter; and it did so. Therefore, in the process of refining its methods, nineteenth-century psychology discarded its essence, thereby alienating humans from their experience, their selves and their existence in much the same way that the essence of wheat is discarded in its refinement; the reasons were the same: expediency and convenience.[102] So by 1890, when William James published his overview of psychology, he could accurately state that most psychology was 'soulless'.

Soulless psychology in the twentieth century
William James (1842–1910), who is acknowledged as the father of American psychology, described the psychology of his time in his *Principles of Psychology* (1890). Along with the empiricists and positivists, he refused to postulate a metaphysical entity such as soul, mind or self.

He used the terms *mind* and *self* simply to refer to the phenomenal center of human experience that provides its perceived unity, that which experienced 'the stream of consciousness'. Conceiving of psychology as natural science, he expressly criticised the idea of a soul because it implied something substantial to which the individual has no empirical access. He maintained that *soul* adds nothing to our understanding and is superfluous for scientific purposes. After James, American psychologists felt little need to refer to a soul.[103]

Nevertheless, like James, many American psychologists at the turn of the century believed that psychology could and should study the mind: the phenomenal contents of an individual's experience. However, some twenty-five years later, the psychologist John B. Watson (1878–1958) rejected all references to mind. His express aim was to rid psychology of all residual 'religious' concepts like mind or consciousness that he considered little different from soul. He argued that a truly scientific psychology could not be based on anything that was not publicly verifiable and should be based solely on observable behaviour. In 1914 he wrote:

Psychology, as the behaviorist views it, is a purely objective experimental branch of natural science which needs consciousness as little as do the sciences of chemistry and physics[104]

apparently unaware that physicists were beginning to realise that it is not possible to formulate the laws of physics in a fully consistent way without reference to consciousness.[105]

This, then, is Newtonian psychology par excellence, a psychology without consciousness that reduces all behavior to mechanistic sequences of conditioned responses and asserts that the only scientific understanding of human nature is one that remains within the framework of classical physics and biology; a psychology, furthermore that reflects our culture's preoccupation with manipulative technology designed for domination and control.[106]

In reducing the study of man to those of his aspects that are 'objective facts' — his physical behaviours — and precluding any examination of his experience, psychology had taken away from man what is essentially and fundamentally his humanness. By so doing, what had come to be known as **behaviourism** had reduced man to an object or thing, and from this it was but a small step to accepting the idea that man is a machine and nothing but a machine.[107]

In adopting the mechanistic formulations of nineteenth-century physical science, early twentieth-century psychology did precisely that. It conceived of man as like an engine, and in trying to identify his mechanisms or laws of behaviour, psychologists implicitly became engineers. Adopting a suitably clockwork metaphor, psychology set itself the task of finding out how humans 'tick', without any reference to mind, much less to soul or spirit. Psychology's engineering function was explicitly addressed however by some psychologists[108–10] who proposed that it should engineer a technology of behaviour that would make people behave in socially acceptable ways and maintain established patterns of social life and its institutions. Hence the psychologist should not merely be a student of human behaviour, a spectator, but should attempt to control it in the same way that physical scientists seek to manipulate natural phenomena. Supported by the reigning philosophy of science of that time, logical positivism, behaviourism dominated psychology throughout the machine age of the early twentieth century and its influence remains to the present day. Progressively, psychology focused only on objective aspects of human functioning and by the mid-twentieth century it had become predominantly the scientific analysis of behaviour. Virtually all references to the soul had disappeared from textbooks on psychology. Psychology, in:

> trying to imitate the natural sciences and laboratory methods of weighing and counting, dealt with everything except the soul. It tried to understand those aspects of man which can be examined in the laboratory, and claimed that conscience, value judgements, and knowledge of good and evil are metaphysical concepts, outside the problems of psychology; it was often more concerned with insignificant problems which fitted the alleged scientific method than with devising new methods to study the

significant problems of man. Psychology thus became a science lacking its main subject matter, the soul.[111]

Bereft of its soul or psyche, psychology had become an empty or hollow discipline, leading one commentator to observe that psychology 'having first bargained away its soul and then gone out of its mind, seems, as it faces an untimely end, to have lost all consciousness.'[112] Certainly, in as much as it was no longer faithful to its original subject matter, the soul, psychology could be said not to be psychology at all. Moreover, it was highly questionable whether it could be considered 'science'. Discoveries in physics undermined the materialist, mechanistic model on which science was based. As the physicist Sir James Jeans pointed out, 'the stream of knowledge is heading towards a non-mechanical reality; the universe begins to look more like a great thought than like a great machine.'[113] Not only did investigations of the subatomic realm in the early years of the twentieth century completely undermine the notion of a clockwork universe, but they also revealed a world-view astonishingly consistent with that of the mystics of antiquity. These developments in thinking demanded a conceptual transition 'from the mechanics of behaviour — man the robot — to the properly human aspects of man the pilot'.[114]

However, for the most part psychology continued to resist this trend. Having struggled to conform to the mechanistic model of nineteenth-century physics, psychology was reluctant to abandon it, although physics had long since done so in favour of a radically new paradigm. Only gradually did it move away from the extreme mechanistic view of behaviourism to an acceptance that human beings cannot be adequately understood without reference to some internal mental processes. These processes were given the collective label of 'cognition' and were assimilated into the framework of physical science as 'brain function'. Hence, by the end of the twentieth century the psyche was generally seen as a merely epiphenomenal by-product of organic processes in the brain. Psychologists were no longer students of the soul in any sense but neuroscientists.

As for a modern scientific psychology which starts from the point of spirit as such, there simply is none. No-one today would venture to found a scientific psychology on the postulate of a psyche.[115]

Ironically, therefore, while the concept of soul has had a long history in Western thought it no longer has any place in modern psychology, as is reflected by the 'ubiquitous absence'[116] of the term in psychological literature. 'The term psyche remains only as an empty prefix, an ever present reminder of a bygone era in thinking about human nature, standing as a semantic equivalent of the ghost of Hamlet's father, complaining about his premature death. Psychologists of virtually all stripes have agreed that the term soul does not belong in psychology.'[117]

2

SAVIOURS OF THE SOUL

The origins of medicine are shrouded in mystery but ancient mythology suggests that the art of healing throughout the world is rooted in mysticism and magic. However, through the ages magic has been so obscured by 'the lush growth of superstition'[1] and uninformed thought that, in the Western world at least, its true nature has been lost.

Fundamentally magic asserts that the universe is a unity with no part separate or separable from any other. All that exists in the universe or cosmos is an expression of this underlying oneness that subsists through all things. Nothing exists except as an integral part of our timeless and eternal universe. The human soul or essence is therefore part of this greater whole and humankind a replica of it, a microcosm of the macrocosm.

Magic can be considered to be applied or practical mysticism in that mystical vision, awareness and sensitivity enable the individual to penetrate the mysteries and secrets of the universe and to work with its forces to produce desired effects. Those able to do so, often using spells, incantations, invocations and various rituals, are variously known as magicians, sorcerors or shamans.

Shamans

The term 'shaman' was first introduced to the West in the seventeenth century when Siberian tribes known as the Tungus were first encountered. Their tribal life centred on individuals known as the *shaman*, *saman* or *haman* to whom various magical powers were attributed. These included mastery of natural lore, healing the sick, telepathy, clairvoyance, divination of the future, dream interpretation, mastery of fire, rain-making and communion with spirits. Shamans were not simply practitioners of magic and medicine believed to perform miracles and cure but also priests and poets. They coexisted alongside other priests, magicians and healers but were distinguished from them because they were specialists of the soul — they alone could 'see' it and know its form and destiny — and they were able to journey in non-ordinary reality in pursuance of it. This was achieved by way of ecstasy, a trance-like state during which the soul of the shaman was believed to leave the body and ascend into the heavens or descend into the underworld in order to gain information to help members of the community in various ways. The 'ecstatic journey of the soul' is the defining characteristic of the shaman. In it he or she 'dies' and with his or her soul visits the spiritual realm or 'Beyond'. 'The shaman is the classic investigator of the realm of death; he explores the routes of travel to and in the Beyond and thereby produces a map of the postmortem terrain.'[2] In this domain the shaman contacts those who have died and spiritual beings who provide advice relating to life on earth. Communication in this realm is not by language but through feeling and telepathy.

> Because there are, in the Beyond, neither material barriers nor corporeal limits, but only pure consciousness in the form of the soul, it is perfectly possible to participate directly in the 'other' and to spontaneously penetrate the psychic atmosphere of another person or being.[3]

Hence, the shaman is a messenger between the world of the living and that of non-material existence, or the dead. Through the shaman, members of the tribe can hear the spirits speak and comment on the present and future. 'Their shaman affords them contact to the land of shadows and a dialogue with the dead.'[4] In this way members of tribal cultures have a close relationship with death and the death realm.

The shaman's journey into this other dimension is extremely dangerous, and fraught with perils. The shaman may not return from it. His or her body may remain without a soul, as a corpse. Hence the shaman is a hero and as such is celebrated in the traditions of the people and immortalised in their myths and poems.

The shaman's journeys or soul-excursions could be for various purposes:

diagnosing or treating illnesses; for divination or prophecy; for acquisition of power through interaction with spirits, power animals, guardians or other spiritual entities; for establishing guides or teachers in non-ordinary reality from whom the shaman may solicit advice on tribal or individual problems; or for contacting the spirits of the dead.[5]

In primitive societies the shaman's ability to act as an intermediary between worlds was seen as critical to communal life and human survival. It fell to the shaman to guard and defend the 'soul' of the community, and keep its members in touch with it, nurturing, protecting and restoring the soul to those who have lost sight of or contact with it. This process was generally conceived as a quest in which the shaman journeyed through the underworld in search of the person's lost soul.

The very ancient shamanic cultures of the world all conceived of three 'worlds' — the upper, middle and lower — that can be visited by a shaman in a 'journey', which is a metaphor for the shamanic trance state. 'This metaphor of a journey to the Beyond is a classical image of which practically all cultures make use to bring the travels of the consciousness of shamans or saints within the range of people's understanding. In the last resort all such attempts to present subtle experiences encountered in a transpersonal dimension in terms of metaphors common to our three-dimensional world are inadequate. However, they are the only method available to us for verbalizing the inexpressible.'[6]

The different 'worlds' identified are also metaphors for the realms, domains, planes or levels of consciousness visited or dwelt in by the shaman during such altered states.[7] Similarly, 'loss of soul' is a metaphor for detachment from feelings and the essential self. It means 'to lose contact with the thread and purpose of life, to stray from the path of inner harmony that is right and true for each of us as individuals, to violate our own inherent nature'.[8]

> The shamanic notion of soul loss is a metaphor for soul's tendency to elude the grasp of consciousness as well as its more primal detachment from feelings. The soul cannot be lost in a literal sense because it is always present with us. However, we

do lose contact with its movements within our daily lives, and this loss of relationship results in bodily and mental illness, rigidification, the absence of passion, and the estrangement from nature. It is the nature of soul to be lost to that aspect of mind that strives to control it.[9]

The sense of self and contact with feelings is lost because of the influence of the conscious, rational mind. As a result the soul is lost sight of, hence 'what is essential is invisible to the eye.'[10] Salvation of the soul involves re-establishing connection with and experience of one's essence.

The shaman's fundamental role in the community depended above all on insight: the ability to 'see' what is invisible to others and to provide direct and reliable information from this hidden domain. Hence shamans 'all seem able to see through the filters of culture, language and sense systems to other aspects of the real world — to non-ordinary reality'.[11]

> The shaman is part of the age-old tradition of the Perennial Philosophy — the mystical teaching of the unity of all things and all beings. In the realm of magic everything is interrelated; nothing exists in isolation. Here rules the principle of *pars pro toto*. This level of consciousness, like a gigantic telephone exchange, affords access to all other levels of awareness. All mystical paths are agreed that such a way of experiencing requires a suspension of normal awareness and rational thought by way of special techniques and mind training.[12]

The shaman's art calls for supreme control of awareness, thought and feeling, culminating in a separation of the soul from the body. It requires 'the deconditioning and annihilation of our customary modes of perception, the interruption of biopsychic functions'.[13] The shaman achieved this by withdrawing consciousness from the everyday world and shifting it to the inner world, which is accessed, explored and interpreted by way of visual images. By provoking powerful images in themselves and others, shamans bypassed the conscious mind and were able to commune with the energies of the unconscious mind. They did so by imagining these energies in various ways as human or animal spirits. Thus characterised, these were cultivated as 'inner guides' to help them explore the inner world of others. Various techniques were used which have the effect of transferring consciousness from the outer sensory world to the inner. These included sensory and sleep deprivation, fatigue, fasting, and breath control. Hallucinatory and stimulant drugs, drumming, dancing, rhythmic movement, chanting incantations and other rituals were also sometimes used to intensify perception, intuition and imagination in preparation for what in the manner of the Native American Indians might be termed a 'vision quest' or 'dream of knowledge': a journey that is visually a fact-finding mission aimed at discovering the cause of sickness, injury, drought, famine and other ills. All of these techniques essentially put the shaman beyond ordinary conscious processes, out of his or her mind in the normal sense, and in touch with what might be thought of as living energies conveying information and ideas. In these ways the shaman 'sees', albeit in the 'mind's eye', what others cannot. Mastery of methods for divining the inner world is traditionally the aim and purpose of shamanism, and applying the knowledge derived from such insight in the mundane world constitutes the science or knowledge on which the practices of shamanism, including healing or medicine, are based.

Shamanic healing

> Everything that concerns the soul and its adventure, here on earth and in the beyond, is the exclusive province of the shaman. Through his own preinitiatory and initiatory experiences, he knows the drama of the human soul, its instability, its precariousness; in addition, he knows the forces that threaten it and the regions to which it can be carried away. If shamanic cure involves ecstasy it is precisely because illness is regarded as a corruption or alienation of the soul.[14]

Throughout the world, shamans, and most indigenous peoples, regard all disease as originating and gaining meaning from affliction or loss of the soul. The former involves introduction of a pathogenic object and treatment is directed to expelling the cause of the trouble. However, whereas in the modern sense illness is typically viewed as an external agent entering the body, something to be destroyed or protected against, to the shaman illness-producing agents constitute a threat only if the person's protective mantle or soul body develops a weakness. Hence it is loss of personal power that allows intrusion in the first place.

Many magical notions derive from the idea of a subtle energy or soul body. In all ethnic groups this is generally conceived as a second, non-material or spiritual body possessed by all living entities, including animals and plants. It can separate from the body and therefore come and go during dreams, illness and in other states, before finally departing at death to a spirit world. It can lodge in other bodies and take possession of them, or be taken possession of by alien forces or disease. As the causes of illness reside in the soul body, healing must therefore concentrate on harmonising it.

> The Beyond, in which the soul lives, is subject to laws and conditions of space, time, and causality known in our world, but at the same time embodied in the qualities and capabilities of the soul. Since all material forms not only possess a soul body but at the same time are bearers of the spiritual essence ... our soul is directly connected with them: the soul and the ensouled universe are one.[15]

By altering the structure of their consciousness, people of all cultures acquire access to the soul body, to the Beyond, and to a non-material cosmic reservoir of energy.[16] Shamanic treatment therefore emphasises augmenting the personal power or energies of the sick person by tapping into cosmic forces and making them available to the soul body.

In the case of soul loss, effort is directed to finding and restoring the soul and re-establishing an individual's connection with it. In such cases the shaman is absolutely necessary as only he or she can 'see' the soul and only the shaman is able to travel in the soul body of the individual to other realms of existence in order to locate it. In this sense therefore shamanism can be regarded as a controlled act of mental dissociation. All shamanic healing is thus spiritual rather than physical. Its aim is primarily to preserve and nurture the soul and to restore its balance or harmony. Hence all healing involved attending to the soul, the literal meaning of the term 'psychotherapy'.

However, the shaman did not work exclusively in the context of disease. Shamanism is *applied animism*, or animism in practice. 'In animistic cultures nature is believed to be alive with gods and spirits, and because all aspects of the universe are perceived as intertwined, the shaman is required as an intermediary between different planes of being.'[17] He or she not only combated disease but also demons and the power of evil, defending life, health, fertility and the world of 'light' against death, disease, sterility, disaster and the 'world of darkness'.[18] Healing overlapped with all aspects of secular and sacred life. Nevertheless, as the specialist of the soul the shaman who understands the mysteries of life and death is also capable of causing harm.

Shamanism is a visionary tradition, an ancient practice of using altered states of consciousness to contact the gods and spirits of the natural world. As such it is a religious phenomenon. Strictly speaking, shamanism is a religious phenomenon of Siberia and central Asia but similar magico-religious practices have been described and documented in North and Central America, the Arctic, Polynesia, India, Tibet, China, Japan, Australasia, Indonesia and Africa. Archaeological evidence and studies which suggest that shamanism was influential within ancient Celtic cultures confirm that these practices are many thousands of years old, widespread and remarkably similar throughout the world. Moreover they survive in various parts of the world in the present day.

Analysis of these practices in 42 cultures confirms that ecstasy is the central and characteristic feature of shamanism. Indeed shamanism has been defined as 'archaic techniques of ecstasy'[19] which is a specific altered state of consciousness or trance. This has been termed the 'shamanic state of consciousness' or SSC[20] and is considered to give access to a clairvoyant reality, a timeless unified dimension, where neither time nor space can prevent information exchange. Shamans can control the trance dimension, entering into this altered state of consciousness or expanded awareness at will in order to access knowledge, insights and information from ordinarily inaccessible realms of the cosmos and waking from it with full knowledge of magical cures and healing procedures.

As an elite with access to knowledge inaccessible to others, shamans exercised, and still exercise, a powerful influence on religious ideology, mythology and rituals world wide and on the practices of healing. Where the fate of the soul is not an issue, the shaman is not absolutely necessary, so their practices have always existed alongside more mechanical and technological forms of medicine. Typically in shamanic cultures a healing hierarchy exists with specialists in physical manipulation and prescription succeeded by diagnostic specialists and then those who use their imagination to intervene with the supernatural.

The shamanic tradition of healing in the West
Although the origins of Western medicine are shrouded in mythology, shamanic practices and healing hierarchies are nonetheless discernible.

Medicine in ancient Egypt
Homer considered the Egyptians to be more skilled in healing than any other people, and pictographs and hieroglyphics in ancient temples such as Kom Ombo bear witness to the sophistication of their medicine. The earliest written evidence of Egyptian medicine appears in papyri of the second millennium BC but such records encode far older traditions dating from the fourth millennium BC when thought and speech were recognised as ruling parts of the soul. The seat of the soul was the heart and so what can be considered Egyptian medical theory comprised a speculative heart-based physiology. This pictured 'a vascular system likened to the Nile and its canals, and as with that water-system, the point was to keep it free of obstruction'.[21]

However, Egyptian physical medicine was rooted in the magical vision of a harmoniously interrelated universe suffused with the divine. Man was viewed as a microcosm of the macrocosm and expected to reflect its order and harmony. This was achieved through a balancing of subtle energies: cosmic 'uranian' forces and subterranean 'telluric' forces.

Uranian forces were seen as an expression of God and were symbolised as light radiating down from the sun, Ra, which is broken down into rays corresponding to the colour spectrum, each manifesting a different facet of the divine and influencing different qualities of life. The most important aim of man was to realise the light and thereby the divine, to become 'enlightened' by opening up to the light, channelling and distributing it, and merging it with earth energies. These telluric forces were characterised as spontaneous upward movement and symbolised by a rearing serpent. Those who had successfully raised this latent serpent energy to merge with the uranian forces are depicted in Egyptian art with a snake emerging from their forehead, which was thought to be the seat of divine consciousness. In so far as man achieved this union, he was the mediator of heaven and earth, and the aim of magic was to produce this connection, thereby 'bringing down the light', transferring and reflecting its power. Essentially, therefore, Egyptian medicine was spiritual, concerned with harmonising the soul or man's essential nature with universal forces, and only secondarily with physical disease which was seen as a reflection of fundamental disharmony.

The secrets of this ancient wisdom were passed on only to the highest order of priests for sole use in the service of man and his spiritual development. Magic and religion were inextricably linked with each other and with medicine, which although essentially practical was sacerdotal, addressing the whole person in soul, mind and body.

The vital energies were thought to be absorbed and regulated by a finer etheric or spiritual 'body' that enveloped the physical body. The temple priests sought to direct these forces by passing their hands over the body, and are often depicted thus in *bas relief*. The priests recognised the therapeutic value of colour and employed variously coloured sanctuaries in treatment. They also recognised the relationship of colour to other vibrational forms and understood that rhythm — the expression of movement in life and the pulse of everything that exists — has the potential for creating harmony and healing, or disintegration and destruction. The laws of rhythm were among the most closely guarded secrets passed on from father to son and master to pupil by secret oral tradition. Rhythmical invocations and incantations, music and movement all played a substantial part in the rites of magic, religion and healing.

In addition to the temple priests there were also healers of various grades. The lowest level were practitioners of physical manipulation, such as bone setters, and the highest comprised those who could access and direct natural forces. Dreams were of great importance in healing because of the insight they provided into the condition of the soul and those healers with the ability to provoke and interpret dreams in both diagnosis and treatment were the most highly regarded.

The first known Egyptian physician, represented as Thoth (known by the Greeks as Hermes Trismegistus), was the god of medicine and the moon. The knowledge of healing which was passed down in the occult traditions, or mystery schools, of the ancient world and used in the training of physician-priests was thought to originate from him. The most renowned healer, Imhotep (born *circa* 3000 BC) proclaimed as a master of magic, poetry, divination and rain-making, clearly displays the shamanic origins of Egyptian medicine. On his death he was elevated first to the status of a demi-god. Then, *circa* 525 BC, he was designated the son of Ptah, the god of healing and so became a full deity of medicine. In his name the ancient traditions of healing were passed on and found their way into classical Greek culture.

Medicine in ancient Greece

Like the Hebrew, Aborigine and most ancient peoples of the world, the early Greeks believed in a past Golden Age, a long lost Arcadia, when man lived in perfect harmony with nature. The Greek poet Hesiod, writing *circa* 700 BC, described Arcadian life as free from ills, hard toil and oppressive disease. Loss of the Golden Age was attributed to the first woman, Pandora, who opened a jar and released 10,000 woes, leaving only Hope behind.

Similarly, in Hebrew tradition, as revealed in *The Book of Genesis*, the first woman, Eve, was tempted by the Devil to eat forbidden fruit. As punishment for this original sin, she and Adam were banished from the Garden of Eden or Paradise and condemned to a life of toil, suffering and pain. Similar legends throughout the world explain how suffering, disease and death became the human condition.

The dream of the Greeks was to restore this Golden Age and to live in perfect harmony with nature. Until the sixth century BC their aim was *physis*, the attempt to perceive the essential nature of all things. It was synonymous with mysticism and its practical applications which were consistent with magic. All knowledge concerned understanding the meaning and purpose of natural phenomena and living in accordance with the natural order. Human problems were seen as disharmony or dis-ease of the soul — literally *psychopathology* — and as fundamentally spiritual in nature. Physical disorders were largely regarded as symptomatic of this fundamental disharmony. Socrates insisted that physicians should not attempt to heal the body without first treating the soul. Curing the soul was essential. Treatment was therefore directed to the cure of the soul, *psychotherapy*, through restoration of its balance and harmony. Accordingly, man had to be attuned to and in harmony with both spiritual and physical realities to be healthy or whole. The legacy of this idea is found in the terms 'health' and 'healing' which originate in the German *heilen* meaning to make whole. This is closely related to the Old English words *hael* (whole) and *haelen* (heal) from which the English 'hale' (as in the phrase 'hale and hearty') and the Welsh *hoil* derive. These terms are very similar to the German *heilig* and the Old English *halig*, both meaning holy. Etymologically, therefore, to be healthy is to be whole or holy, which clearly embraces both spiritual and physical features and not merely the latter.

Any distinction between spiritual and physical realities would have been meaningless to the ancient Greeks as they had no word for matter, viewing all forms of existence as manifestations of *physis* and endowed with life and spirituality. All things were thought to be comprised of gods and spirits and the universe was deemed to be a kind of organism sustained by *pneuma* or cosmic breath, in much the same way that the human body is sustained by air. Until the sixth century BC gods and spirits were central to all thinking about the universe, so healing was essentially a spiritual phenomenon associated with the deities.

Various gods were seen as principally responsible for healing but it is in the cult of Asclepios (known to the Romans as Aesculapius) that similarities with Egyptian medicine can most clearly be seen. Like Imhotep, Asclepios has uncertain origins. Evidently, though, a mortal physician of that name was revered as the founder of medicine who on his death became first a demi-god then a full deity. The followers of the latter, the Asclepiads, were temple priests and, like their Egyptian counterparts, they worshipped the rising sun. Moreover, Asclepios was typically depicted with the *caduceus* or rustic staff around which is curled a serpent representing earth energy. This later became the emblem of the Hippocratic school of medicine and subsequently Western medicine. Like the Egyptians, the Asclepiads also made use of dreams in diagnosis and treatment, and therapeutic use of movement and music. By the fifth century BC the cult of Asclepios had spread widely.

However, the most revered of the healing deities was Hygeia, who can be thought of as the goddess of preventative medicine. She was concerned with the promotion of health and personified the wisdom that health lies in understanding how to live in harmony with oneself and the environment. The tradition that grew up in her name focused on special diets, baths, ablutions, exercise and dance and methods such as listening to music and attending theatre, which were considered highly therapeutic.

Hippocrates, who subsequently established a medical school that flourished at the end of the fifth century BC, is commonly regarded as the father of Western medicine. He integrated medicine into the universal laws of nature as they were then conceived, thereby unifying medicine and philosophy. Yet all that is known of him is legend.

Like early thinkers such as Anaximander, Alcmaeon and Empedocles, Hippocrates subscribed to the view that health lay in balancing opposite qualities, heat, coldness, wetness and dryness, associated with four basic elements, earth, air, fire and water. In his treatise on the 'Nature of Man' Hippocrates extended the doctrine to physiology by associating these with four humours or bodily fluids: blood; phlegm; yellow bile, or choler; and black bile or melancholy. These humours arose in various bodily organs, and were affected by thoughts, feelings, emotions and behaviours, climate, polluted water, over- and under-activity, lack of sunlight and other environmental factors. The mixture of these humours determined the moral and physical characteristics of individuals, and to some extent the diseases to which they were subject. The proper balance of humours constituted health, and so Hippocratic healing involved restoring equilibrium within these fluid essences by regulation of psychological and environmental variables, and lifestyle. Indeed *diatetica* (dietetics), the cornerstone of the healing art, involved the entire lifestyle.

Like the shaman, the Hippocratic physician was a diviner of natural signs and an expert in natural lore. He used all his senses to measure and define the environment, taking account of its position in relation to the stars, sunrise and wind direction, the conditions of soil and water, and the weather. Students of medicine were required to study the effects of natural cycles, such as the seasons, on health. The physician recognised the wholeness of things and did not view disease as an isolated phenomenon. This principle is embodied in the Hippocratic doctrine:

> There is one common flow, one common breathing: all things are in sympathy.

So too is the idea of a life force inherent in all living organisms, which Hippocrates recognised as nature's healing power — the *vix medicatrix naturae*. He placed great emphasis on this, insisting that as 'our natures are the physicians of our diseases' the healing process is only designed to assist the body's own self-healing, providing assistance to the natural forces by creating the most favourable conditions for such a process. Accordingly the physician was the servant of nature. Physicians trained in the Hippocratic tradition did not try to cure patients without educating them in the nature, origin and development of their illness. They clearly saw their role as helping nature to heal itself; restoring the balance disturbed by disease but not interfering with nature. The physician was a therapist, literally, from the Greek *therapeia* (attendance), an attendant to the healing process.

There is little doubt that Hippocratic philosophy was inspired by mystic vision. It is therefore somewhat ironic that Hippocrates is regarded as the father of modern Western medicine because in the main his views diametrically oppose much modern medical theory and practice. However, in the Hippocratic tradition there emerges for the first time awareness that health and illness are natural biological phenomena rather than the work of gods and spirits. They are the reactions of an organism to its environment, lifestyle and other factors, and can be influenced by therapeutic procedures and by wise management of one's life. As such it represents a break with the magico-religious tradition of ancient medicine, healing by rational methods of treatment rather than the magical cures of the temple. Under its influence health became the ideal of culture.

Plato upheld the Hippocratic doctrine, claiming that diseases originated in the body from physical causes and humours, or bodily fluids. Some were hereditary and others the result of 'rebellion of the soul', or inner conflict. Because body and soul were involved in disorder he believed that all treatment should be psychosomatic, involving physical exercises for the body, training of the emotions through the theatre and the arts, and training of the intellect.

Galenism

The humoural doctrine of Hippocratic medicine was subsequently systematised and codified by Galen (*circa* 130–200 AD), the Greek physician to the Roman emperor Marcus Aurelius. He was the leading physician of the ancient world and one of the most influential physicians of all time. Like Hippocrates and Aristotle, Galen was trained in the Asclepian tradition and like them he attributed varieties of human temperament to different admixtures of the humours. He described four personality types, each associated with the dominance of one of the humours. Too much black bile resulted in a tendency to depression and melancholia, while dominance of yellow bile produced a choleric, bad-tempered bitter character; the phlegmatic personality resulting from excess phlegm was characteristically apathetic; and the sanguine type produced by the dominance of blood was cheerful and ruddy. Accordingly, emotional aspects of personality, such as depression, hostility, apathy and optimism were directly linked to health. The theory of humours and the doctrine of four temperaments were included in the immense body of technical treatises written by Galen that formed the basis of a system of medicine known as Galenism. This dominated the Western world throughout the Middle Ages and persisted into modern times, upheld by both philosophers and scientists who asserted that the 'old view is essentially correct.'[22] The ancient doctrine was modified, extended and refined by some psychologists in the twentieth century. 'There is a continuity between ancient and modern theories, and the doctrine of temperament, originating in medicine, has been incorporated into modern differential psychology and become part of the theory of personality.'[23]

Medicine in the Middle Ages

Medicine was central to the ancient civilisations of Egypt, Greece and Rome. The Greeks had developed delicate surgical skills and herbal treatments and elevated the art of healing to great heights but, as Christianity spread, all that was pagan, including its medical practices, was obliterated. This is ironic because Christ himself bestowed a healing mission on his Apostles and gave evidence of his divine powers by miraculous acts of healing. Christ's instructions to his disciples to care for the sick eventually led to the establishment of hospitals and healing ministries, and many people converted to Christianity in the hope of being cured.

However, 'sober ecclesiastics condemned this vulgar zeal for healing marvels, presenting Christ as the physician of the soul.'[24] The early Church distinguished the body from the soul, and considered it inferior. The soul was eternal and the flesh weak. Implicitly it subordinated medicine to religion and the doctor to the priest. The doctor attended merely to the body, while the priest attended to the cure of souls. In elevating the immaterial soul the mortal body was disparaged and commonly viewed as the prison of the soul. Some elements in the Church, dismissing the teaching that man had been created in God's image, viewed the flesh as the Devil's domain. Disease was therefore caused by Satan and could not be exorcised by pagan methods of healing. These were condemned in favour of brutal practices such as mortifying the flesh, which were seen as a way of freeing the soul from the clutches of Satan. Glorification of the suffering associated with its release remained a powerful force within Christianity until the late Middle Ages when new emphasis came to be placed on the soul's incarnation in the flesh. Consequently Christianity has been blamed for bringing about the Dark Ages of health care and the practice of medicine to an all time low.[25]

Certainly throughout the Middle Ages pagans and all visionary movements were intensely persecuted by the Church, and under its influence serious study and the practice of medicine were discontinued. Healing was subject to ecclesiastical regulation and monks and clerics commonly practised medicine. Monasteries became key healing centres and healing shrines flourished. Every organ of the body and each complaint acquired a particular saint whose help was invoked in effecting cure. Damian and Cosmas supplanted Asclepius as the patron saints of medicine. Traditional forms of healing were preserved only by secret oral tradition, healing rites being regarded as mysteries to be shared only with initiates. Consequently most healing practices can only be deduced from documents relating to witch trials, reflecting the fact that in Europe healing was largely the province of wise women or witches who were purged relentlessly by the Church as heretics and purveyors of magic. As a result, much of their knowledge was lost, with dire consequences for medicine.

In the ancient world women were generally believed to hold the secrets of life within their very being. During the Middle Ages those women with superior knowledge were known as witches. They were probably the most advanced scientists of the period. Many of their practices were clearly shamanic in origin, most notably their 'flight' on broomsticks, which more properly can be thought of as flights of imagination or fantasy, or journeys in altered states of consciousness. They were wholly shamanic in their regard for the unity of all things, in their attempts to use the forces of nature for healing and their use of spells and herbal remedies. Paracelsus (1493–1541), who was one of the most enduring influences in the development of medicine, attributed to his conversations with wise women his understanding of the laws and practices of healing and the role of the healer. The thinking of Paracelsus rested on a mystically inspired 'interpenetrative holistic cosmology'.[26] His ideals of bringing all things into perfect harmony were diffused at all levels of medical practice.

However, Paracelsus brought about a significant reformation in medicine. At the time when Copernicus and Kepler were challenging the religious and scientific orthodoxy of the earth as the centre of the universe, Paracelsus challenged Galen's humoural doctrine that was at the centre of the medical orthodoxy and called for its complete abandonment. 'For centuries, of course, Galen had been God: the Arabs had synthesized his works and the medieval West had translated these into Latin.'[27] From the fourteenth century Europe's cultural and intellectual life had undergone a dramatic rebirth. Renaissance humanism and mysticism fostered interest in the human soul, 'the spiritual fulcrum in a cosmos governed by supernatural forces'.[28] Art drew attention to the body, seen to have been created for the sake of the soul, and in an intellectual climate that revered the classics and all things Greek, the dream of the renaissance humanists was to restore medicine to its Greek purity. There was a revival of ancient medicine and Galenism was venerated. However, Galen's doctrine discouraged empirical observation and so had never led to a systematic collection of observed relationships between lifestyle, thought patterns, emotions and illness. In the course of centuries the doctrine had become dogmatic, encouraging principally speculation on the nature and consequences of the hypothetical humours rather than the further development of knowledge and practice. Consequently, Galenic medicine had become stagnant. Furthermore renaissance anatomy had revealed that the structures of the body were not strictly as Galen as stated, and that Galenic ideas about the function of bodily organs were also flawed.

In contrast to Galen, Paracelsus advocated a system of healing based on observation and experience. He pioneered the use of specific treatments to remedy particular disease and introduced into the *materia medica* chemical compounds, such as mercury and antimony, and distilled essences of herbs and opium. As the originator of some of the most effective drugs in the Victorian pharmacopoeia he is credited with laying the foundations of modern chemistry and chemotherapy although in fact the science of chemistry originated in alchemy, which for many centuries had been concerned with the study of materials. The writings of Paracelsus, when published in the second half of the sixteenth century, influenced the courts of Europe and continued to exert a strong influence until the nineteenth century. However, developments in thinking during the seventeenth century overtook Paracelsus' holistic views.

The emergence of medical science in the seventeenth century

Descartes viewed the body and soul as distinct. As matter, the body was extended, corpuscular and quantifiable. The soul, which he equated with mind, was insubstantial, immortal and the source of consciousness. He proposed a mechanical model of the human animal, drawing analogies with clocks and automata. Animals did not possess souls and so were viewed simply as automata.

> Descartes thus radically rethought the metaphysics of physiology and medicine — his mechanistic account of the nervous system included a model of the reflex concept. But he never worked out, or at least to his critics' satisfaction, how mind and body could actually interact; for critics, his speculative localization of the link in the pineal gland, a unitary structure seated in the mid-brain just behind the main ventricle,

merely compounded the problem. Mind had been made a mysterious ghost in the machine, while his notion of the passions as mediating mind and body was more holistic than his mind/body dualism seemed to sanction. Overall, however, Cartesianism's significance for bio-medicine was enormous. Descartes regarded the body exactly as he viewed the world, as a mechanism. Dismissing Aristotelian–Galenic elements and humours even more radically than Paracelsus, he postulated that matter in motion would explain both the human body and the system of nature at large. That was an audacious challenge.[29]

Descartes' dualistic philosophy introduced a schism between soul and body which when viewed against the history of medicine is quite aberrant. Before Descartes, most healers addressed themselves to the interplay between body and soul and treated their patients within the context of both psychophysical and spiritual realities. In traditional tribal medicine and in Western practice from its beginnings in the work of Hippocrates the psychological component in illness had been recognised,[30] and the need to attend to the patient's soul was a basic premise of healing. The effect of this negation of soul on medicine was devastating. It meant that the soul no longer had a place within medicine, which as a result became a purely physical science focused on the body.

> The Cartesian formulation led to the view that the body reflected the machine-like characteristics of the universe itself — machine-like bodies inhabiting a machine-like world. Disease thus arose as a disorder of mechanism. Something went awry in the machine.[31]

The Cartesian view provided scientists of the time with a mandate to examine bodies by anatomical dissection. Until that time the Church, whose primary function was to preserve the soul, would not sanction such an invasion, but if, as Descartes maintained, body and soul were separate it followed that the soul could not be harmed if bodies were dissected. 'This proved to be the handiest of arrangements for an infant bioscience as for the Church. It gave scientists a green light to begin investigating bodies in earnest, searching for mechanisms of causation of disease; and the Church could take comfort that, in so doing, no violence would be done to the soul.'[32] The Church was therefore largely responsible for the ensuing anatomical and structural emphasis within Western medicine.[33] 'Opening up bodies — dead human cadavers, living animal ones — had become the prescription for true medical knowledge,'[34] and to Descartes medicine was the key to the natural world. However, before the construction of the microscope in the seventeenth century it was not possible for philosophers or physicians to do much more than indulge in speculation.

Descartes supported his new philosophy by reference to the discovery of blood circulation by William Harvey (1578–1657). Although Harvey 'saw through Aristotelian spectacles',[35] his discovery had subverted further still the medical legacy of ancient Greece.

> Harvey did not, as sometimes supposed, conceive of the body in a 'modern' mechanical fashion: it was not a machine, but was moved by vital forces. In discussing the circulation, his terms and ideas were Aristotelian ... With Aristotle he shared a teleological view of the body and the belief that its workings depended upon the distinctive soul.[36]

However, Harvey's discovery led to the development of a new physiology. It, and the revelation by dissection of anatomical structures unknown to ancient authority, led to the realisation that medical science had to be placed on a different footing than formerly. For the first time it became possible to envisage life not as a mysterious extra-material power, but as explicable in terms of physical forces. Descartes and later materialist philosophers were determined that their 'new philosophy' should replace the Aristotelian cosmos of qualities and elements with one composed of matter in motion obeying mathematical laws.

The new philosophy had crucial implications for understanding the soul and mind–body relations. The implications of Cartesian philosophy for mental illness were enormous. Descartes' dualistic philosophy ruled out primary mental disease: madness could not reside in the immortal soul or mind but had to be in the body. This inspired a search for the site of madness within the organism, and specifically, within the brain.

The progress of medicine in the eighteenth century

> Until well into the eighteenth century, in spite of the revolution in the approach of the life sciences which began in the previous century, traditional views inherited from the ancient world were still largely prevalent. The system of living things was a static system, in which each form of life held its appointed place in 'the great chain of being' ordained by the Creator. Life itself was explained in terms of an animating vital principle which differentiated it from non-living matter. The workings of the brain and nervous system had hardly begun to be understood, and even their basic structures were far from clearly delineated.[37]

However, once firmly established in biology, the mechanistic view advanced by Descartes dominated the attitudes of biologists and physicians towards health and illness and resulted in the so-called bio-medical model which forms the conceptual basis of modern scientific medicine. Consequent with this emphasis on the body, all that was not physical was excluded from Western medicine. All that was intuitive and irrational was purged. Intuition, feelings, sensitivity, imagination and spirituality simply had no place in a universe composed of cogs and springs, or in scientific method. These impediments to the new scientific order were discarded as medicine progressively focused on probing, detecting, isolating, analysing, controlling and usually destroying the 'problem', which was seen as an invasion, defect or aberration quite separate from the person. In this way diseases were 'isolated' and the use of physical measurement prepared for the belief in the real existence of diseases and their autonomy from the perception of both doctor and patient. This led to a tendency for disease to be spoken of as a thing and not as part of the total life process. In this way the person became separated from the sickness and the doctor's interest shifted from the sick to the sickness. Hospitals became laboratories for the study of disease processes rather than institutions for the care of the sick and nearly all discourse on health actually came to be about disease, a focus which is essentially negative.   Birth of the Clinic,

However, the Cartesian philosophy was not universally accepted, especially within eighteenth-century medicine. Georg Ernst Stahl (1660–1734) denounced its materialism and advocated an animism that proposed a God-given soul or *anima* as the prime mover of all living things. This anima was the agent of consciousness and physiological regulation and disease was the soul's attempt to expel morbid matter and re-establish bodily order. Friedrich Hoffmann (1660–1742) supported this view of disease while also accepting the body as a mathematically understandable machine. Very few physicians reduced man wholly to mechanism. An exception was Julian Offray de La Mattrie (1709–51) who insisted that the body was a machine that winds its own springs and thus has no need of a soul.

Not only natural philosophers but also scientists of the era insisted that there was more to bodies than cogs, wheels and pulleys. Experiments revealed the limitations of the mechanical model and reinforced the remarkable abilities of living things. René Réaumur (1683–1757), for example, demonstrated the ability of lobsters to grow new claws after amputation, and in 1768 Lazzarro Spallanzani (1729–99) showed that salamanders, snails and tadpoles could regenerate their tails. These discoveries transcended clockwork: 'There was more to life than the mechanical philosophy had dreamt of. But how was this to be explained in an era no longer prepared to entertain miracles or Galenic innate virtues?'[38]

Experimentation prompted new accounts of vitality and the relations between body and soul. A towering figure in this movement was Albrecht von Haller (1708–77).[39] On the basis of animal experiments, von Haller graded organs and ascribed to them inherent sensitivities independent of any soul principle. His views were opposed by Robert Whytt who, in 1751, reiterated the role of the soul. His soul, unlike that of Descartes, was energetic, sentient at a non-conscious level (thus automatic) and spatially extended in the body. The sentience of the soul was fundamental to his notion of bodily coordination.

However, experimentation also advanced knowledge of the structures and functions of living organisms. The workings of the lymphatic system and the lacteals were discovered, and in the eighteenth and nineteenth centuries the operation of the nervous system and brain became better understood. With the development of the microscope and the laboratory, nineteenth-century scientists explored the nature of body tissue and pioneered cell biology. Discoveries in organic chemistry yielded knew knowledge about respiration, nutrition, and digestion that led to the development of endocrinology.

Nineteenth-century medicine

During the nineteenth century spectacular progress was made in understanding infectious diseases. Bacteriology, which originated in the work of the Frenchman Louis Pasteur and Robert Koch in Germany, established the role of pathogenic micro-organisms and led to dramatic new cures. The life sciences made it clear that living organisms are composed of ordinary chemical elements organised in complex ways. Further discoveries suggested the close interdependence of body and mind. It became clear that the mind was dependent on the stability of the bodily environment and any disturbance, whether physical or chemical, could affect its workings. This led to the view, contrary to ancient belief, that the psyche does not build itself a body, but matter, by chemical action, produces the psyche. Therefore mind must be thought of as epiphenomenon of matter, and human beings as 'physical machines that have learned to think'.[40] 'To grant the substantiality of the soul or psyche (was) repugnant to the spirit of the age, for to do so would be heresy.'[41]

However, **mesmerism**, the forerunner of hypnotherapy, showed that the mind also has an influence on the functions of the body. It seemed increasingly clear that mind and body were part of one single system, and the term 'psychosomatic' was introduced to express this unity. In the light of these developments Descartes' separation of the mind and body needed rethinking. Always problematic, Cartesian dualism was increasingly unattractive as animistic and vitalistic ideas were eliminated from the life sciences. From a purely scientific standpoint the reduction of the operations of the mind to the functions of the brain was attractive. However, the reductionist view that psychology is rooted in the physiology of the nervous system and that the operations of mind are functions of the brain was not universally accepted. The neurophysiologist Sir Charles Sherrington believed that there was 'an inalienable residue enshrined in the ancient concept of the soul, which could not be reduced to physiology',[42] and the argument between mechanism and vitalism continued throughout the eighteenth and nineteenth centuries. But by the twentieth century the perfect correlation between behaviour and neural function was taken for granted.

> Whereas most traditional healing systems have sought to understand the relations between the sick person to the wider cosmos and to make readjustments between individual and world, or society and world, the western medical tradition explains sickness principally in terms of the body itself — its own cosmos. Greek medicine dismissed supernatural powers, though not macrocosmic, environmental influences; and from the Renaissance the flourishing anatomical and physiological programmes created a new confidence among researchers that everything that needed to be known could essentially be discovered by probing more deeply and ever more minutely into the flesh, its systems, tissues, cells, its DNA.
>
> This has proved an infinitely productive inquiry, generating first knowledge and then power, including on some occasions the power to conquer disease.[43]

Nevertheless, despite these developments and the emerging science of pharamacology, nineteenth-century medicine could do little about disease and death. Bio-medical understanding exceeded breakthroughs in curative medicine. The eventual decline in lethal diseases such as cholera, dysentry, scarlet fever, diphtheria, typhoid, tuberculosis, whooping cough and measles, owed more to improvements in sanitation, nutrition, water purification, food hygiene, housing, sewage processing, working conditions, standards of living, smaller families and other social improvements than to medicine or the development of sulphonamide drugs, antibiotics and mass immunisation. It was only as a result of these developments, which owed little to medicine *per se* but were claimed as evidence of medical progress, that Western scientific medicine could become truly powerful.

(handwritten margin note: imp. public health)

The twentieth-century challenge to medical 'science'

Consistent with the reductionist, determinist orientation of modern medicine the thrust of medical scientists throughout the twentieth century was to understand disease processes at the molecular level on the assumption that it will eventually be possible to locate the aberrant molecules in all disease. In the meantime medicine settled for repairing, removing or replacing those parts it could not as yet more successfully engineer. By the end of the twentieth century the mechanics of medicine were increasingly evident in various developments in spare part surgery, the mechanisation of childbirth and engineering of every kind, genetic, biochemical, neurological and structural. However, 'the emergence of this high-tech scientific medicine may be a prime example of what William Blake denounced as "single vision". The kind of myopia which (literally and metaphorically) comes from looking doggedly down a microscope.'[44] Indeed, it soon became clear that in the pursuit of this vision the whole picture had been lost.

> We have now discovered that it was intellectually unjustified presumption on our forefathers' part to assume that man has a soul; that that soul has substance, is of divine nature and therefore immortal; that there is power inherent in it which builds up the body, supports its life, heals its ills and enables the soul to live independently of the body; that there are incorporeal spirits with which the soul associates; and that beyond our empirical present there is a spiritual world from which the soul receives knowledge of spiritual things whose origins cannot be discovered in this visible world.
>
> But people who are not above the general level of consciousness have not yet discovered that it is just as presumptuous and fantastic for us to assume that matter produces spirit ... that apes give rise to human beings ... that the brain cells manufacture thoughts, and that all this could not possibly be other than this.[45]

Ironically, while during the twentieth century psychology and medicine struggled to conform to the mechanistic model of nineteenth-century physics, physics has long since abandoned this paradigm as outmoded and inappropriate. Investigations of the subatomic realm in the early years of the twentieth century completely undermined the Cartesian/Newtonian notion of a clockwork universe.

By the end of the century every basic tenet of the Newtonian view of how the world behaves had been abandoned in favour of a radically different view. This revealed more than simply a better model of the physical world. Scientific discoveries demanded a radically different reformulation of the most fundamental aspects of reality. Physicists began to approach their subject in totally unexpected and novel ways that seemed to turn common sense on its head and to have more in common with mysticism than materialism. In so doing they also demonstrated that 'it is more in keeping with the history of thought to describe science as the myths about the world which have yet to be proved wrong.'[46]

Relativity theory

All the principal ideas of the Newtonian world-view were shattered by developments in physics in the early twentieth century, notably relativity theory and atomic physics. Notions of absolute space and time, elementary solid particles of which matter is composed, the strictly causal nature of physical phenomena and the ideal of an objective description of nature simply did not apply in the new domains penetrated by physics. According to relativity theory time and space are linked and all measurements involving space and time lose their absolute significance. Previously time had been regarded as absolute, fixed, universal and independent of material bodies or observers. Relativity theory suggested that time is dynamical, able to stretch, shrink, warp and even stop altogether, and clock rates, rather than being absolute, are relative to the state of motion and gravitational situation of the observer. Space and time thus become merely elements of language used by an observer to describe his or her environment, and as such are used by observers in different ways.

Cause and effect

Without direct experience it is difficult to conceive of or describe four-dimensional space–time. To do so requires a picture or 'map' covering the whole span of time and the whole region of space. These space–time diagrams are four-dimensional patterns in space–time representing a network of interrelated events that have no definite direction of time attached to them. Consequently there is no 'before' or 'after' in the processes they picture and no linear relationship of cause or effect, unless direction is imposed on the picture by the 'map' being read in a certain way, such as from bottom to top. All events are interconnected, but the connections are not causal in the Newtonian sense. The ordering of events will differ depending on how a person accesses the 'map' or picture, so there will be no universal flow of time as in the Newtonian model. Different observers will order events differently, that is, take a different view of the picture, if they move with different velocities relative to the observed events. Two events that are seen as occurring simultaneously by one observer may occur in different temporal sequence for other observers.

One casualty of this 'elastic' time is the division of time into past, present and future. In relativity theory everyone has a personal time, locked to his or her state of motion. Accordingly the concept of time — a universal standard of public time — is an illusion and what people mean by 'now' depends on how they are moving. Therefore the idea of subjective time, with its emphasis on 'now', has no objective meaning. It follows from this that if there is no universal 'now', then in some sense the past and the future exist and are equally real in the present. Events are simply there in space–time and do not happen, so the apparent 'flow' of time is illusory. It would seem, therefore that what moves is the human mind rather than time.

While this reality can be described mathematically, ordinary language refers to conventional Newtonian notions of time so it is very difficult to convey these concepts. In fact the conventional concepts of space and time are so basic to our thinking about the universe that the view of them demanded by relativity theory requires modification of the whole framework used to describe the universe. Moreover, as unification of space and time necessarily unifies other apparently unrelated features, it demands a fundamental change in the way the universe is perceived.

The General Theory of Relativity

The General Theory of Relativity put forward by Albert Einstein (1879–1955) in 1915 completely abolished the concepts of absolute space and time and suggested that the whole structure of space–time depends on the distribution of matter in the universe. Thus, the concept of empty space loses its meaning. The upheaval in understanding the universe demanded by relativity theory goes still further. Mass and energy are simply different manifestations of the same thing, mass being a bound form of energy. Mass is no longer associated with material substance and is not seen as consisting of any basic 'stuff' but as bundles or 'quanta' of energy.

Energy is associated with activity and processes and this implies that the nature of matter is intrinsically dynamic. It can therefore no longer be pictured as being composed of units like tiny billiard balls or grains of sand, as in the Newtonian view. Such images are inappropriate not only because they represent the constituents of matter as separate but also because they are static three-dimensional images. Their forces now have to be understood dynamically as forms in space and time, as dynamic patterns of activity which have both a spatial and a temporal aspect. The former makes them appear as objects with a certain mass, and the latter makes them appear as processes involving the equivalent energy. As they are different aspects of the same space–time reality, the being of matter and its activity cannot be separated.

The equivalence of mass and energy has since been verified innumerable times by physicists and has forced fundamental modifications of existing notions about matter. These are embodied in quantum theory and its mathematical formulation, quantum mechanics, which set out the laws of the subatomic realm as conceived by physicists in the early twentieth century.

Quantum reality

Newtonian physics is based on the concept of solid material bodies moving in empty space. This idea is so deeply ingrained in Western thought that it is extremely difficult to imagine a physical reality where it doesn't apply. Yet this is precisely what twentieth-century physics demands. Not only is the concept of matter drastically altered, but also the concept of force, which is now seen to originate in dynamic energy patterns continually changing into each other, so that it unifies concepts formerly held to be distinct.

When the atom was first split in 1909 it became clear that atoms are nothing like the solid objects conceived by Newton but are vast regions of empty space in which extremely small particles — electrons — move around the nucleus, bound by electromagnetic forces. The distinction between matter and empty space had to be abandoned when it became evident that an unlimited number of particles endlessly come into being spontaneously out of the void, and vanish into it again. Hence the vacuum is far from empty. Moreover, experiments showed that matter is completely mutable. All particles can be transmuted into other particles; they can be created from and vanish back into energy. The universe thus appears as a dynamic web of inseparable energy patterns.

Subatomic particles were also found to make jumps or quantum leaps from one orbit to another without leaving any trace or path. Therefore at the subatomic level matter does not exist with certainty in definite places, nor do subatomic events occur at definite times and in definite ways. Rather matter shows tendencies to exist and subatomic events show tendencies to occur. These tendencies are expressed mathematically as probabilities in the form of waves. These are not three-dimensional waves like those of sound or water but waves of abstract probabilities, or probablity amplitudes. Hence particles can at the same time be waves depending on how they are observed. Consequently subatomic events can never be predicted with certainty, only as a likelihood of their happening. Such a perspective completely overturns the common-sense view that electrons really exist in definite places with definite trajectories. However, this common-sense view has been shown to be false.

Indeed developments in physics have dispensed completely with the idea of a fixed observable reality and a predictable universe by showing that reality is not only not independent of, but also shaped by, the observer. The observer is necessary to observe the properties of subatomic phenomena and to bring certain of these about. In short, the electron does not have objective properties independent of mind. Given that it is not possible to predict future events exactly if the present state of the universe cannot be measured precisely, it follows that the ideal of measurable objectivity in science is quite unfounded.

These conclusions seem quite bizarre because the apparently concrete matter of daily experience dissolves into 'a maelstrom of fleeting ghostly images'.[47] The physicist Neils Bohr observed that those who are not shocked by quantum theory have not understood it. Even Einstein found it disturbing because if quantum theory is correct and everything in the universe is interrelated and interconnected, it implies that action at a distance — instantaneous change in widely separated systems — is possible, and this represented the unthinkable to physicists of his era. Einstein regarded the idea as 'ghostly and absurd' and devised an argument to prove that this was impossible, but in the 1960s it was experimentally demonstrated that action at a distance can occur, and subsequently it was established beyond doubt that quantum theory is right and Einstein, in his efforts to disprove this theory, was wrong.

These findings resonate with ancient belief in the fundamental unity of all things. Throughout history, influences, sympathies and correspondences have been invoked as explanations for events that seem unaffected by causal laws. The doctrine of the 'sympathy of all things' can be traced back to Hippocrates. It remained a recurrent theme in the teachings of Pythagoreans, neoplatonists and philosophers of the Renaissance, until the eighteenth century when, following the Newtonian revolution, 'causality was enthroned as the aboslute ruler of matter and mind.'[48] It was this reign that quantum theory brought to an abrupt end, because:

> ... if all actions are in the form of discrete quanta, the interactions between different entities (eg: electrons) constitute a single structure of indivisible links, so that the entire universe has to be thought of as an unbroken whole. In this whole, each element that we can extract in thought shows basic properties (wave or particle etc.) that depend on its overall environment in a way that is more reminiscent of how the organs constituting living things are related, than it is of how the parts of a machine interact. Further the non-local, non-causal nature of the relationships of elements distant from each other violates the requirements of separateness and independence of fundamental constituents that is basic to any mechanistic approach.[49]

The conclusion to be drawn from modern physics is therefore that at a deep and fundamental level the apparently separate parts of the universe are connected in an intimate and immediate way.

The full implications of this quantum weirdness cannot be dismissed as mere theoretical speculation. Despite its bizarre implications quantum theory is primarily a practical branch of physics that has yielded among other things the laser, the electron microscope, the transistor, the superconductor, nuclear power and the bases of modern chemistry and biology. In its everyday applications it is a very down-to-earth subject with a vast body of supporting evidence not only from commercial gadgetry but also from careful and sophisticated scientific experiments.

Similarities between modern physics and ancient views of the universe

The new physics arising from twentieth-century descriptions and investigations of the subatomic realm presents a totally different world-view from that portrayed by Newton. This can be characterised as organic, holistic and ecological because it suggests a basic oneness of the universe. It highlights the inadequacy of Newtonian mechanistic notions of order, that is, the way in which the universe is thought to be arranged. This can be described as 'explicate' in that each of its elements lies only in its own regions of space and time and outside the regions appertaining to other things. It is in this sense that events are conceived as separate and independent, and understandable in terms of regular arrangements of objects as in rows or events in sequence. The undivided wholeness implied by the new physics, in which all parts of the universe, including the observer and his instruments, merge and unite in one interdependent totality, demands a radically new concept of order. It has been suggested[50, 51] that the universe is organised like a hologram, each part of which contains information about the whole so that if the hologram is broken the whole can be reconstructed from each of the pieces. Such a view was expressed in the second century AD by Plotinus, who insisted that each being contains in itself the whole intelligent world. Therefore 'all is everywhere.'

The hologram cannot be understood in terms of explicate order. It has to be understood in terms of a total order contained implicitly in each region of time and space. Here 'implicit' (from the verb 'to implicate' meaning to fold inwards) is used in the sense that each region contains a total structure enfolded within it. However, while a hologram is a static record of this order, the order itself is conveyed in a complex movement of electromagnetic fields in the form of light

waves termed 'holomovement'[52] and, as such, constitutes life energy.
It is an unbroken and undivided totality from which particular aspects
such as sound and light or electrons can be abstracted but which are
essentially inseparable. This energy, which in its totality cannot be
limited in any specifiable way nor bound by any particular measure,
is indefinable and immeasurable. Hence, according to this theory,
everything is movement and the world of manifest reality a secondary
derivation from this primary order of the universe.

The notion that hard reality is an abstraction from the 'blur' of
basic reality is a central tenet of mysticism and common to the
teachings of mystics and sages throughout the ages and all parts of the
world. In describing a holographic universe, physicists are, like the
mystics of antiquity, depicting a world in which what appears to be
stable, tangible and 'out there' is not really there at all but is an
illusion, a magic show. Accordingly, reality is thus not what the eyes
perceive. It has been proposed[53] that the brain may act like a lens,
mathematically transforming the blur of primary reality into hard
reality, and that otherwise we would know only a world of
undifferentiated energy, without space and time, such as that
described by mystics throughout history.

It has been suggested[54] that we do not ordinarily see true reality
because habitually we notice secondary or mundane reality that is
emphasised in thought and language, both of which are
predominantly linear and sequential.

> All of our methods for interrogating nature depend upon
> language — and it is the very nature of language to refer to
> things. We therefore think in terms of things. How can we
> possibly think about nonthings, no-things, nothing? In our very
> *forms* of thought we instinctively divide the world into subjects
> and objects, thinkers and things, mind and matter. This division
> seems so natural that it has been presumed a basic maxim of
> objective science.[55]

While there is little doubt about the influence of language on thought
and perception, it is inaccurate to suppose, as stated above, that we
instinctively think about the world in these ways. Rather we learn to.
Both linguistic and cognitive development result from objects being

named and pointed out. In this way they emerge as discrete entities from a diffuse, homogenous background and it is through this process that a child learns about its world. Western culture as a whole is habituated to a description of a manifest 'out there' reality because it has been conditioned to think in this way, and there is a tendency to feel that primary experience is of this order. However, prior to the development of rational, linear thinking and the emphasis on reason in Western culture this was not the case, as is clear from the mystical tradition of thinking. This would seem to support the view that habituation to the secondary or mundane reality is not only a developmental process but also an evolutionary one, which emerged alongside the development of language and language-related functions,[56] and explains the prevalence of mystical thinking in primitive and pre-literate cultures.

Mystical and magical traditions emphasise that true seeing or direct perception of reality can be achieved by developing insight, literally a looking inwards. This idea is consistent with the holographic notion that the universe is implicit within each of its parts. Accordingly, the truth of the universe — ultimate truth — lies within the person rather than in the 'external' world.

Like the mystics of old, contemporary scientists have suggested that this ultimate reality can be accessed by various means, notably psychedelic drugs such as those traditionally used in shamanic ritual. These prevent us from 'thinking straight' in the linear manner of conscious rational thought and so bypass ordinary consciousness enabling direct perception of the holographic universe.

Transformation theory

Support for a holographic universe comes from a theory advanced by Nobel Prize-winning chemist Ilya Prigogine. Transformation theory suggests the way in which various forms emerge from the primary order and are manifested in time and space and establishes the connectedness of living and non-living forms, thus bridging the critical gap between living things and the apparently lifeless universe in which they arise.

Transformation theory concerns dissipative structures, that is, all living things and some non-living things, such as certain chemical reactions, which maintain their form by a continuing dissipation of energy. As such they constitute a flowing wholeness which is highly complex and always in process. The more complex a structure is the more energy it requires to maintain its coherence and, paradoxically, the more coherent it is, the greater its instability. This instability, Prigogine suggests, is the key to transformation because the dissipation of energy creates the potential for sudden reordering. The continuous movement of energy through the system results in fluctuations. Minor fluctuations do not affect the structural integrity of the system but if they reach a critical size they 'perturb' it by increasing the number of novel interactions within it. Elements of the old pattern come into contact with each other in new ways and make new connections and in this way the parts reorganise into a new whole. Accordingly, nature has the potential to create new forms by allowing a shake-up of old forms and this capacity is the key to growth and creativity. Dissipative structures insulated from disturbance are protected from change and become stagnant; this is as true for forms of knowledge or science as for any other system. This suggests that paradigm shifts are essential for the development of thought, because only through the chaos they introduce can order emerge.

> Dissipative structures are found at all levels in nature. The same ordering principles that operate at the microscopic levels of nature permeate human life at the social and cultural levels. There is a principle of connectedness here, implying a oneness between man and nature. Nature is part of us, and we are part of it ... We *are* nature; and as such it is not surprising that we are discovering common principles that describe not only how *molecules* behave, but how *we* behave.[57]

Such a view is fully consistent with that of the ancients, as is the central tenet of transformation theory: the meaning of the whole is traceable to the behaviour of its parts, which reverberate throughout the entire system. Here again there are parallels with the views of mysticism.

The insights provided by transformation theory, which have been confirmed experimentally, are far from new. The ancient Greeks recognised and valued therapy because of its power to shake up or perturb. They believed that the evocation of unsettling emotions such as fear and anger cause a profound change to take place and an emotional purging which Aristotle termed 'catharsis'.

In the light of the many similarities between the insights of modern science and ancient wisdom, mysticism cannot be dismissed as trivial or as a mere anthropological curiosity. Rather, it has to be admitted to any scientific framework that purports to be a complete understanding of reality. Indeed it is now recognised that the new physics, and to some extent modern chemistry, restates, albeit in the language of mathematics, the mystical descriptions of reality common to ancient traditions throughout the world. 'The collapse of materialistic and mechanical explanations within the physical sciences has certainly helped to promote an animistic revival, and forced us to consider the possibility that within the luxuriant profusion of animistic ideas there may indeed be a central core of truth.'[58]

Although initially shocked by comparisons between the descriptions of mysticism and physics, physicists have increasingly come to accept that mysticism provides a consistent and relevant background to Western science that unifies and harmonises scientific discoveries and man's spiritual aims and beliefs. In so doing they have come to appreciate that it is less a matter of choosing between alternative views than of embracing what is complementary among them.

For many people this idea is difficult to accept because they have been conditioned to believe that Western science is superior to other forms of knowledge. This is particularly true in relation to Western medical science. The world-view underpinning Western medicine is generally unquestioned. It is assumed to be correct and to be the only view possible in the light of modern discoveries and knowledge. Accordingly, medicine grounded in the physical sciences is held to be the only way of mediating between people and disease. Alternative views, whether those of earlier epochs or other cultures, and medical approaches derived from them, where recognised at all, tend to be dismissed and even despised as primitive, defective, inferior, and although untested, disparaged in practice. Western medicine is a belief system so fixed, so inherent, that any truth to the contrary is dismissed as virtual blasphemy.[59]

The institution of medicine itself reflects this resistance to external challenges by adhering steadfastly to an outmoded model of how the *[handwritten marginal note: But Buddhist (& others) even if they do not believe in these attitudes]*

world behaves, almost totally ignoring the insights of modern physics. The result is that modern Western medicine has 'a set of guiding beliefs that are as antiquated as body humors, leeching and bleeding'.[60] Notions of life, death, health and disease rest solidly on seventeenth-century principles and medicine has resisted any redefinition of these notions, remaining governed by mechanistic thinking. So 'three centuries after Descartes, the science of medicine is still based, as George Engel writes, "on the notion of the body as a machine, of disease as the consequence of breakdown of the machine, and of the doctor's task as repair of the machine."'[61]

Physician Larry Dossey[62] has summarised the assumptions of modern medicine as follows. The body is a material object existing in a specific space and a finite time, which is composed of past, present and future. Birth and death occur in this sequence. These events never recur after happening once, and they are the poles of one life, demarcating existence. Events in life, including disease, happen in this timeframe. Disease occurs because of some malfunction at the level of molecules comprising the individual body, and disease, like the body it inhabits, is confined in space and time and located in the body and experience of an isolated individual. It is an unshared experience. Since illness is the result of objective disturbances in the body, treatment must be objective and, since disease is a physical malfunction in a physical context, it requires physical interventions, such as drugs, surgery or medical technology, after diagnosis that relies on objective factual information. Disease is a bodily affair, standing apart from psychological events and spiritual experiences which are ignored. All treatment is viewed as a matter for emotionally neutral, scientifically trained professionals. Inevitably despite the best efforts of these professionals, the body dies and life ceases with the death of the material body. Twentieth-century 'science', however, demands a radical re-examination of these principles and practices.

Dossey points out that a fundamental problem facing Western medicine is that of reconciling ordinary descriptions of bodies, health and disease as separable and distinct entities within the context of the quantum description of the universe, where everything in it is an inseparable entity. Principles of relatedness, oneness and unity have to be addressed rather than those of fragmentation and isolation. In the new view, the body is dynamically related to the universe and other bodies through actual physical exchange. It ceases to be a mere object surrounded by empty space and, rather than being composed of discrete atoms, comprises patterns and processes that account for its total renewal down to the last atom every few years. Ultimately, the body is an illusion, as is its separateness from other bodies. Accordingly, health is a shared phenomenon and treatment can never be directed to only one individual.

In unflowing non-linear time, past, present and future become arbitrary and the ordinary ways of marking life and death become suspect. It becomes clear that there is no ultimate end from which we can be saved by doctors. As all bodies are coextensive through actual dynamical physical processes, the idea of individual death becomes absurd. In the new view, life is not a property of single bodies but of the universe at large, connected as are all living bodies to all living things that share information. 'Crisp, causal events that were once thought to characterise each and every human disease fade into endless reverberating chains of happenings.'[63] In the new view, discrete causes never occur in individual bodies for the simple reason that discrete, individual bodies do not themselves exist. The goal of traditional Western medicine of an utterly objective treatment that can be aimed at the causal end of every disease is unrealistic according to the modern view: it is not possible to stand apart from nature and intervene dispassionately and objectively. Furthermore, in the modern view, rather than attempting to eliminate the subjective, it is encouraged. The spiritual goal of transcending the physical at the heart of most Western religion also needs rethinking. 'Our greatest spiritual achievement may lie in total integration of the spiritual and the physical — in realising these two aspects are in fact one.'[64]

Many physicians and medical scientists have been reluctant to address the issues raised by Dossey. 'It is almost a modern embarrassment to have to admit to the importance of human factors in disease causation when all along the answers have been expected to arise from the cryptic depths of molecular biology.'[65] Such reformulations are profoundly unsettling to those attached to the old scientific model of medicine, especially to those who had not realised how vulnerable it was. However, according to transformation theory, without some shake-up of its foundations, medicine cannot evolve and progress. The implications for Western medicine of continuing to resist the challenge they offer are considerable because 'flawed images of the body lead to flawed therapies for the body.'[66]

The need for revision of fundamental principles and practices has been grasped by the so-called new biology of the late twentieth century which is fully consistent with the new understanding of reality. It emphasises the unitary ontological nature of a material world in which biological and social factors are neither separable, nor antithetical; not alternatives but complementary. Hence, organisms and the environment can no longer be considered in isolation from each other. They are interrelated and complimentary so there is no universal physical fact of nature whose effect or even relevance to an organism is not in part a consequence of the nature of the organism itself. This new biology calls for a radical reappraisal of our thinking about 'being in the world' and has important implications for medical science.

When translated into practice these new conceptions of reality require bodies, health and diseases to be viewed, rather than as discrete entities, as dynamic processes which need to be understood in terms of patterns of relationships within the organism and its environment and not in terms of its separate parts. Health and illness need to be viewed in relation to the wholeness or integration of these processes rather than in terms of symptoms or the lack of them. Accordingly, mind has to be regarded as a primary factor in health and illness and therefore 'psychosomatic' illness becomes a matter for all health-care professionals, who are themselves therapeutic partners in the healing process rather than 'external' to it. Essentially the new description of reality demands, as Hippocrates did, that physicians understand the whole of things, including the soul.

Indeed, the world-view that has emerged from the physical sciences in the West in the twentieth century is strikingly similar to those of ancient traditions and those of other cultures where these traditional views survive and form the basis of their systems of medicine. Fundamental to these traditions is an understanding of the soul.

3

SEERS OF THE SOUL

From the renaissance onward, our culture has acknowledged the soul less and less as a nonmaterial life-principle. With the rise of economic materialism and a mechanistic, purely object-oriented science, our modern culture has come to look increasingly upon the psyche as a conglomerate of biological, physiological and sociocultural factors. The idea of an indivisible life-giving soul — or entity of consciousness — independent of the body, soon came to be seen as no more than a primitive and superstitious notion without any content of reality. Yet this notion of the soul has from the very beginning been part of the philosophical and psychological state of man; it has been present through the centuries and epochs.[1]

Western civilisation is 'an island in an ocean of animism' and the soul remains at the core of thinking about the universe in most cultures.[2] This is particularly true of those cultures where perspectives on the universe are based on a philosophical tradition quite different from that of the West.

Thinking in many cultures remains close to its mystical origins because the distortions introduced into the mystic tradition of ancient times by classical Greek civilisation are not present in cultures that largely lack its influence. This is particularly true of Eastern cultures.

Several common themes can be identified in Eastern traditions of thought. They are holistic in recognising the interrelatedness of all things; they are relativistic, focusing on the illusory nature of time and form; and they all share an awareness of subtle energies in the universe. Human beings are viewed as being imbued with these universal forces and as manifesting them on three levels: physical, emotional and spiritual. The traditions of the East all aim at achieving a balance of these forces within man, and between man and the environment. This integration or wholeness is synonymous with holiness and health. Typically, therefore, Eastern traditions of thinking are characterised as philosophical or religious. However, on closer examination they resemble neither philosophy nor religion as these are understood in the West. Rather, 'the psychological window is the best one from which to view the traditional wisdom of the East.'[3] These traditions have thus been referred to as 'traditional esoteric psychologies'[4] or 'spiritual psychologies'.[5]

Traditions of thought in India

> For thousands of years Indian thinkers have concentrated their studies upon the nature of man, and with few exceptions, the different schools of thought have agreed that there is an inner self or soul of man, and that it is eternal and indestructible.[6]

Accordingly, the study of the soul, or psychology, has been the focus of Indian culture. Whereas the Bible and the Koran emphasise the greatness of God, Indian scriptures emphasise the nature of the soul. Vedanta, the philosophy expounded in the earliest Hindu scriptures, comprises the knowledge of all the various sects that exist in India. Its chief concern is the human soul and divine spirit. Vedanta derives from the *Vedas*, ancient teachings preserved by oral tradition for many centuries, specifically the *Ved-anta* or 'Veda's end' (composed *circa* 800–300 BC), also called the *Upanishads* or 'private sessions'. In the Upanishads there is never any doubt about the soul and its immortality.[7] The first Upanishad declares belief in the indestructible, eternal soul:

> The soul is 'not this, not that'
> It is intangible, for it cannot be grasped,
> Indestructible, for it cannot be destroyed,
> Detached for it cannot be attached.
> It is unbound, does not tremble and cannot be hurt.[8]

In early scriptures the embodied soul is described as *jiva*, the vital breath or animating principle, that which breathes in all things. In later scriptures the nature of the soul was held to consist of Being-Awareness-Bliss — the nature of Brahman.

In Western culture the universe is seen as being composed of parts distinctly separate from each other — nature, man, animals, birds, trees, plants, minerals and so on — created as such by God in the beginning of time. The thinkers of ancient India regarded the idea of such separateness as erroneous. They considered that a connection existed among all these phenomena, a unity that pervaded the whole universe, including God. This one great, impersonal, absolute power, an immutable, ultimate and essentially indescribable reality that permeates and transcends all things is known in Sanskrit, the ancient sacred language of India, as *Brahman*. It is pure consciousness, the first principle from which all things derive, by which all are supported and into which they eventually disappear. Brahman is the ground of all existence, the eternal substrate of the universe, and is considered to be the Universal Soul.

> That which is the finest essence
> The whole universe has it as its soul.
> That is Reality. That is the Soul. That thou art.[9]

Hence, the inmost essence of human beings is at one with the ultimate essence of the universe. This is the doctrine of non-duality, *advaita* ('not-two-ness'). Moreover:

> This great unborn Soul is the same which abides as the intelligent (soul) in all living creatures.[10]

A frequent metaphor for Brahman is 'ocean', which denotes inexhaustible potentiality. Like Brahman, the greater part of the ocean is never visible or known, and the rising and disappearing waves represent the ephemeral lives of innumerable living creatures that come into existence for a while and are then reabsorbed into it. According to ancient teachings[11] the individual soul returns to and is temporarily absorbed by Brahman in deep sleep. The waking state is therefore a return from Brahman.

Etymologically, the word 'Brahman' denotes an entity whose powers cannot be measured. Reason, rationality, analysis and dissection, with their implicit notions of measurement so esteemed in the West, are seen as *avidja*, or ignorance, which is not so much a not-knowing as a not-seeing of the reality of the world. As such they are the very antithesis of knowledge or philosophy (*darsana*, or seeing, in Sanskrit), the aim of which is to understand the unity of all things or Natural Law.

According to Natural Law, all phenomenal existence is transitory, impermanent and in the process of change, a ceaseless cycle of beginning and ending which in Sanskrit is termed *samsara*, literally meaning a 'going around in circles'. Just as man is subject to cycles of birth and rebirth, the universe itself is thought to go through cycles of dissolution and re-creation spanning vast periods of time in a process that is indivisible and irreducible. Therefore all reduction to objective facts and forms constitutes illusion or *maya*. *Maya* comes from the Sanskrit root *ma*, meaning to measure. So *maya* literally means 'world-as-measured', divided up into things and events. As such, it is illusion. Yet, paradoxically, *maya* is also reality in that this illusion constitutes reality.

Not a mere intellectual understanding, Vedanta is a practical philosophy in which reality must be directly known and this knowledge applied in daily life. Vedanta teaches that while human beings live in a body and have feelings and thoughts, their essential identity is the soul or *atman*, a manifestation of Brahman, the timeless Ultimate Reality, Universal Consciousness or World Soul. Human life has no other purpose than learning to know the self for what it really is. Like the ancient Egyptians and Greeks, the Hebrews, Aborigines and other tribal cultures, Hindus and also other sects of India such as Buddhists and Jains teach of a golden age of the past, an age of truth, when humans directly knew and lived in accordance with the Ultimate Reality. However, Ultimate Reality is no longer known directly because human consciousness is layered by *kosas*, or sheaths. In order to reach the true self, the state of total oneness, five levels of consciousness have to be accessed. Each of these levels or *kosas* is considered to sheath a more subtle level beneath it and to dissolve through repeated contemplation. As the layers dissolve the individual progresses towards an increasingly profound awareness of reality.

From outermost to the most subtle level of consciousness, the *kosas* are:

- *Annamayakosa* — the physical body made from food. This level of consciousness is that of chemistry and physiology, the main focus of modern Western medicine.

- *Pranamayakosa* — the sphere of the five senses, the emotions and the subtle energy called *prana*.

- *Manomayakosa* — the lower mental body composed of thought. Its desires, motives, resolutions and wishes form the complex called mind.

The second and third *kosas* are the levels of consciousness addressed by Western psychology. 'This is the great challenge of modern man: to see beyond this stage of development and, with the help of the more penetrating insight afforded by the next stage, to transcend it.'[12]

- *Vijnanamayakosa* — the aspect of mind that can discern higher moral principles and can see beyond the separate individual to the universal and eternal

- *Anandamayakosa* — the stage of constant bliss beyond feelings, thoughts and mind.

Beyond this final stage, *atman* is reached:

> ... the unseen basis, the real self, one's divinity — the soul which is the reality within the five sheaths, the outer of which is the body. It is the spark of God within, one's innermost reality. It is the substance of the objective world, the reality behind the appearance, the universal and immanent in every being ... the *atma* is imperishable. It does not die like the body and mind. It is the essential reality of the individual, the witness — unaffected by all this change in time and space, the immanent spirit in the body, complex abode, the mystery that is beyond that complex, the motivating force of the impulses and tensions and the intentions of that complex.[13]

Hence Vedanta teaches that humans can, by personal effort and the use of inner knowledge, attain union with the divine while on earth. Its aim is to harmonise all. This is possible because Brahman or Ultimate Reality and the individual soul, *atman*, (literally meaning 'breath'), though seemingly apart, are, in actuality one, as is conveyed in the teaching:

> The real is one. It is the mind that makes it appear many.

This illusion, *maya*, disappears when knowledge of Brahman is attained. Understanding *maya* — the illusory nature of reality — is therefore of key importance. The 'three strands which constitute the rope of maya with which men become bound to the phenomenal world'[14] are termed *gunas*, and symbolised in the Indian 'trick' in which a rope appears to be a snake. The *gunas*, known as *Rajas*, *Tamas* and *Sattva*, are held to be present in various degrees in all phenomena, including mind, intellect and ego.

- *Rajas* is characterised by energy and manifests in ceaseless activity. It creates attachment and suffering.

- *Tamas*, which manifests in inactivity, dullness, inadvertence and stupidity, is the mother of illusion and represents the veiling power of maya.

- ·*Sattva*, which manifests as spiritual qualities, strikes a balance between the opposing characteristics of Rajas and Tamas.

Although these *gunas* are present in all things, one sometimes preponderates over the other. According to Vedanta, when these three *gunas* are in balance the universe remains in a state of non-manifestation or dissolution; and when this equilibrium is disturbed through a preponderance of any one *guna*, the creation of the material world occurs.

The first element to evolve at the beginning of a cycle is *akasha*, often incorrectly translated as ether, space or sky. It is the intangible material substance that pervades the whole universe, filling all space between worlds and molecules. It is the substance from which all else is formed. Often referred to as *prana* or breath, it is seen as the primal life-giving force and thought of as a subtle biological conductor in the body.

Gradually four other elements manifest — air, fire, water and earth — but these are not the elements perceived by the sense organs. Initially subtle, they become grosser through a process of combination and from the gross and subtle elements emerge physical objects, the body, mind, intellect, mind-stuff and ego. Vedanta speaks of five elemental features in the universe: sound; touch; form; taste; smell.

After these material forms are projected through *maya*, the material cause of the universe, Brahman, the efficient cause of the universe enters as life and consciousness and animates them. Divinity thereby pervades all things and this belief forms the basis of Indian morality. *Prana* is material and immaterial, endowed with intelligence and likened to the spirit. The flow of this psychic energy is the totality of the entire self and is equivalent with vitality.

According to Hindu tradition, cosmic energy is distributed down through the body to the base of the spine where it mixes with dense, dormant earth energy represented by the coiled serpent *Kundalini*. This symbolises the stored energy or potential of the organism. It is seen as the task of the individual to mix, balance and refine these energies and direct them upwards. The ascent occurs along the two major pathways or *nadis*, the *Ida* on the left and the *Pingala* on the right, which criss-cross around the central *Shushumna*. This is represented symbolically as twin serpents coiling upwards around a central staff and, as such, is similar to the caduceus of ancient Greece. As the ascent occurs, the various energies are blended and transmuted, creating a variety of experiences and profound changes in awareness. The ultimate goal is not only to raise the energy vertically but also to open and balance the energy in flowing harmony through the total body/mind/soul system. It is directed to achieving a state of harmony, wholeness or holiness, and oneness with the Ultimate Reality or Soul, synonymous with health. In this sense Indian culture is concerned with health and healing, which are essentially spiritual in nature.

Vedanta recognises that the human mind is incapable of imagining the Ultimate Reality with which it seeks union. So it turns towards the highest it can conceive, either a God or gods with attributes that are projections of human virtues, or God-like men, exemplars, who strengthen and purify by example. The dynamic unity of the universe, for example, is personified in the God Shiva, the cosmic dancer, who sustains the manifold phenomena of the universe, unifying them by immersing them in his rhythm and making them partake in the cosmic dance. Such deities are worshipped in the hope that through devotion the worshipper can become like them.

Vedanta does not condemn cults of this kind. Rather, it reminds the worshipper that gods or exemplars must not come between him or her and the knowledge that they are all essential projections of the same Ultimate Reality. It teaches that in worshipping those in whom eternal nature is revealed, they are revering their own divine nature, which is more or less obscured. Vedanta has thus sustained many cults of gods and divine incarnations and as a result Hinduism is often, mistakenly, seen as polytheistic. It is rather that to the Hindu there is one truth called by many names. Essentially Vedanta teaches that 'men should have faith in themselves first.'

Jainism

Jains have been a feature of Indian culture for 2,500 years and their beliefs predate the Buddha. The term 'Jain' derives from *jina*, meaning 'conqueror', the name bestowed on twenty-four great teachers or exemplars who taught through example that human beings are capable of conquering the bondage of physical existence and achieving feedom from rebirth by various ascetic practices. Jains believe the whole world can be divided into *jiwa* — sentient souls — and *ajiva*, the non-sentient and material which has become associated with *jiwa* and prevents it realising its true nature, which is immortal, omniscient and absolutely complete in itself.[15] *Jiva* exists in all living matter. It is the 'knower' and agent of activity in living things. It is the principle of life, the vivifying soul quite distinct from the body, although it fills all the body and can feel all sensation. There is no common source from which *jiva* originates and each *jiva* has been eternally associated with *ajiva*, so there is 'fall' of the *jiva* into an impure state. The association between the two is without beginning, like the universe, but is changeable through karma, which in the Jain view is a subtle form of matter that clings to the *jiva* obscuring its innate capacities. This causes the *jiva* to be reborn into an infinite series of physical existences from which it can be freed by an ascetic life and introspection, by which the soul can be directly perceived. This is true knowledge or awareness, and such 'enlightened souls' eventually gain *nirvana*, or liberation: a state of calm bliss.

The ancient teachings of India indicate that the soul may be apprehended in various ways. However, as in other Eastern cultures, meditation is regarded as a fundamental means by which the true self, the soul, is known. Many different forms of meditation are practised but common to these is an introversion of attention, a looking inwards to the inner self rather than outwards to the ephemera of the outside world. The aim of meditation is progressively to relinquish the ordinary thoughts, ideas and images with which the sense of self is identified, so as to attain a state of pure being or consciousness and an experience of unity with the whole of creation. This state, known as *samadhi* or 'still mind' in the Indian tradition, can be likened to an inner silence or void in which experience as it is usually known ceases.

Buddhism

Meditation is a central feature of Buddhism, which is an evolving tradition extending over 2500 years, and has been the dominant philosophical force at some time for over half the world's population. It originated around the sixth century BC — the century in which ancient Greek thinking underwent such a profound change — in the teachings of the Indian sage Siddartha Gautama, the Buddha or Awakened One. He was so called because he had 'woken up' to the true nature of reality and knew the basic truths of the universe.

The cardinal principles expounded by the Buddha are regarded by his followers as fundamental truths that explain the human condition. His teaching rests on two fundamental concepts: *anicca* and *anatta*, respectively the impermanence and insubstantiality of all things. He asserted that the individual lives in process or continuous motion, *samsara*, with the result that life is experienced as change or flux. The impersonal law operating within this process and governing growth and development is *karma*, the law of causation, or cause and effect. The doctrine of karma holds that everything performed during life has moral significance and will influence the fate of the individual in subsequent incarnations. Consequently all living beings exist under conditions they have inherited by virtue of past deeds. This Cosmic

Law shapes all deeds on Earth, but without eliminating free will, because humans can decide their actions, and therefore their karma.

Westerners often misconceive karma as a deterministic view of humans as activated by controllable, external forces that gives rise to and justifies a resigned attitude to life. However, in Buddha's teachings the mind has a dual aspect in that it can be directed outwards or inwards. When the mind is turned inwards it is the cause of freedom and release, but when turned outwards it is the cause of bondage.

Buddha identified the outward looking aspect of mind with ego, self or rational mind, and he likened it to a monkey that plays tricks on humans by creating illusion or *maya*. The fundamental illusion it creates is of itself as a separate substantive entity. According to Buddha, individuality is merely the result of the basic unifying tendency of life, *ahamkara*. This is found in every living creature and maintains its individual structure. In humans this principle calls itself 'I' and confers self-consciousness. It also constructs a separate, permanent ego that is in contrast to the rest of the world. In Buddhism this idea of a separate self is considered an intellectual invention that corresponds to no reality. The term 'I' is therefore merely a useful linguistic device for designating the ever-changing combination of mental and physical qualities, or *skandhas*, that gives rise to individuality. There is no 'I' behind thoughts, memories, sensations and perceptions and without them there is no sense of 'I'. The 'I' derives its existence from these mental states. Hence the person's apparent individuality is not real in any fixed sense but is actually only a succession of instants of consciousness. The only continuous thread is *bhava*, or continuity of consciousness over time. The 'self' is therefore a process in time, not a single solid thing or fact. In an absolute sense of a permanent substance, it is an illusion, a false notion. Nevertheless, while refuting its metaphysical reality, Buddha conceded its existence as the subject of action in a practical or moral sense.

In Buddhism, the illusion of a separate self is original sin. It is the cause of evil, death and all human suffering. The separate ego regards itself as subject and views everything else as objects — it is the knower in contrast to objects that are known. 'It is an artificial attitude that makes sections in the stream of change, and calls them things. Identity of objects is an unreality.'[16] Buddha insisted that thinking of things rather than of processes in an absolute flux comes about only by shutting our eyes to the succession of events. Hence Buddha termed this human tendency to obscure and veil the true nature of the universe as ignorance or not seeing: *avidja*. The self or ego is thus blind to the true nature of reality. It not only creates a false objective reality but also creates its own bondage and suffering by its attachment to and apparent inability to grow beyond the appearance of things. For Buddha, the ego's attachment to power and possessions, to having, holding, possessing, being this or that, is the source of all suffering, or *dukka*. It arises because humans live in process and therefore experience the impermanence of things, or change, whether physical, psychological or emotional. Humans are aware of change and its consequences — illness, ageing, death, loss, changing relationships and separation — and suffer anxiety and fear as a result. Human hunger for security and permanence, represented as resistance to change, are manifestations of suffering and clinging to the familiar is a defence against change that provides a false sense of security, as is clinging to the ego, self-identity or the sense of self. Nevertheless, change is intrinsic to the human condition and therefore the human condition is the cause of sorrow.

Buddha asserted the Oneness of all life as truth. He insisted that it can be fully realised only when false notions of a separate self whose destiny can be considered apart from the whole are forever annihilated. Relief from suffering can only be achieved by complete freedom from the sense of a separate self that is its source. Buddha taught that freedom from the illusion of separateness could be achieved only by gaining insight into the true nature of reality and grasping the basic truths of *anicca* and *anatta*. This insight comes about literally through a change of perspective, from looking inwards. He therefore identified the inward-looking or introspective mind with essence or authentic being and encouraged its development through meditation. Whereas the outward-looking mind creates bondage through its attachment to things, persons and life itself, the introspective aspect of mind has the ability to transcend all attachments and become free from desires and needs. It therefore has the potential to transform karma into the pursuit of wisdom and enlightenment.

Buddhism, like Hinduism, focuses on the self-liberating power of the introverted mind. It advocates the person freeing themselves from the illusion of self or ego and fusing with the Ultimate Reality or unity of the universe, which is indivisible, timeless and formless.

Buddha's teaching of non-ego, known as *anatta* or *anatman*, is often interpreted as a denial of soul (*atman*). Whether early Buddhists believed in an indefinable soul like other Hindu philosophies has been much debated. 'Some writers consider that Buddhism does not exclude belief in a universal Soul ... Recent studies of Buddhism as practised, even in the most conservative countries ... reveal that modern Buddhists, both monks and laymen, think of themselves as having a fairly stable existence and speak of their personal survival in terms which clearly imply belief in something not unlike a soul.'[17] Clearly Buddhists were strongly opposed to the notion of the soul 'as a sort of manikin inside the body, or a being in any way identifiable with any of the constituent parts of the body or mind'.[18] However, rather than claim that the Buddha denied the existence of the soul, it is truer to say[19] that Buddha was silent concerning it. Buddhists use *atman* to refer to 'self' rather than soul. If soul is equated with self, in the sense of the substrate of changing states of consciousness or of a thing, as the bearer of attributes, they certainly dismiss it as an illusion. However, if soul is taken to mean the sum of the states that constitute mental existence, or mind, Buddhist teaching is certainly not soulless.

Buddha acknowledged the continuity of consciousness over time, or *bhava*, which can be likened to the perennial flow of a river. Just as music is not simply a series of notes but also the silences between notes, so consciousness is not comprised merely of a series of mental states, but also the void between them. *Bhava* refers to the void between the items in the series. It is the natural condition of mind uninterrupted by thought. The void is not nothingness or annihilation but the very source of life. It is the field of being out of which all thought and all forms emerge: the field of infinite possibilities. The void is 'a fullness of nonmaterial intelligence'[20] and can therefore be conceived as the universal mind or cosmic consciousness.

Buddhists use the term *bhavanga* to refer to the unbroken flow of unconscious life within the individual mind and it is seen as the cause of the unbroken continuity of the individual in various existences. Impressions and experiences said to be stored in *bhavanga* may occasionally approach the threshold of full consciousness,[21] so *bhavanga* is used to explain memory, intuition, states of consciousness, such as sleep, dreaming and trance, and the relationship between these states and higher consciousness.

Bhavanga is also used to explain survival after death, *karma* and reincarnation. The doctrines of karma and reincarnation serve to emphasise the continuity of *bhavanga* from one life to another. The bhavanga of an individual at the time of his or her death is thought to be linked to the *bhavanga* at the time of rebirth and thereby establish continuity between lives. At rebirth *bhavanga* is said to receive the dying thoughts and in this way the consciousness and moral tone of a person's life is influenced by his or her previous life. Karma, the motive force for action, revives in the dying person memories of his or her actions, good and bad, and these are distilled into the dying thought in the form of a mental image. In this way the person perceives his or her future fate at the moment of death.

With its interpretation as both a factor and a cause of existence, *bhavanga* is, in this sense, the 'soul' of Buddhism. Certainly without such a concept difficulties are encountered when explaining the doctrine of reincarnation which affirms not only life after death but life before birth, or pre-existence.[22]

Tibetan Buddhism

As Buddhism spread from India it found different forms of expression and so it differs in various cultures. Nevertheless, this diversity rests on a basic unity that exists in spite of many denominational differences in interpretation and practice. The expanded and deeper truths of Buddhism are pursued in traditional Tibetan Buddhism.

The ancient and sacred *Bardo Thodol*, or *Tibetan Book of the Dead*, is not a ceremonial of burial but a set of instructions for the dead and dying and contains the quintessence of Tibetan Buddhist psychology. Like the *Egyptian Book of the Dead* it is meant to guide the 'aggregate of energies'[23] of the dead person through the changing phenomena of the *Bardo*, that state of existence described symbolically as an intermediate state of forty-nine days duration between death and rebirth. The *Bardo Thodol* reflects the belief that the art of dying is as important as the art of living and that right dying is initiation, 'conferring, as does the initiatory death-rite, the power to control consciously the process of death and regeneration'.[24]

In the original German version of his *Psychological Commentary* on the *Tibetan Book of the Dead*, Carl Jung (1875–1961) used the German word *Seele* as it had been used by German mystics to refer to Ultimate Reality. Although translated in English as 'soul' it is not synonymous. As used by Jung, it refers to the essence or matrix of everything, the collective unconscious or universal mind, from which the flow of unconscious life within the individual mind, or *bhavanga*, emerges. 'Psyche' and 'soul' are used in this sense here, not only as the essential nature and condition of all metaphysical reality or being, but *as* that reality. The *Bardo Thodol* commences with this great truth, saying to the dead person 'Now thou art experiencing the Radiance of the Clear Light of Pure Reality. Recognise it. O nobly-born, thy present intellect, in real nature void, not formed into anything as regards characteristics or colour, naturally void, is the very Reality, the All-Good.'[25] This realisation is the *Dharma-Kaya* state of perfect enlightenment. On this clear and particularly bright light, held to be visible at some point to all the dying, the person is urged to concentrate every possible mental and psychic mental force.[26]

As Jung points out, it is highly sensible of the *Bardo Thodol* to make clear to the dead the primacy of the soul, 'for that is one thing that life does not make clear to us. We are so hemmed in by things which jostle and oppress us that we never get a chance, in the midst of all these "given" things, to wonder by whom they are "given". It is from this world of "given" things that the dead man liberates himself; and the purpose of the instructions is to help him towards this liberation.'[27]

According to Buddhist tradition, death discarnates the 'soul', just as birth incarnates it, so death itself is only an initiation into another life. Death is not an absolute ending, but the separation of the psyche from the gross body. The former then enters a new life, while the latter, having lost the principle of animation, decays. The purpose of the *Bardo* is to restore to the soul the divinity it lost at birth. As such, the *Bardo* was originally conceived as much as a guide for the living as for the dead. The whole aim of its teaching is to cause the dreamer to awaken into the true nature of reality, freed from all illusions.

The *Bardo Thodol* is undoubtedly one of the most remarkable works to emerge from the East. 'As a mystic manual for guidance through the Otherworld of many illusions and realms, whose frontiers are death and birth, it resembles the *Egyptian Book of the Dead* sufficiently to suggest some ultimate cultural relationship between the two.'[28] Certainly the similarities between the teachings, particularly as it relates to judgement, are so much alike in essentials as to suggest a common origin. The death rites of both cultures are also similar to the European medieval tradition of *ars moriendi* — the art of dying. Common to them all is the description of the psychic states experienced during and after death as the soul leaves the body and sets out on its journey to another realm of existence.

Given these similarities it is more likely that these traditions all originate in shamanism rather than through contact between these disparate cultures in ancient times. It has been suggested[29] that many features of conventional funeral rites, as well as several themes of the mythology of death, can be traced back to the ecstatic experiences of shamans, who described as precisely as possible both during and after their trance the places they visited and the people or beings they met on their journeys to the Beyond, and in so doing, gave a form and order to the unknown and frightening world of the dead.

Zen

Buddhism reached China in or some time before the first century AD and from its introduction one form was unique in purpose and method. It focused on meditation or *Djana* in Sanskrit, and the Chinese version of this, *Chu'an*, was subsequently rendered as *Zen* when passed on via Korea to Japan, where it was formally established in the thirteenth century. The character of Zen has largely been influenced by its cross-cultural evolution. It is essentially 'a unique blend of Indian mysticism and Chinese naturalism sieved through the rather special mesh of the Japanese character'.[30]

Zen is based on specific teachings of the Buddha, specifically:

Look within, thou art the Buddha.

Accordingly, it emphasises the development of insight through meditation. Its aim is enlightenment, the realisation of the Ultimate Reality beyond words or reasoning. In Zen the universe is one indissolvable substance, one total whole of which man is but a part.

Satori — awakening to this reality — involves abandonment of the ever-present intrusive self or ego.

> Each one of us is but a cell, as it were, in the body of the Great Self, a cell that comes into being, performs its functions and passes away, transformed into another manifestation. Though we have temporary individuality, that temporary limited individuality is not either a true self or our true self. Our true self is the Great Self, our true body is the Body of Reality.[31]

Zen denies that understanding of the universe can be achieved by conceptual thought or ever fully communicated, but it can best be accessed and expressed through wordless activities. Wisdom is derived from Intuitive awareness or insightful understanding achieved by close attention to the performance of mundane activities. Zen teaching is therefore concentrated on 'intuitive experience'. For the student of the *Rinzai* School of Zen, brought to Japan in 1191 by the Japanese monk Ersai, the path to enlightenment may involve archery; judo; *kendo* (fencing); *ikebana* (flower-arranging); the ceremonial preparation of tea; gardening; *haiku*, the Japanese 17-syllable poem; and calligraphy. All are used as ways to the One.

In the *Soto* School of Zen, introduced by the monk Dogen in 1227, intuitive insight is achieved primarily by *zazen* or seated meditation, which is directed to riddles or *koans* that defy reason and rational analysis, their aim being complete destruction of the rational intellect.

Although the aim of Zen and its basic approach is stated in Buddhism, it and Japanese culture were profoundly influenced by Chinese philosophy and thought. The priests who were the indigenous physicians of ancient Japan were completely displaced by Chinese medicine by the ninth century BC and, according to a *Book of Laws* published in 702 BC, medicine and education were already regulated along Chinese lines.

Taoism

China has two classic philosophies, Taoism and Confucianism. These are said to represent the two sides of Chinese character, the mystical and the practical respectively. Central to both these philosophies is belief in the intuitive wisdom of human beings which only needs awakening to serve as a support and guide to conduct. Both teach trust in human beings and in humanity, are present-centred and concerned with the Tao, which in the pre-Confucian world was implicitly and explicitly a symbol for the ideas of men, or the world of ideas.

The concept of Tao is one of the oldest and certainly the most fundamental in all Chinese thought from its emergence out of prehistoric myths up until the twentieth century. The ancient concept of Tao is implicit in every system of Chinese thought. The Chinese have always recognised a magical link between man and the cosmos and have viewed this unity as a sacred metabolic system. In the Chinese view the cosmos is an organic entity that spontaneously, out of itself, evolved the manifest and unmanifest worlds. The cosmic source, without beginning or end, is the *Tao* or *Dao*, roughly translated in English as 'the Way'.

The character for Tao, composed of a foot and head suggests the idea of walking and thinking, of knowing the correct path and following it. In combining the idea of foot and head it personifies wholeness, from head to foot as it were, and since the head is often equated with Heaven and the foot with Earth, it also implies cosmic wholeness. The Tao is at once the primal principle of the universe and the way to achieve personal realisation of it.[32]

The most important principle of the Tao relates to consciousness, which is expressed in analogies to light. The Tao is symbolised by white light, and the *Hui Ming Ching* — the Book of Consciousness and Light — contains instructions as to the way of producing light within the self.

Taoism, or the Teachings of the Way, was formally expounded in the doctrines of Lao Tzu in about 6000 BC and later expanded by Chuang Tsu. Other than the *Tao Te Ching* or Book of Changes, which forms the basis of classical Taoism and is attributed to both Lao Tzu and Chung Tsu, there is no other authentic text.

At the centre of Taoist thinking is the concept of *chi, ch'i* or *qi* (known as *ki* in Japan). This is often translated inaccurately as gas or ether but refers to the vital energy or breath that animates the cosmos. It inflates the earth, moves wind and water (*feng* and *shui*) and breathes life into plants and animals. It pulses throughout the cosmos, motivating all things. It was first described by the Emperor Fu Hsi around 2900 BC and likened to dragon veins running in invisible lines from sky to earth — a similar notion to the concept of energy found in ancient Egypt. The movement of this energy between two poles or extremes known as *yin* and *yang* is the activating force of all phenomena (and is comparable with the Platonic concept of energy). Everything has *chi*, but the rate and quality of this movement or vibration between the two poles of *yin* and *yang* vary in different phenomena, giving rise to their distinctive character.

Yin and *yang* are tendencies in the movement of energy. *Yin*, which literally means 'dark side', is the term used for the tendency towards expansion or centrifugality emanating from the planet Earth and is associated with sedation, passivity and negative force and is characterised as feminine. Earth energy is thus *yin chi*. *Yang*, or the sunny side, is the tendency towards contraction or centripetality, energy acting on the planet Earth from beyond. It is symbolised as the force of Heaven, associated with activity and positive energy and characterised as masculine. *Yang chi* is cosmic energy.

When the contracting force reaches its limit, it changes direction and begins to expand, and vice versa. At the extremes, therefore, it changes into its opposite, and it is this constant flux between extremes that can be observed in all things from the smallest molecule to the pulsation of the galaxies. It is the rhythm of life and can be perceived within the human body in the movement of the heart and lungs and in the peristaltic waves of the intestines. Often the transition from *yin* to *yang*, or vice versa, occurs in a spirallic manner. This is discernible in the spirallic formation of the human embryo and in the structure of muscle and bone. The movement is typically characterised as two fishes, a symbol that implies the dynamic principle of constant movement, but also the unity of opposites. 'The *yin yang* principle is therefore not what we would ordinarily call a dualism, but rather an explicit duality expressing an implicit unity.'[33] Indeed, Taoism asserts that although human experience of the world is characterised by continual movement or change, there is within this change a pattern that is non-random and has a kind of structural unity, constancy or fixity. This is the Ultimate Reality or background against which the two opposite but complimentary *yin–yang* forces are reconciled and as such it gives coherence, continuity and unity to all things. This unity or One was identified by Lao Tzu as the indivisible, inaudible and unfathomable Tao. 'It is the same One, past and present; it embraces form and formless alike, being as well as non-being. The One is therefore a unification of duality and multiplicity. It is eternally without action, yet there is nothing it does not do.'[34]

The forty-second chapter of the doctrines of Lao Tsu provides the definitive statement on the origin of the universe:

> The Tao gave birth to One. (*T'ai chi*)
> The One gave birth to the Two. (*yin and yang*)
> The Two gave birth to the Three.
> The Three gave birth to the myriad creatures.[35]

The meaning of the text is expressed in the Taoist ritual of *Fen-teng*, or 'dividing the new fire'.

> From a new fire struck from a flint is lit a first candle, representing the immanent, visible Tao, *T'ai chi* or primordial breath within the (head) microcosm of man. From the *T'ai chi* is lit a second candle, representing primordial spirit, or soul within man, the chest or heart of the microcosm. A third candle is lit symbolic of vital essence, the gut or intuitive level within man. These three candles represent *T'ai chi*, the immanent, moving Tao of nature, *yang* and *yin* ... On the spiritual level the Tao is seen to be ever gestating, mediating and indwelling within man.[36]

The person is thus seen as infused with the powers of the universe — as a microcosmic image of the macrocosm. Like the cosmos as a whole, the body is seen as being in a state of continual, multiple and interdependent fluctuations whose patterns are described in terms of the flow of *chi*. This cosmological view is central to the *Tao Te Ching*. It teaches that the task of the sage is to create a conscious harmony between himself and the cosmos. By following the path of nature, he can attain eternal union.

According to Taoism, as in Hinduism, within any situation a particular balance may be discerned between the energies that comprise the unity. In nature this balance is deemed to be correct, but in human affairs it is influenced by individual choice and volition. The person is therefore the mediator of these great universal powers, the centre of a personal universe, and is seen as needing to maintain a balance between its forces physically, mentally and emotionally.

Taoism therefore emphasises attainment of *wu-wei*. By doing nothing (*wu-wei*) and saying nothing (*puh-yeh*) the condition of equilibrium or balance (*hu-wu*) is achieved. *Wu-wei* is having effect without acting: a state of being rather than doing. Essentially this elusive concept means triumphing over the insistent ego, letting things happen in accordance with their own innate laws instead of trying to impose personal wishes as if *they* were the laws of life.[37]

Being infused with all the powers of the universe, human beings must necessarily look to themselves for wisdom rather than to some external source or authority. The aim of finding one's centre and balancing these forces is achieved by looking inwards, that is, through insight. The more off-centre or unbalanced the individual, the more dangerous the opposing forces become, because at the extremes they become antagonistic and destructive. Complete awareness, wakefulness or mindfulness transcends and dissolves all extremes promoting union with the universal Tao, which is seen as synonymous with wholeness or health. Inner development is therefore a precondition of health, and when healthy a person resonates with the vibrations of the environment so that his or her *chi* is in harmony with that of the surroundings. All physical and emotional illness is seen as resulting from imbalance in the flow of *chi*. Traditionally Chinese medicine therefore aims at maximising the harmonious flow of *chi* in and around the body and balancing *yin* and *yang*.

Upon death, the soul is thought to sink downwards into the realm of *yin*, where it is purged of its darkness and its sins for a period before release to the heavens. During this period the soul can cause sickness in the family or other calamity if unattended by the prayers of the living. Traditionally the role of the shaman was to descend to the underworld to enquire about the needs of the unattended or sickness-causing soul and Buddhist ritual was thought to be effective in freeing the soul from the underworld and enabling it to ascend to the heavens.

Sufism

Sufism is the mystical tradition of Islam. It shares with other forms of mysticism both a belief in and a striving to merge with a Higher Reality, an infinite realm, a boundless unity quite different from the realm of appearances. The human soul is viewed as exiled from the spiritual realm when it enters the physical body and becomes imprisoned in the material world. The body by itself is inert, and cannot fulfil its own urges. Power to do so comes from the soul, which has several levels, seven in all:

- *the mineral soul* is basically static and inert

- *the vegetable soul* acts simply to respond to the environment and ingest nourishment

- *the animal soul* acts through desires, passions and movement

- *the human soul* is responsible for cognition, self-awareness and future planning

- *the angelic soul* acts through prayer and devotion

- *the secret soul* is similar to the angelic soul, but acts at a deeper level

- *the Soul of the secret of secrets* is the divine in each individual; it is infinite, beyond time and space and transcends all material creation.

> These various souls are not actually distinct from each other. They are somewhat like facets of a single gem. They share within each other, and each is evolving. In each individual, the souls are integrated in either the human soul or one of the higher level souls.[38]

Human experience is determined by which soul is dominant at any time; in dreams each soul functions differently. The dreams of the vegetable and animal souls are concerned with wish fulfilment, whereas those produced by the human soul are what Jung termed 'high dreams' that include complex archetypal images and symbols. The dreams of the secret soul are actual spiritual experiences and the dreams of the Soul of the secret of secrets are direct messages from the divine.

As in other forms of mysticism, Sufism holds that the soul, the divine spark in each person, longs for union with its source and is capable of achieving it, not through intelligence but by intuition, and by way of love. Love is the soul's guiding light in this spiritual quest because only love can free the soul from the bondage of selfishness and sensuality.

The aim of Sufism is to lead the individual to wisdom — insight into the unity of all things and the essentially spiritual nature of the universe — not through intellectual or rational analysis but by experiential understanding of existence. The focus of Sufism is solely on individual experience. There is no dogma, and its practices are variable, although basically they involve meditation on tales, parables or poetry. The greatest of the Sufi poets, known as Rumi, was Mowlana Jalal al-Din Mohummad Balkhi, a thirteenth-century sage, who is believed to have taught his followers the ecstatic circular dance from which they gained their 'whirling dervishes' reputation. This dance is a form of dynamic meditation in which the dancer 'loses' him- or herself and communes with the unity of all things. The dance is also a metaphor. The outward dimension of Islam, the *sharia*, has been likened to the circumference of a circle, and its inner truth, *haqiqa*, to the circle's centre. The line from the circumference to the centre represents the spiritual path, *tariqa*, that proceeds from observance of rituals to inner conviction and from belief to vision. Strictly speaking, the word *Sufi*, like the Sanskrit word *yogi*, refers only to those who have achieved this spiritual union, although it is commonly applied to those aspiring towards it.[39]

In Sufi literature, the state of being which the spiritual seeker aspires to is often likened to a clear mirror that reflects reality without distortion. By contrast, the truth of existence is obscured to the ordinary person, whose mind is likened to a mirror that has become clouded by the development and demands of the ego, the socially conditioned self and intellectual attachment to it. This 'self-intellect' or knowing-self is only partial, a limited aspect of one's totality, universal self or soul, to which it is blind. Rumi explains that the intellectual self, proud in its knowledge, becomes conceited and deviates from the real self. This leads to a division between the intellect and the real self, between reason and intuition. The voice of the real self may be resisted by the self-intellect, but the extent to which this occurs varies from one individual to another.

> Some people find it self-evident; others obscure; some experience it as an intimate part of themselves; to others it is inaccessible. When the mind is receptive, it may appear suddenly without the individual's realization, only to disappear a moment later ... One may become ambivalent and retreat into self-intellect again, another may hear the voice but ignore it, while another may attend to it and become aware of his or her own state of being ... A dominant ego nurtured by everyday society can easily drown out a dim inner voice and inhibit the rise of a universal self.'[40]

Whatever the case, Sufis believe that egoism and the strife that inevitably arise as a result are folly and that the essence of the universe is spiritual. Attaining a state where the individual functions harmoniously with the universe is the aim of Sufism. Fundamentally, therefore, the spiritual path that is Sufism involves liberation from the cultural, or socially conditioned, self and ways of thinking and following a quest for the essential self, or soul. Because throughout life mental blocks have hindered perception of the real self that is the object of this quest, Sufis perceive the task as removing these barriers and becoming a mirror of the universe. The task is so perilous that seekers are advised to enlist the services of a guide who has undergone the experience and knows the hazards. As awareness cannot be attained from knowledge transmitted by others, the guide cannot teach by instruction, only by setting up situations in which the seeker experiences what he or she needs.

> Soul receives from soul that knowledge, therefore not by book or from tongue,
> If knowledge of mysteries comes after emptiness of mind, that is illumination of heart.[41]

The resulting state of harmony with the universe is synonymous with wholeness or health.

Similarities among the traditional psychologies of the East

There are clear similarities in the concepts underpinning the psychologies of the East. They all share an emphasis on an invisible, immaterial reality out of which all forms emerge and into which they all disappear. This Ultimate Reality or ground of being immanent in all things, referred to by many different names, is the unifying principle of life. Though spoken of as One, or unity, it is not static but a flowing wholeness, an endless process or movement. Awareness of and union with the flow of the universe is considered to be synonymous with perfect health, and as such is a goal to be striven towards. This goal is attainable through introspection and immediate experience, both of which can occur only when the rational or outward-looking mind is transcended or circumvented. Only with the mind 'emptied' of its usual thoughts and preoccupations can it become mindful of the true nature of reality, which is wordless, formless, timeless, endless and limitless. Only then can the mind enter into the realm of infinite possibilities that is the Universal or Cosmic mind, the universal intelligence that is the source of all existence.

Although Eastern psychologies describe Ultimate Reality as a void in which there are no things — its *no-thing-ness* — it is not nothingness. 'The void is all inclusive, having no opposite, there is nothing which it excludes or opposes. It is a living void because all forms come out of it.'[42] Nor is the void empty. It is the vehicle for subtle energies such as *chi* and *prana*. Western thinkers typically have considerable difficulty in translating these terms because they are prisoners of a dualistic conception of the world that divides reality into matter and spirit, space and form. Within the West, where matter is viewed as a concrete phenomenon that forms the building blocks of the material world, there is no place for a concept that describes both matter and space simultaneously. Yet this is precisely the case with *chi* and *prana*, which in some circumstances become form and in others remain space. 'If material force (*chi*) integrates, its visibility becomes effective and physical form appear. If material form does not integrate, its visibility is not effective, and there is no physical form.'[43] This principle is similar to that enshrined in quantum physics. Indeed, the concepts of *chi* and *prana* reflect an intuitive awareness and understanding of quantum reality long before there were scientific instruments with which to observe it. 'Though accepted as scientific fact, such knowledge of the insubstantiality of substance plays little part in the living of our everyday lives or the thinking of our everyday thoughts'[44] in the West, whereas it is central to thinking in Eastern cultures.

Eastern systems of thought are rooted in a common vision of the universe — a view that is now finding accord with the view of contemporary Western science. The convergence of ideas in modern physics and ancient mysticism appears to have come about because Western scientists, extroverts looking outwards to the cosmos, and introverted mystics looking within themselves, have discovered the same truth: that the universe is one great unity; that the process of this whole is an energy dance; and that everything is an energy phenomenon. Both conceive this energy not as some underlying substance or 'stuff' but as dynamic patterns of activity, movement or change (hence the Greek *energeia*, activity), to be understood in terms of vibrations, pulsation, flow, rhythm, synchrony, resonance and as relative to time.[45]

The understanding that time and energy are relative and reciprocal, interdependent aspects of one and the same phenomenon, found expression throughout the ancient world in mythologies where various gods representing movement were personifications of both time and world-creating energy. In Hindu tradition the god Krishna reveals his divine role as creator and destroyer of the world with the words 'know that I am Time.' The god Shiva bears the titles *Maha Kala*, or great time, and *Kala Rudra*, all-consuming time, and is depicted as the cosmic dancer who symbolises the energy of the universe.[46] In the ancient Egyptian, Greek, Roman, Indian, Iranian and Mayan cultures time is energy, or change in nature. Within contemporary physics the same 'truth' is encountered, expressed in the symbols of mathematics rather than those of myth. The modern statement of this relationship is Einstein's formula $E=mc^2$, where energy is equivalent with matter (or nature as we know it), changing over time.

The relativity of all things, which is a feature of Eastern thinking, is markedly at odds with Western thinking with its origins in Greek natural philosophy which was based largely on geometric considerations and was essentially static. Its influence on Western thought may be one reason why the West has great conceptual difficulties with the relativistic models of modern physics. Certainly, as is now more generally appreciated, Eastern thought corresponds much better in general with modern scientific thinking than Greek philosophy does. Western thinking has been shaped by classical physics and a paradigm that represents the universe as a material and mechanical system in which matter is inert and unconscious and creative intelligence an unimportant by-product of material development.[47] Only objective and measurable phenomena are considered real. Eastern traditions of thought see consciousness and intelligence as fundamental qualities of existence and acknowledge a hierarchy of realities ranging from those that are manifest to those ordinarily hidden.

> Twentieth century physicists have transcended the Newtonian–Cartesian model: they no longer speak of a world of substance, but rather of process, event, and relation; they now regard the objective world as inseparable from the observer. Scientists no longer view the universe as the intricate mechanical clockwork of Newton but as a network of events and relations. And they consider mind, intelligence, and perhaps consciousness, to be integral constituents of existence rather than mere derivatives of matter.[48]

Recognition in recent years that the world view that has emerged from Western physical sciences during the twentieth century is strikingly similar to ancient oriental traditions has led to an appreciation that certain of the non-Western psychologies represent descriptions of nature, including human nature, that may be as or more sophisticated than those of the West. This open-mindedness is a relatively new phenomenon. It has been preceded by a long period in which only Western science and psychology were deemed worthy of consideration. Alternative views, where recognised at all, tended to be dismissed and even despised as primitive, defective, inadequate and inferior.

> Why have eastern psychologies been so misunderstood and underestimated? The major factor is probably simple ignorance. We appear to have dismissed the eastern traditions in large part

through ignorance and ethnocentricity, much like the nineteenth-century British envoy to India who made himself famous by remarking that he had never felt the need to learn the Indian language because he knew that the Indians had nothing worthwhile to say. Moreover, we have commonly assumed that only one psychology, almost invariably our own, described 'the truth' and that competing models were false.[49]

Eastern descriptions of human nature and potentials often run counter to basic Western assumptions and beliefs. Understanding their concepts and principles presents very real difficulties for people educated in the rational, intellectual, egocentric tradition of Western culture. Only recently have the limitations inherent in the verbal, logical approach of the West have been identified and the necessity of taking into account Western assumptions and world-views when examining other cultures accepted. Among the fundamental problems for Westerners is that in Eastern psychologies there is no 'ghost in the machine', and those Western psychologies based on assumptions of ego identity are viewed as though based on illusion:

> Asian psychologies point out that upon close examination, the ego is nowhere to be found. Rather, the sense of a continuous solid ego, when examined minutely as in Buddhist insight meditation, dissolves into (or in phenomenological terminology is deconstructed into) insubstantiality. Just as a movie presents an apparently continuous image, so too our lack of precise attention and careful introspection allows us to mistake a flux of individual thoughts, emotions and fantasies for a solid continuous ego.[50]

The Christian emphasis on the importance of redemption of the soul, which in the West is commonly seen as synonymous with the self or ego, and the general Western emphasis on individuality and the cult of personality, have made Eastern psychologies' repudiation of the idea of specific definite egos perhaps the most difficult of all its concepts to grasp. Yet many Western thinkers such as William James, Bertrand Russell, Schopenhauer, Henri Bergson and David Hume have reached similar conclusions.

However, the dismissal of Eastern psychologies is perhaps based less on the ethnocentriciy of the West than its cognocentricity. A fundamental difference between Eastern and Western psychologies is that the Western psychology is descriptive of only one state of consciousness while Eastern systems claim to be 'the products of, descriptive of, and only fully comprehended in multiple states of consciousness'.[51] Higher levels of consciousness long recognised in the East are rarely addressed in Western psychology, which has 'stopped short in describing the span of consciousness at the level of the "healthy functioning ego", ignoring any higher dimension that may exist.'[52] It takes into consideration only what is experienced in an ordinary state of consciousness, by which is meant rational, verbal consciousness. Higher or altered states of consciousness are viewed as pathological.

> From a multi-states-of-consciousness model, the traditional Western approach is recognised as a relativistically useful model provided that, because of the limitations imposed by state-specific relevancy, learning and understanding, it is not applied inappropriately to perspectives and states of consciousness and identity outside its scope. If it is so applied, then misinterpretations and misunderstandings may result.[53]

Classic examples of such misunderstandings include the pathologising of mystical experiences that was almost the norm until recently, particularly among psychoanalysts and psychiatrists. Misunderstandings still occur quite frequently because psychiatrists may be unable to comprehend and accept their patients' spiritual experiences.[54]

> The field of the normal man's sense perceptions is, as can be demonstrated, narrowly circumscribed and extremely limited. There are objects and colours he cannot see, sounds he cannot hear, odours he cannot smell, tastes he cannot taste and feelings he cannot feel. And beyond his work-a-day consciousness, which he assumes to be his only consciousness, there are other consciousnesses, of which *yogins* and saints have cognizance, and of which psychologists are beginning to glean, but as yet very little, understanding.[55]

Certainly because of its cognocentric, or single state, view Western psychology has difficulty accommodating religious experience. Its preoccupation with the material 'has fostered a world view in which man is merely a highly developed animal, and the spiritual side of human nature expressed in religion, spirituality and mysticism is either ignored or termed pathological'.[56] In this way 'we have pathologised the experience of every saint, prophet and shaman throughout history.'[57] In contrast, Eastern psychologies are essentially spiritual. They point to a view and understanding of religion that is radically different from those in the West. This is akin to that described as the 'perennial philosophy'[58] and more recently as the 'perennial psychology'.[59] They can be viewed as multi-state disciplines designed to provide strategies for the induction of transcendent states of consciousness, and guidance on the perspectives, insights, understandings and world-views afforded by these states.

Inasmuch as Western psychology is no longer faithful to its original subject matter, the soul, it can be claimed that it is not true psychology at all, while many Western psychologists would deny that the esoteric spiritual traditions of the East constitute psychology in anything other than the loosest sense. The point at issue here is considerably more than mere etymological dispute. It is a question of what constitutes the proper subject matter of psychology and this reflects the different traditions of thought — indeed the very 'soul' — of those cultures in which it is embedded.

In the East, where psychology is rooted in mysticism, emphasis is on the spiritual, the subjective and the individual and its dominant ethos is necessarily humanistic whereas, in the West, psychology is rooted in the tradition of science and its emphasis is on the material, objective and general and its predominant ethos is accordingly mechanical and impersonal.

The most fundamental difference between them, however, is one of perspective. East and West represent respectively the polar extremes of mystical insight and scientific outlook. The dichotomy can be seen to correspond with the two aspects of mind as conceived in Indian thought, the inward-looking aspect of which is directed towards the essential nature of man, and the outward-looking aspect directed towards the world of things and external appearances. In the traditions of the Orient both aspects are viewed as complementary facets of one whole or unity, and virtue and harmony are deemed not to consist in an accentuation of one aspect to the detriment of the other, but in maintaining a dynamic balance between them. Nevertheless, it is a human tendency to divide and separate rather than see things in the round, and this produces blindness to half the visual field.[60] In the pursuit of understanding innermost being, the cultures of the East and notably of India have tended to ignore the material world, developing their spiritual, poetic, artistic and mystical traditions and cultivating thereby an attitude to life quite alien to Western eyes. In the West, with its reverence for the intellect and rationality and the outward appearances of things, the inner man has been neglected as science and technology progress. While in the West we have developed one half of the ability and organised external reality to an unparalleled extent, Westerners remain 'blind', or at least hemianopic to the other.[61] This oversight may prove particularly significant in the light of the Eastern injunction against single-minded attachment to the world of appearances which is held to be illusion, human bondage and folly. Certainly at the peak of scientific ascendency and scientific psychology in the mid-twentieth century there was dawning awareness that the attempt to understand the world whilst precluding any attempt to understand human nature might be the ultimate in human folly. There was also growing recognition that reduction (from the Latin *reductio* meaning to take away from) when applied to human beings takes away their essential humanness.

Another fundamental difference between Eastern and Western psychologies is that the former are implicitly and explicitly concerned with healing. This cannot be understood in reductionist terms because in the traditions of the East, body, mind and spirit form an integral whole and any treatment of the body cannot be separated from psychological and spiritual dimensions. Hence the development of medicine goes hand in hand with these psychologies whose goal is to liberate human consciousness to its natural level of being, and sound health is both the condition and creation of this end. Psychology and medicine are one and the same in the East rather than separate disciplines, as they are in the West.

4

DOCTORS OF THE SOUL

In the West where mind and matter still occupy largely different realms, psychology is generally thought to have little part in the promotion of health and disease. In the East there is no separation into body and mind, nor the individual and the universe, they are intimately related in a dynamic manner. So in the traditions of the East, psychology and medicine are essentially one and the same.

Traditional Indian medicine: Ayurveda

Traditional Indian medicine, Ayurveda, embodies the fundamental principle of Vedanta: people should have faith in themselves first. As such it may be considered the archetypal self-help system of healing. The tradition of Ayurveda is some 3000 years old and until the formation of the British Empire, when Western medicine was introduced to India, it was dominant on the Indian subcontinent. Since India gained independence in 1945 there has been a resurgence of interest in this system, and many colleges and universities offer training in this discipline. According to some estimates[1] approximately 80 per cent of India's population rely on Ayurvedic medicine.

Ayurveda has become known in the West only relatively recently through its practice within immigrant Asian communities but in 1980 the World Health Organisation suggested that its principles should be widely known as they offer a holistic health system that integrates orthodox modern Western medicine and complementary approaches.

Ayurveda is Sanskrit for 'the science of life', and it is a section in the last four Vedas, the *Atharva Veda* dating from about 1200 BC. Although its early history is obscure it contains magical spells and charms to cope with a wide range of natural and supernatural conditions, suggesting origins in ancient magic. Moreover, as ancient

India had no writing and no written history, all its teachings were memorised and handed down by the highest caste, the Brahmins, in characteristic occult tradition.

The first school of medicine was established at Banares in 500 BC and in 5 and 6 BC respectively the main texts *Susruta Samhita* and *Charaka Samhita* were written there. Together they constitute a comprehensive system of medicine that is essentially cosmological, for, as in all traditional systems of healing, health is considered a balance between constituent qualities and energies of man and the universe. Fundamental to it is the idea that man must be regarded as whole with no separation between his body, mind and soul. Only one-third of the system is concerned with disease. It is mainly concerned with health and providing a guide to living. As such it is an excellent system of preventative medicine.

Healing in Ayurveda is based on the premise that balance can be achieved through the *tridosha* or *tridhatu*, which differentiates into three elemental energies, or *doshas* — *kapha*, *pitta* and *vata*, or *vayu* — which govern physical processes in the body without themselves being physical:

- *Kapha* is associated with air and is concerned with growth and nutrition, or anabolism.

- *Pitta* is associated with fire and relates to digestion or catabolism.

- *Vata*, or *vayu*, is associated with water and concerned with the nervous system, mind and the distribution of psychic energy. It also controls and regulates the other two elements, which come under the general heading of metabolism. *Vata*, which reflects the psychosomatic component of Ayurveda, is therefore central to health and healing.

All areas of human functioning are located in one or other of these *doshas* or cosmic forces, each of which has two aspects, *purusha*, the material side of man and his conscious state, and *prakriti*, his essence, the unmanifest self, subconscious or spirit. These dynamic processes are intimately connected and move together. The interplay of these forces is described in terms of 25 fundamental qualities or *gunas*.

These are enduring qualities throughout nature and the source of all the characteristics of worldly phenomena. The degree to which the *gunas* associated with a particular *dosha* prevail over the others determines the nature of a person or thing, and people are thought to be constitutionally of one predominant type or other.

From the Ayurvedic standpoint the body's systems exist to balance the *gunas* and achieve dynamic equilibrium of the *doshas*. Illness is viewed as imbalance and so healing relies upon accurate diagnosis of constitutional type, which is achieved partly by observation of the person's attitudes and behaviour. More fundamentally it relies on the intuition of the practitioner. An Ayurvedic doctor does not literally see the *doshas* because although they can be moved, increased and decreased they are fundamentally abstract metabolic principles and as such are invisible. Accordingly, like the shaman, the Ayurvedic physician 'sees' what is invisible to others: the way in which the soul is expressed in a person's being.

Once a person's constitutional type has been established the physician recommends various food, minerals and specific remedies. This is a logical process as the *gunas* required to promote balance are found in all things. Diagnosis and prescription is no simple matter, not only because Ayurveda recognises thousands of sicknesses but also because all remedies are prepared with regard to the patient's individual susceptibilities, seasonal and climatic variations and other environmental considerations. The many similarities between the Ayurvedic and Hippocratic traditions have prompted the suggestion that at some point Pythagoras was influenced by Indian philosophy. It is more likely, however, that the similarities between the traditions arise from their common origin in the mystical, shamanic traditions of the ancient world.

Prakriti, the spirit, is accessed by way of five *doshas* or essence types. The energy system and the five fundamental powers of nature — space, air, fire, water and earth — are seen as intrinsically related and all bodies as different combinations of these natural elements which arise out of the absolute substance *prakriti*. In human bodies these substances combine in special ways to become transformed into seven tissue types or *dhatus*. Excess, under or over use or abuse of these is considered an important cause of imbalance or 'unmeasured' being, and consequent ill health. Alienation of man from his natural environment is seen as the loss of the natural relationship between the senses and the elemental powers of nature at both the individual and social levels. In this way modern man has 'taken leave of his senses'. He needs to return not only to his senses but to right measures, knowledge of which is present in the human heart.

In this Indian concept of measure one finds yet again close similarities with the ancient Greek tradition. The view of the physician–patient relationship is also similar. Ayurveda has always been based on positive interaction between them. The principle of self-help is fundamental to Ayurveda. The need to strive for spiritual self-development is understood and taken for granted by both the patient and Ayurvedic practitioner who combines the role of physician with that of spiritual guide. This is in marked contrast to the relationship between a Western doctor and his patient. The latter is the passive recipient of the practitioner's treatment and without obligation to strive for his own fundamental physical well-being, much less that of his soul, which the physician ignores.

> Ayurveda is steadfast in insisting that medicine should always be centered on the person rather than on disease. It believes that the twin goals of maintaining good health and deliverance from disease can be reached only if the doctor has a thorough understanding of the person. The person in his wholeness is called the 'asylum' (*asrya*) of disease and constitutes the main subject of medical science. In the words of an oft-quoted verse, 'Mind, soul and the body — these three are like a tripod; the world is sustained by their combination: they constitute the substratum for everything. This [combination] is the person (*purusa*): this is sentient and this is the subject matter of this Veda (Ayurveda): it is for this that this Veda (Ayurveda) is brought to light.[2]

The emphasis on the wholeness of the person is reflected in the comprehensiveness of the diagnostic examination conducted by the Ayurvedic physician. The patient in Ayurveda is conceived of as simultaneously living in and partaking of different orders of being, physical, psychological, social and metaphysical, and a systematic knowledge of all these orders and their interrelationships is considered essential in the doctor. This is an inevitable corollary of seeing the person as a microcosm of the universe, as equivalent with creation.

A great deal of research in Ayurveda is carried out and published in the *Journal of Research in Indian Medicine*, although this is still relatively unknown in the West. Some ancient traditional practices of Ayurveda such as vaccination, anaesthesia by inhalation and dietetics have only been practised in the West for the last hundred years or so, and some of its practices, such as those inducing muscle regeneration, were not considered possible in the West until relatively recently. However, in the past decade Ayurveda has become better known and popularised in the West, not only through its practice within immigrant Asian communities but also through the best-selling books of Dr. Deepak Chopra.

Fundamentally Ayurveda is a holistic health care system. One of its best-known practices in the West is yoga. This is much more than a combination of physical and breathing exercises. It is a complete philosophy and self-help system that embraces the whole person in their physical, mental and spiritual aspects

Yoga

The practice of yoga is a training that unifies the parts of the body with the whole of mind and spirit. The word *yoga* is derived from a Sanskrit word meaning to join or to yoke, and it signifies the union of the individual with the Ultimate Reality. Yoga is essentially therefore a spiritual discipline, a means of attaining the highest aims of Vedanta and the Hindu tradition. It is a development of the Upanishads, that portion of the Vedas dating from 1500 BC devoted to philosophy. The metaphysical aspects of yoga are expounded in the *Yogasutra*. This clearly suggests a holographic understanding of the universe, which is described as a set of pearls so arranged that when one pearl is looked into all the others are reflected in it. It is also likened to a web that trembles in its entirety if any of its strands are touched.

There are many different forms of yoga other than the *Hatha* yoga practised in the West that is concerned with bringing the body to the peak of health and efficiency through physical and breathing exercises. Many of these are a refinement of ancient shamanic practices. *Mantra* yoga, for example, is based on the inherent power of sound and vibration as revealed by ancient seers. Its aim is to alter consciousness by rhythmical repetition of divine names or phrases known as mantras. *Laya* yoga is concerned with arousing cosmic energies so as to enable the individual to merge with Ultimate Reality. Similarly, *Kundalini* yoga is concerned with arousing the unlimited divine cosmic energy that exists in every living thing and signifies unlimited potential. It is conceived as the female creative energy, symbolised as a serpent curled half-asleep at the base of the spine. The aim of *Kundalini* yoga is to raise the energy upwards through the body, primarily through meditation and visualisation. *Hatha* yoga was not intended to be pursued in isolation from the other forms. Its function is to prepare the practitioner for meditation, which is considered to be the only way to know Ultimate Reality. Only by overcoming physical obstacles can the person commence the inner journey towards integration or union, which is the aim of yoga.

Similarities between yoga and Kabbalism

There are many similarities in the philosophy and practice of yoga and the Jewish mystical traditions of the Kabbalah and Hasidism. Kabbalah is based on ancient traditions but was revived in the twelfth and thirteenth centuries when it expressed the hopes and needs of Jews exiled from their homeland. Its teachings were absorbed into Hasidism, which developed in the eighteenth century. Exile served as a profound symbol for Jewish mystics and focused not only on their historical and religious experiences but also on the very condition of the cosmos itself and of the existential estrangement of the human soul from the Divine Root. The aim of Kabbalism is the union of the seeker's soul with the divine.[3] Exile is essentially separation or the disruption of what is meant to be unified or harmoniously related. In Hasidism, which means unification, the unity of personal being became the unifying force for the cosmos as a whole. The goal is a life of ecstasy, an unfolding of the soul that flows into the Absolute. It teaches that transformation of the world and its unification is ultimately bound up with the ability to unify one's own being, body and soul, into a unified existence. In Hasidism prayer is a means to unify the soul, to unite it with other souls and raise all these souls to God. In Kabbalism unity is achieved priimarily through meditation on the *Sephirot*, the tree of life, which represents man's relationship to

God. Both implicitly and explicitly, as in yoga, healing or wholeness is the aim of these practices.

Western research on yoga during the twentieth century has shown that yoga has many positive therapeutic benefits in the treatment of psychosomatic and organic disorders, notably in the management of hypertension, the major cause of death in the West, where it has been shown to have beneficial effects similar to the tranquilliser, diazepam.[4] It has also proved effective in the treatment of venous and lymphatic insufficiency, peripheral artery disease, chronic bronchitis, emphysema and sinusitis.[5]

Buddhist medicine

The Buddha is often referred to as the Supreme Healer because he embodied the qualities of the ideal physician, serene detachment and selfless compassion, and devoted his life to the alleviation of suffering.[6] Buddha taught that:

> ... human beings suffer because of self-delusion, striving to possess that which inevitably must crumble, and because of desire. The Buddha did not stop with a mere diagnosis. He proclaimed that the cure is to reach a higher state of being, wherein self-knowledge has eradicated delusion, attachment and desire. Buddhist psychology asserts that not only all psychological pain is caused by false knowledge and covetousness, but also that physical illness can be traced to these factors.[7]

Buddhism is implicitly and explicitly concerned with healing in that it is directed to the relief of suffering through annihilation of the concept of separateness and the promotion of a sense of oneness with the whole of things, the literal meaning of health and healing.

Underpinning Buddhist healing principles are the teachings expounded in the *Abhidharma*. This is a psychological theory based upon observations of the workings of the human mind in meditation. It describes mind as being comprised of wholesome or healthy, afflictive and neutral factors. Of these, the afflictive or unhealthy factors such as greed, hatred, pride, envy and lack of insight are seen as the ultimate underlying causes both of physical and mental diseases. Three afflictive factors in particular are seen as the roots of all unwholesome states of mind: desire or attachment; hatred, anger or aversion; and ignorance or confusion. These unwholesome or unhealthy states of mind are viewed as the root of all physical illness as they give rise to physiological imbalances in bile and phlegm that activate disease. Such a view is clearly similar to that underpinning the ancient doctrine of humours; but it is also contemporary in that it recognises the role of the mind in triggering disease and as such shares similar understanding with behavioural medicine and psychoneuroimmunology.

Through the practice of meditation, afflictive factors can be identified and eliminated, restoring mental health and physiological harmony and relieving distress. Accordingly, in Buddhism meditation is medicine. Indeed, the Latin root of the word meditation — *mederi* — means to heal. Meditation heals not only by restructuring mental contents but also by promoting wholeness or holiness. It does so because it involves a letting go of the concept of the individual self and absorption in what one is: part of the totality. It is a state of no will, of inaction or non-doing. In that it is a letting go — of notions of the self or ego and its limitations, of the illusion of separateness; of what one believes or would like oneself to be — it is equivalent to relaxation: 'Life in cosmic consciousness is tensionless.'[8]

Since the 1930s there has been abundant evidence that meditation confers a number of health benefits. In 1935 the French cardiologist Thérèse Brosse recorded measures of heart-rate control in Indian meditators indicative of an advanced voluntary capacity to regulate autonomic functions, including metabolic rate. Subsequently it was established[9] that during meditation metabolism decreases and that advanced meditators could produce effects through the control of the autonomic nervous system formerly considered to be beyond voluntary control.

During the 1950s and 1960s research on meditation was facilitated by the development of sophisticated recording devices such as the electroencephalograph or EEG which detects the electrical rhythms generated by the brain. Explorations with the EEG showed that meditation produces changes in brain wave activity suggestive of deep relaxation. During the 1970s much research was conducted on meditation and this confirmed earlier findings that meditation is a thoroughly relaxed state and an effective antidote to anxiety which underpins stress and stress-related illness. Awareness of the possible therapeutic benefits has led to the application of meditation in the treatment of stress and stress-related conditions. Research in the 1980s and 1990s[10, 11] indicated that meditation may confer long-term health benefits and that it is possible to develop a habitual low arousal state.[12]

Other therapeutic benefits claimed for meditation are that traits such as depression and neuroticism change significantly in a positive direction and anxiety is significantly reduced. Significant improvements in self-concept have also been reported along with other benefits consistent with psychotherapy and psychosomatic medicine. Meditation is not only a means for exploring the mind but for transforming it and achieving a state of optimal psychological functioning. As such it resembles what in the West is known as psychotherapy. Indeed, Buddhist healing cannot easily be distinguished from psychotherapy.

Tibetan medicine

Meditation is at the core of Tibetan medicine, which rests fundamentally on the belief in a vital force or energy that moves in channels throughout the body and underlies psychological processes. This energy, *prana*, is an aspect of universal or cosmic energy. It is in continuous flux, permeates all things, yet is undefinable, dissolves at death, is blocked or disrupted in disease and channelled and controlled through meditation.

> As a body man is a microscopic but faithful reflection of the macroscopic reality in which he is embedded and which preserves and nourishes him every second of his life; as a mind, he is a ripple on the surface of a great ocean of consciousness. Health is the proper relationship between the microcosm which is man and the macrocosm which is the universe. Disease is a disruption of this relationship.[13]

The channels over which the energy moves are termed *nadis* in Sanskrit and referred to as *tsas* in Tibet. They comprise a 'kind of psychic nervous system' because the natural functioning of mind depends on the balance of pranic currents.[14] The movement of the energy within the channels is termed *rlung*. Consciousness is carried by the currents of *rlung* as it changes from moment to moment. Five major subdivisions or currents of *rlung* are distinguished on the basis of their location, area of circulation and function. These represent the distinctive *pranic* currents that support the psychophysical organism. The life-sustaining current located at the crown of the head provides the physical basis for mind and is broken down into five secondary currents each of which serves as the basis for the consciousness associated with the five senses. It also serves on a more subtle level as the basis for conceptual mental consciousness and on an even more subtle level is the aspect of *prana* that supports the very subtle mind or soul that passes from one life through the intermediate *Bardo* state to the next life. The ascending current located at the chest but circulating in the throat and head regions supports speech, eating and aids mental tone. The pervasive (diffusive) current located at the heart helps flexion and extension of the limbs, muscular action, physical growth and coordination of bodily and mental functions, including thinking. The metabolic (fire-accompanying) current located in the stomach regulates digestion. The descending current located in the pelvic area regulates eliminatory and reproductive functions. Thus *rlung* serves as the basis for nervous, hormonal and organic functioning and also as the foundation for mental and sense consciousness. In this way, *rlung* encompasses mind and body. Accordingly, mental disturbance is reflected in the alteration of the flow of *rlung* and disturbance of *rlung* anywhere within the organism is said to produce correlative mental or emotional disturbances.

Conversely *rlung* is at the root of all physical illness. It is one of three physical processes or *nyes-pa*, whose harmonious interaction is necessary for life from the cellular to the organismic level. When these *nyes-pa*, crudely translated as wind, bile and phlegm, are in balance, physical and mental health are maintained but when they are increased or decreased, they give rise to disease. Initial disorders are thought to arise from disturbances in the flow of *prana* through its natural channels. Repeated aggravation leads to an increase in *rlung* beyond its normal range, which if continued leads it to overflow its natural channels and disrupt the other *nyes-pa*. Similarly disruption, that is, increase or decrease, in the flow of the other *nyes-pa* will affect the circulation of *rlung*, causing imbalance and disease. Causes of *rlung* imbalance can include poor diet, improper behaviour, seasonal factors or poisoning, but ultimately imbalances in any of the three *nyes-pa* are attributed to psychological causes. Indeed the three *nyes-pa*, which can be translated as 'defects' or 'faults' arise in the three afflictive mental factors that are the root of all unhealthy states of mind. Thus, the medical theories of Tibetan traditions are tied to the psychological principles set out in the *Abhidharma*, disease states being seen as 'crystallizations of dominant states of mind'.

Tibetan medicine is fundamentally concerned with maintaining the balance of the *nyes-pa* and promoting the flow of *rlung*. This is nowhere more important than with regard to the death experience. Death can be described as the sequential dissolution of the various aspects of *rlung*. In death all the *pranic* currents of the body ultimately dissolve into the subtle life-sustaining current that serves as the basis for consciousness of the intermediate *bardo* state between physical death and rebirth.

Practitioners of Tibetan tantric Buddhism seek through meditation to consciously mirror the death experience by deliberately bringing about the same dissolution of vital currents that occurs at death. This involves gaining mastery over the currents of *prana*, mimicking the many alterations of consciousness that tantric theory describes as occurring at death. Perfection of this yoga allows mastery over death, the transformation of the very subtle life-sustaining *prana* into the clear light of the void. These descriptions lie at the core of the *Tibetan Book of the Dead*.

At a more mundane level meditation is concerned with the dissolution of the ego. In Tibetan Buddhism ego is viewed as a limitation of human reality and as such is not only a mental and spiritual problem but also a physical one. This is because holding on to a rigid self-image, struggling to censor and manipulate experience to meet its demands, is hard work involving physical tension and pain. So Tibetan Buddhism promotes a series of exercises in relaxation to deal with life's anxieties. The Tibetan approach to healing therefore reflects the belief that optimum well-being is a relaxed, balanced, open state. Human illness, however minor, is seen as a cosmic event.

The aim of Tibetan medicine is to restore harmony and balance. Healing is essentially spiritual and the leading physicians are *lamas* or monks. However, although Tibetans have developed a complex system of medicine with elaborate techniques and sophisticated pharmacology, it has never resembled its Western counterpart. Diagnosis and care in traditional Tibetan medicine operate on several levels. Physical, emotional and spiritual and ecological aspects of disorders are considered. The physician looks into the life situation of the patient and may diagnose disease as some expression of disturbance in the psychosocial environment such as bereavement, personal misfortune or sudden change in routine. Emotional nourishment may be prescribed as the remedy for some conditions. In so doing Tibetan medicine anticipated contemporary Western attention to stress and life-change by several thousand years.

In most cases extensive physiological diagnosis is conducted. The doctor examines the body, takes the pulse, analyses urine, faeces, sleep and eating patterns. When medicines are called for, herbs, flowers, fruit, roots, honey and minerals are used as infusions, poultices and vapours. The patient is always an active rather than passive participant in cure.

The feeling tone of the healing experience is extremely important, perhaps more important than the specifics of medical practice. A certain caring and trust has to be present and mutually experienced. Compassion is the supreme virtue of the medical practitioner, but the state of mind of the patient is equally important. The optimum emotional state for healing includes such qualities as compassion for the self; awareness or mindfulness; a realistic understanding of karma in illness; cheerfulness; optimism; and a basic confidence in the naturalness of the healing process.

Chinese medicine

Traditional Chinese medicine was founded around 2900 BC by the half-mythical Fu Hsi who first described *chi* and the two complementary principles of the universe, *yin* and *yang*. His successor, Huang Ti (*circa* 2600 BC) introduced into medicine the principles of ancient natural philosophy that regarded the human being as an image of the cosmos. Conversations between Huang Ti and his minister Ch'i Po form the content of the *Nei Ching*, variously known as the *Theory of Internal Diseases*, or the *Yellow Emperor's Classic (or Treatise) on Internal Medicine*. This oral tradition thousands of years old is still in use today.

According to the principles established in the *Nei Ching* there are definite pathways of *chi* in the body known as *ching mo* or meridians, and these are associated with different bodily functions or organs. *Chi* flows along these in much the same way as blood and lymph circulate through the body, keeping the organism alive; its obstruction gives rise to ill health. Treatment focuses on normalising energy flow and restoring the balance of *yin* and *yang*. It requires understanding of a number of energy cycles, principally the Shen Cycle, or Cycle of the Spirit.

The Shen Cycle

In Chinese thought the symbol of the Tao is represented as a circle containing *yin* and *yang* and all opposites. The clockwise flow of this circle forms the Shen or Spirit Cycle. Healthy people are viewed as flowing with the Tao, through the Shen and other cycles, whereas unhealthy people are seen to resist and fight it. The natural flow of the Shen Cycle is linked to five seasons — summer, late summer, autumn, winter and spring — and each of these is associated with five elements — fire, earth, metal, water and wood. Each of these elements also has various other associations or correspondences — a colour, climate, direction, sound, odour, power, life aspect, time of day, emotion, bodily organs, sense organs and a secretion. So, for example, fire is associated with summer, heat, the colour red, the time interval 11 am–3 pm, and a southerly direction. Its associated odour is scorched and its taste bitter. Associated with joyful emotion, its sound is laughter. It is related to the organs and functions of the heart, small intestine and triple heater (which has no Western counterpart), circulation, and sexuality. Its sense organ is the tongue and its secretion perspiration. Each element also corresponds with specific meats, fruits, vegetables and grains.

Implicit in the Shen Cycle is another cycle, the K'o, the cycle of mastery and control. It is associated with emotions, thoughts and behaviour, the mastery of which involves understanding the K'o and the fundamental principle of opposites. Emotions arise in pairs of opposites — empathy and fear, joy and sorrow, anger and sympathy — and each of these can be controlled by its opposite. Hence joy is the antidote to sorrow. The emotions determine thoughts and behaviours because normally a person's emotions dictate his or her response in a given situation. These emotions also effect particular elements and organs, and consequently physical health.

When emotion is too intense or prolonged, disease may ensue. It can be discerned initially as a distortion of energy balance within the individual, and eventually in distortion of the organs or functions themselves. Conversely, if an organ becomes diseased there is corresponding imbalance in the emotion associated with that organ. All disease is therefore considered psychosomatic in that it affects both mind and body. Excess anger allows energy to rise up in stiff shoulders, headache, tinnitus and sinusitis. The Chinese regard prolonged or unresolved anger leading to resignation, resentment, frustration or bitterness as probably the most destructive to health — a view now echoed by many practitioners of Western medicine — and as particularly damaging to the liver. Fear predominantly affects the water element, the kidneys and bladder. A sudden fright may affect the kidneys or heart but chronic anxiety is considered to permeate a person's entire system and be more damaging. Worry and over-concentration are held to damage the spleen, grief the lungs. At the centre of the Chinese system of medicine is the realisation that imbalance of an individual's emotions inevitably leads to imbalance of physical functioning.

Understanding of the Shen and K'o cycles and their correspondences and associations forms the basis of diagnosis in Chinese medicine, which is both complex and subtle. The medical practitioner uses all of these, including colour, sound of the voice, predominant emotion and smell, to diagnose imbalance, predisposition to imbalance, its type and extent. In addition, the practitioner takes the pulses and enquires into the person's dreams.

Treatment in Chinese medicine

In Traditional Chinese medicine one practitioner treats the whole person in body, mind and spirit. There are no psychiatrists, psychotherapists or psychologists. Treatment may involve dietary changes, herbs, mantra therapy, lessons in the Way of life, acupuncture, or moxibustion, where heat is generated over an acupuncture point by burning leaves of the plant *Artemis Vulgaris* or Mugwort.

Traditional Japanese medicine corresponds very closely to that of

China. Acupuncture and shiatsu, or finger pressure, are widely used. Shiatsu originates in massage techniques developed over two thousand years but was first developed as a special therapy by Toru Nami Koshi, who established the Shiatsu Institute in 1925. Various styles of shiatsu are practised, all of which share the common aims of relaxation, improvement of blood and lymphatic flow, alleviation of aches and pains and the heightening of bodily awareness. Anma, the precursor of shiatsu, is a generic term for the use of hands on certain points of the body to promote healing and well-being. It embraces several different forms including daily massage, pressure, kneading and stretching. Do-in and Ge Jo involve self-stimulation of areas of pressure, friction, and percussion and breathing techniques.

Reiki (meaning universal life energy) was developed as a method of healing in the nineteenth century by the Japanese monk Dr Mikao Usui, who claimed to have found in ancient Buddhist scriptures the 'Key' or formula for healing. He discovered how to use its symbols intuitively through intensive meditation upon them. This system of healing involves channelling and balancing energy within oneself and interpersonally by way of these symbols and the laying on of hands. It emphasises the importance of creating a trusting, loving environment in which healing can take place.

Sufi medicine
Within Sufism inner conflict is considered the source of all maladies. It is implicitly a system of healing in that it is directed to reducing the conflict and attaining a tensionless state where the individual functions harmoniously with the universe and experiences life in contentment, creativity and relatedness to all. Like Ayurveda, it is essentially a system of self-healing, as is indicated in Rumi's directive 'You already have the precious mixture that will make you well. Use it.' In explaining the healing arts of the spiritual physician, Rumi demonstrated an impressive talent as a clinician and his works reflect a profound insight into the interplay of natural and cultural forces in sickness and health that rivals that of the most sophisticated contemporary physicians.

Similarities among oriental healing traditions
Clear similarities can be identified in the healing traditions of China

and Japan and those of India and Tibet. They are, despite differences in terminology, essentially the same. The correspondence is not exact owing to the different cultural contexts in which they arose but it is nonetheless clear that they deal with the same fundamental reality. They all recognise the universe as a subtle energy system that is reflected within the human body. The channels for subtle energy in the body, *nadis* and meridians, correspond quite closely. Their correspondences have been mapped using descriptions in the Upanishads, traditional Chinese medical texts and clinical practice.[15] Similar energy systems appear to have been discovered by masseurs who noted a series of energy flows while feeling for reactions in the body during massage and also by Taoists and practitioners of yoga who recognised the channels of vital energy intuitively and extra-sensorily during meditation and developed treatment systems accordingly.

The *nadi* and meridian theories were brought into contact with each other some 2500 years ago in Nepal and Tibet,[16] and communication and mutual supplementation appears to have occurred quite easily owing to their similarity. At about this time the Shen and K'o Cycles emerged in Chinese thought. These departed from the traditional *yin–yang* dualism by dividing all aspects of the universe into five elements and the body into three regions, physical, emotional and spiritual, each controlled by a different energy system. These ideas are essentially the same as those found in the Indian concept of *prana* dividing into five winds or *vayus*, and the body into four regions. Although the number of divisions differs the basic concept is much the same.

Since antiquity, understanding energy has been the very core of traditional healing practices throughout the world. Traditional approaches to healing in both the East and West can thus be considered energy medicine. They share a belief in the existence of subtle energies in and around the person, the mobilisation and balancing of which are seen as fundamental to health, with illness being the result of their stagnation or disruption. In ancient Hippocratic medicine the patient was called *asthenis*, meaning a person who lacked vital energy; the doctor was *iatros*, the healer who re-established the *sthenos* or vital energy of the person. In contrast, modern Western medicine has moved away from this model towards the pathology of life, omitting the source of health which is the vital energy.[17] Most concepts of energy in the West were conceived when its science was formulated in purely objective mechanistic terms and so life energy is frequently conceived as some kind of substance that flows through the organism.

Eastern concepts of energy are markedly different and akin to those of pre-scientific Western civilisations, notably ancient Egypt and Greece. Energy is conceived not as any 'thing' but as continuous movement or change. It is relative and rests on an inner polarity, or regulative function of opposites that flow into one another. This is the vital force. In Aristotle's terms, *entelekhia*, which directs the life of the individual, the soul.

The fundamental concept common to these views is that all matter, including the human body, the mind and all phenomena comprise energy in a particular state of vibration and has both physical and subtle non-physical aspects. Such a view is fully consistent with modern physics. Accordingly wave motion, light, heat, colour and sound are merely different forms of vibration, as are thoughts, images and emotions. Healing approaches based on this view use the various states of vibration to restore energy imbalances within the mind and body. What may be considered 'energy medicine' involves a number of techniques that are believed to influence the organism at a more fundamental level than the physical or psychological symptoms of illness.

> When we realise that in the final analysis our bodies are in fact made up of nothing but energy in constant transformation it is easier to understand how subtle non-physical, energetic influences such as emotions and thoughts can have a direct influence on our physical functioning, just as our physical functioning can have a direct influence on our emotional and mental experiences.[18]

However, even within the scientific community many find it hard to accept the principles of contemporary science, much less accept that these have been mapped out with striking similarity throughout the world since antiquity. Yet this is clearly the case.

The Hopi Indians, who consider themselves the oldest inhabitants of the earth, view the human body and the earth as isomorphic. Both have an axis (in humans, the spine) along which, they maintain, are several vibrating centres or vortices that distribute energy through the body. The first centre at the top of the head receives life energy at birth and is the seat of communication with the creator, the second centre is situated at the brain, the third at the throat, the fourth at the heart, the fifth at the solar plexus. Similar beliefs are common among Native Americans and the Inuit. They are also a feature of early Egyptian, Indian and Tibetan traditions of thought, hence the similarity between Hindu symbols and those of Native American totem poles. However, in addition to the centres described by the Hopi, the Hindu system includes a centre situated below the navel and another located over the sacral bone. These are described as three-dimensional pulsating wheels, known in Sanskrit as *chakras*, which rotate rhythmically from the centre, rather like Catherine wheels, in a way that appears to seers or clairvoyants as the shape of a cone, trumpet or convolvulus flower. According to the direction of spin, they either draw energy in or direct it out of the body, thereby energising or enervating it.

Most of what is written about the chakras is found in the ancient sacred texts of India, the *Arunopnishad*, the *Yoga-Shikka* and the *Bridadarayaka* Upanishads, where they are described as places where the soul rests. In the West the idea of chakra energies is found within the rituals of the ancient Greek mystery schools of Eleusis and Delphi and in the teachings attributed to Hermes Trismegistus (the Egyptian deity, Thoth), who is credited with defining the attributes of the chakras some 50,000 years ago.[19] Many Ancient Egyptian monuments suggest familiarity with the chakras. Evidence that early European mystics were also familiar with them comes from the *Theosophica Practica* issued in 1696 by Gichtel, who was probably a Rosicrucian, and from and the ancient rituals of freemasonry.

The chakras were first described in English in the late nineteenth century and became more widely known in the early twentieth century through the writings of Theosophists, members of the Theosophical Society whose system of belief, theosophy (Greek, meaning Divine Wisdom), was derived from the ancient Indian texts. In the Hindu system the chakras are said to be located at the base of the spine, the gonads, the solar plexus, the heart, the throat and between the eyebrows and the crown of the head, and are traditionally stimulated or 'awakened' by *Raja, Karma, Jnana, Hatha, Laya, Bhakti* and *Mantra* yoga respectively. In addition to these major chakras, a number of minor chakras are variously described in different traditions. According to ancient wisdom, organisms draw vital energies from the atmosphere and earth by way of a subtle, immaterial body or *linga sharirah* — formed from the finer principles of matter — on whose surface the chakras are situated. This is variously known as the 'soul body' in magical traditions; the 'vital body' in certain Rosicrucian schools; the 'astral', 'etheric body' or 'double' in other Western occult traditions; the *ka* in ancient Egypt; the *doppelgänger* in medieval Europe; and the *perispirit* in French spiritism. The subtle body or *linga sharirah* is generally regarded as synonymous with the soul, as surviving physical death and transmigrating to other bodies. In the Theosophical tradition the person is viewed as a soul that possesses not one but several bodies, rather than a body that possesses a soul. In addition to the visible vehicle by which the person acts in the physical world, there are other bodies invisible to normal sight by means of which he or she deals with emotional and mental worlds. This is also the centuries-old claim of many seers and philosophers.

The ancient view is that energy in the form of light is drawn into the body's immaterial counterpart, which acts as a prism, breaking it down into seven energy streams corresponding with the frequency bands of the colour spectrum. Each of these is drawn through resonance to a chakra whose vibrations are of the same frequency. The vibrations become progressively more dense, heavier and lower in frequency along the vertical axis of the body. At its base they merge and arise with earth energies, represented in Indian thought by the coiled serpent *Kundalini* and in Chinese thought by a dragon. The upward spiral motion of these energies around the central axis of the spine is also represented in the caduceus, the traditional symbol of the healing arts since ancient times in the West and the emblem of contemporary Western medicine.

The chakras, which may be thought of as transmitters or transformers of energy, are believed to vibrate at a characteristic frequency as they distribute energy throughout the body. The energy patterns around each chakra, although always changing, are mostly of a certain colour whose vibrations correspond with its basic frequency. The prevailing colour of a chakra indicates how well its energies are being transformed and transmitted at a given time and therefore reflect current experience.

The colours of the chakras were described in the tenth-century yoga text *Gorakshasma-takan*. According to ancient tradition (thought to have been established by Thoth/Hermes)[20] each chakra is also associated with a musical note, a symbolic form and certain elements of the same characteristic vibrational frequency. These vary according to tradition. In the seventeenth century, Gichtel assigned planets to the chakras, suggesting that they are sensitive to planetary influence, thereby providing a physical basis for astrology. More recently the chakras have also been associated with the location and functioning of the major nerve plexuses of the body, each of which is connected to one of the glands of the endocrine system. The slightest imbalance of energy in any chakra is thought to influence the corresponding gland, giving rise to fluctuations in hormones which are secreted directly into the bloodstream, producing immediate changes in mood, appearance, tension, respiration, digestion, intuition and intelligence.

The various traditions hold that by understanding its character, function, associated colour, sound and symbolic form, each chakra can be cleansed, opened and balanced. These beliefs form the basis of most ancient forms of healing, including the colour and sound therapies of ancient Egypt and Greece, the various practices of yoga and the use of 'power' objects such as crystals and stones by shamans and witch doctors. The correct and balanced action of the chakras is expressed as absolute and perfect health on all levels.

A field or realm of existing or potential consciousness, referred to by ancient Hindu, Egyptians and Greeks as a 'body', is also attributed to each chakra. The specific body or viewpoint of each chakra thus dictates a specific attitude towards reality: a prime directive.[21] According to the chakra system, therefore, human nature is sevenfold. The first and second chakras, at the base of the spine and gonads respectively, are mostly directed towards receiving and distributing physical energies and combine to give a person potency, vitality and the will to live. The third, fourth and fifth chakras, situated at the solar plexus, heart and throat, are directed towards and concerned primarily with psychological energies and so with personality and intelligence rather than physical traits, although they underpin physical processes in these areas. The sixth and seventh chakras, located between the eyebrows and at the crown of the head are directed towards and concerned with spiritual energies that express the individual's relationship to the universal energy field or spirit of which the soul is part.

The chakras function as an integrated system, rather than in isolation. If one begins to malfunction, so will others, as they attempt to compensate for imbalances in energy transmission. So the chakra system provides the impetus for the regulated, balanced flow of energy throughout the whole person that is necessary for health. The *nadis*, *tsas* and meridians of traditional Indian, Tibetan and Chinese medicine make up the network of channels or pathways by which energy is directed to every part of the mind/body/spirit complex. Traditionally the flow of energy is not confined within the physical body as this is ordinarily conceived. In the ancient view, the body emits a radiant energy that relates specifically to the location and intensity of energy within it, and reveals how it is functioning. This three-dimensional emanation, which surrounds the body in all directions and extends for some distance beyond its surface, is widely referred to as the aura and represents the sum total of the energy emitted by the chakras.

The aura is normally invisible but discernible by seers and clairvoyants, who since the earliest times have described it as a large shimmering oval, comprising a mass of fine bright fibres or rays arranged in seven bands, each corresponding with the functioning of a chakra. Hence, the aura reveals the physical, psychological and spiritual well-being of the person it envelops.

When the chakras are functioning normally, each will 'open' by spinning clockwise and drawing energy from the universal energy field to be distributed throughout the body. When the transmission of energy has occurred, the colour originating from each should be very pale and translucent.

However, when the chakra spins anti-clockwise it remains closed to incoming energies, which consequently are not distributed within the body and appear as darker, denser patches or blotches of colour in the aura. The space between the body and the first colour emanation of the aura is referred to as the *ovum*. It is not 'empty' as such, but it is colourless and so appears to be blank.

- The first layer of the aura, *the health band*, emanates from the first or base chakra and reflects the overall vitality of the physical body. It is traditionally described as red.

- The second layer of the aura, known as *the emotional or astral band*, emanates from the second chakra in the lower abdomen and reflects physical and sexual activity and gut feelings. It is orange in colour.

- The third layer of the aura, *the mental band*, comes from the solar plexus chakra and reflects mental functions based on intellect and personal power. It is yellow.

- The fourth layer of the aura, or *heart band*, emanates from the heart chakra. It is green and reflects inspiration in all forms.

- The fifth layer of the aura, or *causal band*, comes from the throat chakra and is blue. It reflects the karma of the soul — its progress through successive incarnations.

- The dark blue sixth layer, or *spiritual band*, emanates from the chakra in the centre of the forehead and reflects the person's spiritual development and intuitive awareness.

- The seventh layer or *cosmic band* of the aura reflects the soul principle or cosmic consciousness of the individual located in the crown chakra in the centre of the skull. It is purple in colour.

Each band radiates colours of varying intensity that reveal to those who can discern them the state of a person's health, character, emotional disposition and tendencies, abilities, attitudes, past problems and spiritual development. Traditionally those who understood the principles of the aura/chakra system were seers or clairvoyants and sensitives, mystics who could perceive the subtle energies of the human energy field directly and use it as the basis for diagnosis and healing.

Common themes in Eastern traditions of medicine

In the Eastern traditions of medicine, human beings are viewed essentially as dynamic processes rather than material entities, not analysable into separate parts, and closely linked to the environment. Eastern approaches are therefore organic and ecological. Health is characterised as the harmony of fluid movement, as balance, and all approaches to healing treat the whole person, not only the relation of body, mind and spirit but also of this whole to its entire context. Healing is also energetic. All forms of healing are concerned with insightful awareness into universal energies and how these are being utilised for good or ill. They all involve the person in the entire healing process because they emphasise the need for greater attention on the part of the individual to the pattern of life.

Emphasis is laid on direct, immediate experience of the universe through breathing, postural adjustment, ritual movement, dance and meditation. The aims of the healer are to help the person towards a reordering of his or her world-view and the realisation that he or she is in process, rather than static, part of a whole rather than an isolated entity, and to assist him or her in getting in touch with their being and situation through the awareness of internal and external relationships, thereby achieving health, balance and tranquillity. All the ancient traditions of the East have developed subtle techniques to change individuals' awareness of their existence, their relationship to human society and the natural world, and as such they closely resemble contemporary Western psychotherapy.

5

SEEKERS OF THE SOUL

The displacement of religion by science during the nineteenth century and the consequent 'loss of soul' in the West had important implications not only for religion but also for psychology and medicine. Following the end of the First World War there was a flood of books on religious psychology and the growth of popular psychology primarily as a result of the impact of Freudian ideas 'on mind unsettled by war and social change'.[1] The foundations for religious psychology had been laid earlier by Frederick Temple, later Archbishop of Canterbury, who wrote 'We are in need of, and we are being gradually forced into, a theology based on psychology. The transition, I fear, will not be without pain; but nothing can prevent it.'[2]

During the nineteenth century theologians had turned their attention to the neglected fields of mysticism and religious experience, as had anthropologists in their comparative studies of the origins of religion, and early in the twentieth century Evelyn Underhill's book *Mysticism* (1911) was widely read. The psychological study of religion was first systematised in the USA, the most famous work of this kind being William James' *Varieties of Religious Experience* (1902).

Much of the interest in religion within psychology, and vice versa, arose because of the revival of interest in spiritual healing within the Christian Church towards the end of the nineteenth century. The term 'spiritual' lends itself to much confusion and misunderstanding in materialistic Western cultures that are markedly 'a-spiritual'. The term may be taken as referring to the spirit or soul, and interpreted as relating to churches and religions. Accordingly, spiritual healing tends to be attributed to God or gods and is typically invoked by prayer and other rituals. Healing flourishes in all religions and religious movements, including the Christian Church, and in less orthodox movements such as Christian Science, which was developed at the end of the nineteenth century with the aim of reinstating the healing ministry of early Christianity. However:

> Spirit healing is not the prerogative of any religion or race; it is a common heritage of the whole human family. It is extensively practised in the lamaserys of Tibet, and every Mohammedan priest invokes the healing aid for his supplicants. The gift of healing is no more a perquisite of Christianity than any other religion.[3]

Moreover:

> There is not one set of healing laws for the Spiritualist and another for the Methodist or Christian Science practitioner. There are general laws that govern healing, as there are laws that govern every other effect produced in the universe.[4]

In Britain, within the Anglican community, the Guild of Health was established in 1904 to promote spiritual healing and to study the interaction of the spiritual, mental and physical factors in well-being. It became clear that psychological treatment or psychotherapy has much in common with the healing movements within churches. Healing could be considered a religious problem and religions systems of healing for psychological illness. In Britain, the Guild of Pastoral Psychology was established in 1936 to promote cooperation between ministers of religion and psychologists, although individual ministers had been practising pastoral psychology before then. In the same year the City Temple Psychological Clinic was set up with medical collaboration in Leeds by a Methodist minister, and the Catholic Psychological Society was established with a psychiatrist as its president.

However, such cooperation was the exception rather than the rule. Medicine in the West had become secularised and the spiritual components of disease obscured and then dismissed or denigrated. Disease whose origin could not be attributed to the physical body was incorporated into the framework of physical science by converting soul or psyche into mind and then into brain function, or dismissing it altogether.

> The materialistic prejudice explains away the psyche as a merely epiphenomenal by-product of organic processes in the brain. Accordingly any psychic disturbance must be an organic or physical disorder which is undiscoverable only because of the insufficiency of our actual diagnostic means.[5]

Psychopathology, formerly 'sickness of the soul', came to be seen as mental illness and thus fell within the remit of the brain sciences. Accordingly, human problems were treated as if part of medical science and in accordance with its principles. 'Cure of the soul' — psychotherapy — became the responsibility of psychiatrists. Historically, however, some of the roots of psychiatry were anti-ecclesiastical and as a result many psychiatrists had difficulties with the spiritual realm.[6] Indeed within psychiatry spiritual experience was generally viewed as an indication of pathology.

As the concept of soul gave way to that of brain function, doctors, psychiatrists and psychologists rather than ministers of religion became heir to a 'medical ministry'[7] for which they had no special expertise. They were left to reconcile the spiritual or psychological with the materialistic and medical, a task that was increasingly difficult given that intellectually the West was less and less concerned with spiritual and religious convictions. The result was not a convergence of medicine, psychology and religion but an even greater schism. This is evident in the different views of pioneers of modern psychotherapy such as Sigmund Freud, Carl Gustav Jung and Wilhelm Reich.

Sigmund Freud

Freud (1856–1939) is generally regarded as the founder of modern psychotherapy. More properly he can be thought of as the pioneer of psychological medicine because everything embraced in his approach originated in medical science. Freudian psychotherapy 'bears the unmistakable imprint of the physician's consulting room — a fact that is evident not only in its terminology but also its framework of theory'.[8] It is also discernible in its most distinctive feature, the analyst's couch.

Freudian theory and psychotherapy are replete with postulates taken over from natural science. This is unsurprising as Freud was very much a man of his time and like other nineteenth-century physicians, he saw science as the ultimate authority. Freud insistently subscribed to an irreparable split between science and religion.[9] He was a self-proclaimed atheist and enemy of religion, which he viewed as an illusion preventing people from reaching maturity and independence and as a universal obsessional neurosis.[10] He also had a horror of the occult, by which[11] he meant virtually everything that philosophy, religion and the emerging field of parapsychology had contributed to an understanding of the psyche. Freud wished to establish psychotherapy as a scientific discipline fully consistent with the thinking of the time. So he used the basic concepts of nineteenth-century physics in his descriptions of psychological phenomena and subsequently 'made unjustified and mistaken claims to have established psychology on foundations of any other science, such as physics'.[12] In so doing Freud fooled himself and many of his followers, but in the process he developed 'a model of consciousness which dispensed with spiritual aspirations and made them disreputable'.[13] The emergence of a soulless psychology can therefore be attributed in good measure to his influence.

Confusingly, Freud used the German word for soul, *Seele*, when speaking of what was translated in English as 'psychic apparatus', or the person's inner self. Freud interpreted the term 'psyche' as mind. He developed a theory in which mind is conceived like a machine, made up of various components, the *id*, the *ego* and the *superego*, each driven and regulated by various forces whose integrity is maintained by mechanisms that defend it against breakdown — 'defence mechanisms'. The whole system is fuelled by a basic energy or *libido* (literally, to pour) that flows through the psyche and empowers or drives it. Freud equated this with sexual energy and saw it as originating in bodily processes. He thought that changes in the psychic apparatus resulted from movements of energy from one region to another, while actions were accompanied by discharge of energy. Freud held that energy exists in two forms, mobile and bound. He regarded the former as characteristic of unconscious mental processes, chaotic and unstructured, and the latter as structured, organised and characteristic of conscious mental processes. He believed that unconscious (id) impulses, ideas and emotions strive energetically to become conscious but are prevented from doing so by the restraining forces of the ego. Freud conceived of the id as the dark, inaccessible, largely negative and timeless part of the personality. Known primarily through the images of dreams and fantasy the id, according to Freud, is a 'cauldron of seething excitations'[14] instinctual urges and untamed passions, constantly striving to be satisfied. The 'sensible' and reasonable ego tries to control the id, defending conscious awareness from these feelings by various means including repression, denial and projection. At the same time it also tries to meet the demands of the superego, that is, the values and standards internalised by each individual from parents and society as a whole, and to reconcile its demands with those of the id. The ego mediates between the internal and external pressures and strives to unify the processes of the psyche. When this fails neurosis or disorder occurs. The psychotherapist is rather like an engineer who can look into this complex psychic machinery and identify its problems through careful analysis of its workings and, in principle at least, set it working again. Freud termed this process **psychoanalysis**. It was essentially a diagnostic technique, with the therapist trying to find out how the person 'ticks' just as an engineer might with a machine.

Freud thus conceived of the mind as a structure at war with itself, a concept not dissimilar to that found in Indian and Sufi traditions of thought. The latter advocate looking inwards to gain freedom from the bondage of the conscious mind, ego or self. Freud advocated a cleansing of the mind, or catharsis, by looking inwards with the aim of achieving the desirable *ego state*, a balance between the id and the superego. The early stages of this process involve putting a person in touch with the hinterland of his or her mind, in a way conceived in Eastern traditions as meditation or contemplation. As such, Freud's role as a therapist was little different to that of the shaman or holy man. The methods he employed were remarkably similar, involving as they did evocations and interpretations of imagination as revealed in hypnosis, fantasy, word associations, memories and especially dreams, which Freud considered to be of central importance, declaring them 'the royal road to the unconscious'. Insofar as Freudian psychotherapy 'aims at an artificial introversion for the purpose of making conscious the unconscious components of the subject',[15] it can be likened to the practices or yoga, tantra and traditional magic.

Freud would have been horrified by any comparison of his

approach with these practices. Acceptance of psychoanalysis by the medical profession crucially depended on its being consistent with the scientific thinking of the time and Freud was determined to ensure that it was. Although the structures of the psyche Freud described were abstractions and he resisted any attempt to associate them with specific structures and functions of the brain, they nevertheless had all the properties of material objects. As in Newtonian mechanics, these psychological objects were characterised by their extension, position and motion. The dynamic aspect of Freudian psychotherapy, like that of Newtonian physics, consists in describing how the material objects interact with each other through forces essentially different from 'matter'. These forces, the most fundamental of which are the instinctual drives, notably sexual drive or libido — have definite directions and can reinforce or inhibit each other. 'Thus in the Freudian system the mechanisms and machineries of the mind are all driven by forces modelled after classical mechanics.'[16] As in Newtonian mechanics, the Freudian model is rigorously deterministic with every psychological event producing a definite effect and the whole psychological state being uniquely determined by biology and events in early childhood.

In Freud's view, understanding the dynamics of the unconscious mind was essential in the therapeutic process. To Freud, unfulfilled repressed desires, conflicts between the demands of the id and the superego, and the preponderance of various ego 'defence mechanisms' give rise to pathological or neurotic symptoms and may culminate in mental illness. The psychoanalyst concentrates on identifying obstacles to direct expression of primary forces. Psychoanalysis is therefore principally a method of diagnosis, rather than treatment and, to the extent that the analyst can eliminate obstacles to the expression of primary forces, is concerned with symptom alleviation. As such, it reflects the disease model of Western medicine wherein health is the absence of disease or pathological symptoms. Consistent with the Western medical model, the methods of psychoanalysis are cold and impersonal. Freud advised his followers to cultivate the scientific ideal of objectivity and to be as cold as surgeons in their explorations of the mind. He assumed that observation of patients during analysis could take place 'objectively' with minimal interaction between analysts and patients and insisted that there should be no physical interventions of any kind. Freudian psychotherapy thus reflects the mind–body division characteristic of Western medicine and neglects the body just as emphatically as medical treatment neglects the mind.

Psychoanalysis and the soul

It has been claimed that if Freud had been a religious believer he would not have developed his psychology.[17] This claim is contestable. One of his followers in Europe was the German physician Georg Groddeck. He extended Freud's idea that unconscious conflicts can undergo conversion into physical, symbolic symptoms that bind and contain the anxiety of forbidden desires. Whereas Freud's focus had been on 'mental' disorders arising from unconscious conflicts, Groddeck attended to their conversion into physical symptoms. In his *Meaning of Illness*, published in the 1920s, he described a series of cases that highlighted the symbolic meaning of illness. Although his method was psychoanalytic and the symbols he explored tended to be Freudian and sexual, his work went beyond that of Freud. It yielded a number of seminal ideas, notably that illness is not a random occurrence that comes from outside the person; it comes from within and is an existential messenger telling the person to change his or her way of life. In this view, illness is the creation of some inner vital force that can be known only through its effects. This vital force is expressed through symptoms whose aim is to correct some imbalance. He named this vital force the 'IT'.

> Groddeck's IT is nothing more than what is elsewhere called the soul ... Whatever we call it, however we conceive of it, if diseases are to be given symbolic interpretations, some kind of transcendental force must be postulated as the source of the messages that symptoms carry.[18]

Groddeck's ideas literally embody psychosomatic principles in the true sense of conceiving illness as the means by which the soul expresses its conflicts and inner disharmony within the body. As such they were the forerunner of modern psychosomatic medicine. In the 1950s some theorists saw in Groddeck's original insights the possibility of discovering specific dysfunctional personality traits that might manifest symbolically in the body and thereby explain anomalous chronic illnesses that continued to elude the growing mechanistic and pathology-orientated framework of mainstream Western medicine. However, despite meticulous explorations, the attempt to establish the psychogenic origins of disease failed. No specific psychological cause–effect etiologies were discovered. 'Had they heeded Groddeck's warning that there is no universal meaning in a particular symptom or syndrome, they might have guessed that the problem of symbolic meaning could not be easily resolved in a set of consistent personality traits correlated with each disease.'[19]

More fundamentally, however, to delve into the meaning of disease, as Groddeck did:

> ... is to step inevitably into the realm of life's purpose, to question the existence and nature of a higher Self, that somehow is trying to manifest through individuals ... Seen from this perspective, much illness represents a signal that we are off the trajectory of self harmony, or that we as a collective species are off the path of harmony with the greater whole ... In exploring possible meanings of illness and in examining attempts to decode the language of disease, we enter a realm beyond science.[20]

Traditionally this is the realm of the shaman. Groddeck had entered precisely the sphere Freud strove to avoid merely by reframing the basic force of psychoanalysis within the body and giving it a different name. Freud himself joked that psychoanalysis had to await its creation from a Godless Jew and, by dismissing religion, he put psychiatry and religion at odds. Hence evangelicals treated psychoanalysis as a competing and hostile orthodoxy.[21] Freudian psychology, which omits the psyche in the sense of a soul, 'is suited to people who believe they have no spiritual needs or aspirations'[22] and interest in psychoanalysis throughout Europe coincided with the exodus from the Christian Church. A lasting legacy of Freud has been that spirituality has been treated as a taboo by psychology — 'not even the subject of childhood sexuality presented by Freud at the turn of the century met with such resistance.'[23] As a result:

... orthodox Western psychology has dealt very poorly with the spiritual side of man's nature, choosing to ignore its existence or to label it as pathological. Yet much of the agony of our time stems from a spiritual vacuum. Our culture, our psychology, has ruled out man's spiritual nature, but the cost of this attempted suppression is enormous. If we want to find ourselves, our spiritual side, it is imperative for us to look at the psychologies that have dealt with it.[24]

Psychotherapy as soul searching: the psychology of Carl Gustav Jung

During the early years of the twentieth century Freud attracted a substantial following within the medical profession throughout Europe. One of his most influential supporters was the Swiss psychiatrist Carl Gustav Jung, initially a close collaborator. He shared many of Freud's views on the nature of the unconscious mind, the significance of dreams and other imaginative processes, but Jung became increasingly critical of Freud's approach. Progressively Jung viewed Freudian psychology as a one-sided generalisation of features only relevant to neurotic states of mind rather than a psychology of the healthy mind. Jung preferred to look at people in the light of what is healthy, sound and positive rather than in terms of the negativity that he believed coloured everything written by Freud. Jung argued that because of his fear of metaphysics, which prevented him penetrating the sphere of the occult, it was not possible for Freud's theory to reach anything except an essentially negative evaluation of the unconscious.

Contrasts in their approach are evident at many levels but the major difference between them is Jung's espousal of magical and religious traditions. It was Freud's determination to exclude any consideration of them that led to the breakdown of their relationship. Jung considered Freud's denial of all things spiritual absurd and ironic given the similarity of his methods to those of the occult traditions he so despised. Jung insisted that human beings have always and everywhere spontaneously developed religious forms of expression and that those people who cannot see this are blind to human reality. He considered the spiritual and religious dimensions of human beings essential to any system of psychology and he insisted that a religious attitude or outlook was an element in psychic life whose importance could not be denied. He claimed never to have seen a patient over thirty-five years of age whose problems were not the result of failing to find, or having lost, the sense of meaning or purpose in life that religions through the ages have given their followers; and none had really been treated who did not regain this religious outlook. Jung considered that a truly religious attitude presupposes a healthy mind. Therefore all healing is essentially a spiritual problem and religions are systems of treating psychic illness. Accordingly, the central thrust of his psychotherapy can be understood and described as modern man's search for his soul. His philosophy was that the soul does not take much searching out: 'It is only not there where a nearsighted mind seeks it.'[25]

Jungian psychotherapy is therefore essentially a vision quest. Like shamanism, it is a way of healing and a way of salvation. It has curative power and can release psychic disturbances but it can also lead the individual to knowledge and fulfilment of his or her true self. It is a method of medical treatment and self-education, of value to sick and healthy alike.

Jung's central theoretical concern was to map out both the structure and dynamics of the psyche and to understand its totality as it relates to the wider environment. By 'psyche' Jung meant not only what is generally termed the 'soul' but the totality of all psychic processes, conscious as well as unconscious. Hence psyche is something broader and more comprehensive than the soul which Jung regarded as only a certain 'limited functional complex', and defined as a kind of 'inner personality'; the 'subject' to which the ego-consciousness of the individual is related as the same way as to an outward object. This 'inner personality' is the way in which a person behaves in regard to inner psychic processes, the inner attitude or character displayed towards the unconscious, which he also termed *anima*. It contains all those general human qualities the conscious attitude lacks. So, when Jung spoke of the psyche he was referring to the unconscious soul, the intellect (the power of conscious thought and understanding — the rational aspect of the individual) *and* spirit, which comprises both soul and intellect, forming a bond between them that is a formative principle that constitutes the contrary pole to instinctual biological nature, thereby sustaining the continuous tension of opposites on which psychic life is based. Soul, intellect and spirit denote partial systems of the psychic totality.[26] When Jung referred to this totality he always used the terms 'psyche' or 'psychic'. 'For Jung the psyche is no less real than the body. Though it cannot be touched, it can be directly and fully experienced and observed. It is in a world of its own, governed by laws, structured and endowed with its own means of expression.'[27]

Jung conceived of the psyche as a self-regulating system comprising two opposing but complementary spheres, the conscious and unconscious. He did not consider the latter as an individual feature but as collective and common, not only to the whole of humanity but the entire cosmos. This collective unconscious, common to all beings, is the foundation of what the ancients called the 'sympathy of all things'. According to Jung, the structure of the psyche comprises a personal unconscious beneath the conscious mind consisting of ideas, emotions and memories that have been pushed below the threshold of conscious awareness because of the individual's refusal to acknowledge them. These complexes tend to break away from the general unity and become independent or dissociated. Deeper within this level is the collective unconscious that is not individual but universal and whose contents and modes of behaviour are more or less the same for all individuals. Here reside the primordial or archaic energies that Jung termed 'archetypes'. These are patterns of life energy that have become impressed on the psyche during the course of its evolution, thereby reflecting the life experiences of human beings and their predecessors, which are shared by all humanity, past and present. As such these patterns of psychic activity are unconscious and unknowable directly but may be interpreted as images. Comprehensive pictures of the qualitative aspects of these energies are provided by the symbols of visual imagery. These symbols are mediators between different worlds of experience and transformers of energy.

Jung conceived of the dynamics of the psyche in terms of energy or the life force. He adopted Freud's term 'libido' for this psychic energy. In the manner of Hippocrates he viewed it as a play between pairs of complementary features, each opposite in content and energetic intensity. 'I see in all happening the play of opposites, and derive from this conception my idea of psychic energy.'[28] In the total system the quantity of energy is constant and only its distribution variable. Hence Jung's law of conservation of energy and Plato's concept of the soul as 'that which moves itself' are similar. The specific form in which energy manifests in the psyche is the image that is raised up by imagination from the collective unconsciousness. The creative action of the psyche transforms unconscious content into such images and intuitions that appear in visions, dreams and fantasies. So, when normal conscious energy is turned inwards it proceeds to work on the material of the unconscious. When a person concentrates on a mental picture 'it begins to stir, the image becomes enriched by details, it moves and develops ... and so when we concentrate on inner pictures and when we are careful not to interrupt the natural flow of events, our consciousness will produce a series which makes a complete story.'[29] This enables the person to identify and integrate this material into consciousness and so become more whole or healthy.

As according to Jung the unconscious or soul can only be known indirectly through images and symbols encountered in dreams, fantasies and visions, study of these can provide insights into the energies acting deep within the psyche. The energy patterns of the unconscious can be pictured and depicted in various ways, and personified as gods, goddesses, kings, warriors and angels and so on. Archetypal images which recur throughout fairy tales, mythology, magical and mystery traditions are therefore, according to Jung, essentially metaphors for primordial experience. 'The hidden order which surrounds us cannot be perceived by logic alone and we must pass over to the ships of symbolism to ride through the waters of the soul.'[30] Hence symbolism is the traditional language of the mystic, magician and poet.

Jung recognised the reciprocity of mind and the body and the spirit–mind–body unity as a dynamic life process. He also recognised images as the vehicle for perceiving and experiencing this process and that because the energies they picture are active and alive, images are similarly active and alive and can be interacted with. He advocated exploration of these energies by way of a process he termed *active imagination*. He saw this as training for switching off conscious thought, thereby allowing unconscious content to emerge. He regarded this as important because as long as unconscious information is not understood it keeps intruding as symptoms into consciousness. Therefore the overwhelming of consciousness by the unconscious is more likely when the latter is repressed. Clearly, in active imagination it is possible to see similarities with meditation, in content, practice and aim.

From the Jungian perspective, the aim of psychological development is integration or wholeness. The conscious and unconscious have to be worked on simultaneously so that the parts of the self that are neglected or dissociated can be rediscovered and reintegrated. Jung also recognised that as the self has a dual aspect and can be oriented inwardly or outwardly (as in Indian thought), the reality of both these inner and outer worlds have to be reconciled. He conceived of therapy as a journey along a path of personal development towards integration, or perfect health, a process he termed *individuation* and which he acknowledged as an unattainable ideal. Implicitly he drew attention to an important principle: health should not be conceived as a state but as a process of becoming healthy. The conscious attitude accompanying individuation is essentially one of acceptance, of ceasing to do violence to one's own nature by repressing or overdeveloping any particular aspect. Jung described it as 'waiting for God'.[31] In this respect the principle of balance at the centre of all Eastern healing traditions is evident in Jungian psychology, as is the conviction that healing is a spiritual journey and a religious experience.

Jungian psychotherapy is known as *analytical psychology*. Jung described it somewhat paradoxically as both analytical and complex, in contrast with the reductive method of Freudian psychoanalysis. While the latter was concerned only with the identification and exploration of the component elements of the psyche, Jung was concerned with analysing the elements and reshaping the whole.

Jungian therapy essentially comprises various techniques for deliberately mobilising active imagination. This consists of suspending the critical faculty, allowing emotions, fantasies and waking dream images to emerge from the unconscious, and confronting them as though they are objectively present. In this way the person actively interacts with these energies, albeit within the imagination by personifying them as images and entering into discourse with them. It is not merely looking passively at images as though projected on a screen but rather more like a play in which dialogue goes back and forth between the personified image that has been produced spontaneously and the self that produced it. In this way information and understanding can be gained about the dynamics of the psyche. If inner images are merely looked at nothing happens and it is necessary to enter into the process by way of personal interaction, so 'an alert, wakeful confrontation with the contents of the unconscious is ... the very essence of active imagination'.[32] It is also the essence of shamanism.

According to Jung, what the doctor does is less a question of treatment than of developing the creative possibilities latent within the individual, thereby allowing the soul to express itself. Techniques for encouraging these creative possibilities include painting and drawing fantasies and dreams, meditation upon mandalas (designs, usually circular, symbolising the universe in Indian art) poetry, modelling, sculpture and dance. Much emphasis is laid on the interpretation of these imaginary products, not by the therapist as in the Freudian tradition, but by the individual in collaboration with the therapist. Indeed Jung perceived the therapist as a fellow traveller on the journey of self-realisation and redefined the doctor–patient relationship in such a way as to make it more like that between a master and disciple in the Eastern tradition. So, in the Jungian approach, the human quality of the doctor is crucial. Furthermore, in his view, no one can enlighten others while remaining in the dark about themselves, so the first stage in healing is for the physician to heal him or herself, applying to him or herself the system that he or she is prescribing for others.

Jung's therapeutic approach has many parallels with various ancient and oriental traditions that attempt to lead individuals to self-realisation with the common aim of achieving a point of balance or becoming centred. Indeed Jung was profoundly influenced by and drew heavily upon them in both theory and practice. However, there are differences. Active imagination is not programmed but is completely individualistic. The therapist does not take on the role of guide but merely initiates a process, after which the individual undertakes the work alone, becoming independent of the therapist. In this respect, Jung's therapy has parallels with the magical tradition, especially alchemy.

Jungian therapy as magic

Alchemists considered inorganic matter as alive rather than dead and requiring investigation through the establishment of a relationship with it rather than by technical manipulation. Their vision was unity of soul and spirit with matter and they sought to establish this relationship through dreams, meditation and disciplined fantasy (*phantasia in vera phantastica*), a process very similar to Jung's active imagination, which was described symbolically. Jung realised that the alchemists were imagining the symbolic transformation of the psyche and that they had a deep understanding of the process of psychological growth and healing that he called individuation. Indeed to the alchemists transformation and healing were equivalent.

> What the true alchemists were working on in their retorts and crucibles was the contents of their own unconscious which they projected onto the unknown chemistry of matter. The lead which they were converting into gold was the darkness of the unknown inner world which, through the alchemical opus, they transformed into the divine light of the Self, the gold of their divine nature.[33]

Jung therefore devoted much of his life's work to interpreting the alchemical process in the contemporary language of psychology, thereby providing access to the Western magical tradition of inner transformation or healing.

The occultist W.E. Butler considered Jung the greatest magician of the modern age, because, as he pointed out,[34] the aim of the genuine magician is realisation of the true self and thus the truth of the world that is masked by the earthly personality. Certainly the concept of the personality (from the Greek *persona*, meaning mask) as 'a mask of the soul' is central to Jungian psychology. Jungian therapy embodies two of the most central principles of magic expressed in the maxims *gnothi se auton*: know thyself (the inscription over the entrance to the Temple of the Oracle at Delphi in ancient Greece); and *solve et coagula*: dissolve and reform. Like magic, it accesses the subconscious mind or collective unconscious, referred to in magic and by Jung as the 'treasure house of eternal images',[35] through images and symbols. As the psychic energy that evokes the unconscious is reinforced by primordial forces emanating from spaceless and timeless regions deep within it, changes in consciousness are produced. The resurrection of the 'deeper self' results in regeneration and reconstitution of the personal self.

Jung's system involves several methods whereby this resurgence can be effected just as magic involves various forms of training directed towards this end. In magic, symbolic images are chosen and used by the magician to build up the mental atmosphere that will evoke the deep levels of the mind where archaic images and energies reside. These tend to group around definite nuclei or centres, similar to those Jung named archetypes. Evocation of and interaction with archetypal imagery is a feature of Jungian therapy and in this respect Jungian methods most closely resemble those of the shaman. Indeed the collective unconscious described by Jung would appear to be the terrain of the shaman's venture inwards.[36] It is the underworld or the Beyond where the shaman interacts and communes with living energies, personified as human or animal spirits, which, in exactly the same manner as Jungian archetypes, act as guides to the inner world of the self and others. Jungian therapy, therefore, is very clearly within the shamanic tradition of medicine and many of the therapeutic approaches he inspired have pronounced shamanic aspects. However, Jungian methods differ from those of the shaman because Jung did not prescribe images to be contemplated nor guide the process of active imagination and he did not have a monopoly on the interpretation of dreams, as the patient participated fully in this process.

It was Jung's advocacy of both magic and religion that led to the breakdown of his association with Freud. By far the largest number of psychotherapists in Europe in the early twentieth century were disciples of Freud, which, as Jung observed[37] meant that the great majority of patients were necessarily alienated from a spiritual standpoint. However, Jung's influence on the practice and development of psychotherapy during the twentieth century was considerable, especially in Europe. Moreover, influenced by Jung, numerous scholars from various disciplines have further highlighted the links between mythology and consciousness.

Similarities between Jungian psychology and modern physics
Many of the differences between Freudian and Jungian psychology

parallel those between traditional and modern physics and thus between 'classical' mechanistic, reductionist thinking on the one hand and holistic, organic thinking on the other. Whereas the Freudian system is fixed, mechanistic, rigorously deterministic, causal and dogmatic, Jung's psychology is naturalistic, as is reflected in his statement:'if you think along the lines of nature then you think properly.'[38] In his psychology everything is dynamic, subject to change and, like the psyche itself, subject to the Heraclitan principle that 'everything flows'. Just as there are parallels between his views and those of ancient and Eastern magical and mystical traditions which suggest that thinking in non-classical ways enables understanding of dynamical qualities of interrelation and interconnectedness, there are close similarities between Jungian and modern physical views. In modern physics there can be no direct perception of quantum reality, only inference of the existence of waves and particles from their effects, so in Jung's system the unconscious can only be known indirectly through the images of dreams, fantasies and visions. For Jung the psyche is not confined to space and time. He insisted that only ignorance denies this fact, and that the psyche is under no obligation to live in time and space, as dreams and fantasy reveal. Jung's space–time awareness is also apparent in his concept of synchronicity, the acausal connecting principle, according to which all the experiences of humanity and all events are linked through coincidence in time rather than sequentially or causally. He saw a web of relationships throughout the universe, a fundamental unity of all phenomena. In developing his concept of synchronicity[39] he collaborated with Nobel Prize-winning physicist Wolfgang Pauli. He recognised that sooner or later modern physics and psychology would have to draw together because from their different directions they mapped out the same reality, or transcendent territory. He believed that eventually they would arrive at an agreement between physical and psychological concepts and achieve thereby a mind–body, spirit–matter synthesis. Therefore, if 'there is no Einstein of the mind'[40] clearly Jung comes very close to it. Yet his psychological theory was dismissed as 'mere' mysticism rather than science by most psychologists of the twentieth century who were apparently unaware that physical scientists had already moved into precisely that realm.

The psychosomatic therapy of Wilhelm Reich

Another 'visionary' of the early twentieth century was the Austrian psychoanalyst Wilhelm Reich (1897–1957). His attempt to synthesise psychology and physics led to derision and his social humiliation. As a young man he was a follower of Freud and made significant contributions to the development of psychoanalysis, so much so that we was considered a probable successor to Freud as leader of the psychoanalytic movement. However, he became increasingly interested in aspects of human nature that have traditionally been regarded as within the domain of mysticism, and his unorthodox interests and views eventually led to his expulsion from the psychoanalytic school.

All Reich's ideas originated in Freud's theory of psychic energy or libido. Reich proposed that this sexual energy is constantly built up in the body and needs release. This is the function of the orgasm and if this natural reflex is inhibited for any reason, stasis of the energy occurs giving rise to all kinds of neurotic response and ultimately physical symptoms. Release of the blocked energy through re-establishment of orgasm is the aim of Reichian therapy since this is held to establish the natural flow of energy and eliminate neurosis.

For Reich:

> ... [this] life energy is the vitality of our being; when we are moved, this is what moves. Emotions are e-motions; movements out; but they are not just in our minds but in our bodies, in the charge of energy that builds up and with luck discharges; in the flooding of hormones, the surge of bodily fluids and electrical potential, expanding from deep within us towards the surface, or retreating into the caves of the abdomen or flowing through and out via the heads and hands and legs and pelvis, shifting form easily between muscular or electrical tension, fluid, sound, movement, sensation, emotion.[41]

Reich recognised that when energy cannot flow freely in the body it sets up a chronic imbalance in tissues or organs that allows infection or functional disorder to become established. He also realised that organisms not only defend themselves psychologically against emotional trauma, pain and hurt but also physically by contracting various muscles. Emotion that would otherwise be expressed spontaneously is literally held in muscles, so emotional blocks are also physical blockages. He termed this defensive behaviour pattern 'muscle armouring' and observed that if these tensions are maintained over time they become structural components of a person's character. In other words, they characterise individuals. These 'character structures', as Reich termed them, are reflected in posture and in the whole repertoire of behaviour and often set up patterns of dysfunction and disease. Accordingly, emotional and psychological ways of relating to the world are reflected physically in the body, and vice versa, so for Reich character is as much physical as psychological in nature. Reichian *character analysis* was directed towards identifying and eliminating the muscle armouring so that the energy blocked there could be released and physical and psychological functioning could be normalised.

As, for Reich, the person is united in his or her response to various influences, it makes no sense to separate mind and body in treatment. He treated neurotic symptoms in their psychic and somatic manifestations at the same time. In his view appropriate manipulation of the musculature make it impossible to sustain defences against the spontaneous expression of emotion, and releases it. He became convinced that as emotional problems had physical manifestations they could be addressed by way of physical techniques, breathing exercises and massage. He termed his new therapeutic technique 'vegetotherapy'. It involved direct physical contact between him and his patients and as such broke with the Freudian taboo on touching patients. He found that as he relaxed the energy trapped in muscles this would often be accompanied by recall of the trauma that had led to the initial tension or symptom. He also realised that when they are tense people inhibit their oxygen intake and so those with psychological problems tend habitually to breathe shallowly. He therefore instituted breathing exercises as part of therapy and found that as a result many of his patients reported feeling more vital and alive and experienced a oneness with nature, a mystical harmony that some personified as 'God'. This led Reich to believe that he had discovered a biological energy, or *bioenergy*, which pervades the universe and is the active force responsible for the human longing for orgiastic and mystical union with God. Thus in his search for the biological basis of the Freudian concept of libido he claimed to have discovered the life force, which he called *orgone energy*. He envisaged this streaming through universe and sustaining all life forms. So, although Reich condemned mysticism, which he considered as a flight from physical reality, his own vision was truly mystical. As conceived by him, orgone energy was not merely a biological entity but energy endowed with a spiritual quality, since an essential part of the subjective experience of orgasm is longing to reach beyond oneself and merge with that beyond. Reich considered this to be functionally equivalent with love. In his view, love is the life force that quite literally makes the world go round. It is the basic principle of health in all living creatures and its lack is the cause of disease.

Reich's claim that orgone energy, or the life force, is synonymous with breath, and the other claims he made for it parallel those made for the soul in many cultures, including the pre-scientific West. The aims of his therapy are also similar to ancient and oriental traditions, notably *tantra*, which is concerned with raising *Kundalini* energy through ritualised sexual practices. In many respects Reich's ideas resemble those of Buddhism, notably Tibetan Buddhism. His character analysis led him to view character itself as a disorder: a hardening of the fluid human reality into a fixed and limiting pattern of behaviour. He regarded it as both a physical and a mental problem, the body merely expressing the mind's rigidity, developing character armour as a defence against the fearful uncertainty of life and inevitably against feeling. From this perspective the character or self is unhealthy.

In Reich's terms character is determined by different patterns of muscle armouring, conceived as seven rings of tension lying at right angles to the main axis of the body and dividing it into horizontal segments. The location and nature of these patterns is strikingly similar to the chakra system. Indeed an alternative way of construing the principal character structures of Reichian theory is to regard them as primary functional disturbances of the chakras.

There are also similarities between Reich's later work and the practices of shamans. Reich believed that orgone energy could be accumulated and directed to bring about healing. He believed cancer and other disease to be caused by energy blockages. The devitalised tissues, he claimed, begin to degenerate and form T-bacilli that produce cancer. He claimed that orgone energy accumulated in boxes which he designed and developed could be used in the treatment of these disorders. He also believed that energy accumulated in this way could affect natural processes other than healing and claimed to have demonstrated rain-making in this way. In the scientific climate of the time, Reich was viewed at best as attempting to express in scientific terms what mystics through the ages had conveyed in poetry, and at worst as a deluded 'quack'. His opponents represented a powerful lobby who campaigned against the use of his orgone boxes, and because Reich refused to withdraw them from sale he was eventually imprisoned for alleged fraud. He died in prison in 1957 but his ideas did not die with him. On the contrary, they gained an enthusiastic following and his influence on psychotherapy and other healing approaches has since proved to be considerable and under-estimated. Bioenergetic and 'bodywork' therapies, such as *Bioenergetic Analysis* developed by Dr. Alexander Lowen, the *Core Energetics* of Dr. John Piarrakos, David Boadella's *Psychosynthesis*, Gerda Boyeson's *Biodynamic Therapy* and Ida Rolf's *Structural Integration* were all inspired by Reichian principles and practices.

Soul murder — the impact of behaviourism

The hostility towards Reich leading to his incarceration and death in prison needs to be understood in context. In trying to gain acceptance as a bona fide scientific discipline psychology had been trying to distance itself from the 'irrational' aspects of its subject matter since the early years of the twentieth century. Reich and his followers were therefore a source of profound embarrassment. Psychology had reconciled the apparent incompatibility of science and psyche by denying the existence of the latter and conceiving of human beings solely in terms of their objective behaviour. The 'mindless' soulless approach of behaviourism was considered more consistent with the aims and methods of science and it overtook the psychologies of Freud and Jung and subsequently dominated the discipline for the first half of the twentieth century. Psychotherapy was substituted with behaviour therapy that viewed psychological disorders as learned maladaptive behaviour patterns. Its goal was to rectify these and to restore individuals to normal functioning. It was simplistic in approach and also demeaning in the view of human beings it projected because irrespective of whether they are viewed literally or metaphorically as machines the net result is that they are reduced to something less than human. 'Clearly, the very essence of being human is the capacity for subjectivity, for inner living, inner experiencing, and inner intending.'[42] In extinguishing the essence of human beings — the soul, psyche, or self in whatever way these terms had been construed — it had obliterated their humanity. Behaviourism had effectively and without remorse 'murdered the man it claimed to study'.[43]

Insofar as behaviourism had dispossessed psychology of its soul it could indeed be charged with 'soul murder'.[44] As a result, for much of the twentieth century the word 'soul' could not be found in psychological textbooks, general or otherwise, and it had largely disappeared from theological literature. Even in translations of scripture 'psyche' is substituted with other words.[45] However, the word 'self' increasingly featured in psychiatric literature. Under the influence of psychoanalytic theorists, for whom it is of central importance, the self had become the domain of psychiatrists.[46] Although used in the sense of a cluster of functions rather than in any more substantive sense as an underlying principle, the term 'self' carried much of the meaning formerly associated with soul.[47] Arguably, therefore, 'Self in its more functional sense is the modern substitute for soul in its more historic, philosophical and theological sense.'[48]

Self substitutes for soul

However, this shift in emphasis from soul to self has implications other than merely a change of terminology. Fundamentally, it is a shift of attention from the metaphysics of the soul to an analysis of subject. Description of the soul is a totally objective account of the constituents of human nature. It applies universally to all human beings, whatever their state of mind or degree of development may be. 'We have souls whether we are awake or asleep, saints or sinners, geniuses or imbeciles.'[49] On the other hand, analysis of the subject varies according to the level of consciousness of the subject. The study of subject or self attends to operations. It discerns different levels of consciousness, examines the different operations on the several levels and their relationship to one another.[50] Subject and soul are therefore two quite different topics. The study of the soul — traditionally called a metaphysical account — is an attempt to be objective, to get at what is universal. The study of the subject is an enquiry into subjectivity — of oneself as conscious. Hence the terms 'soul' and 'self' imply different perspectives. Whereas the term 'soul' is used when looking at a subject's essence, the use of the term 'self' implies subjectivity — the attempt to see particular experiences from the perspectives of the subject. Both approaches are needed:

> To study soul is to explore human nature. To study self or its subjective experiences may show more about the development of the soul in general.

'It may well be that ... one of the most important nutrients for the soul (its powers and capacities) are certain kinds of relational experiences that enhance certain kinds of self-experiences.'[51] Focus on self is on experience through introspective, phenomenological enquiry.

However, even when distinguished in this way from soul the term 'self' is problematic. It involves two features that are confused and need to be separated. On the one hand, 'self' is utilised to refer to psychological structure, which is an organisation of experience. On the other hand, it is used to refer to an existential agent that is the initiator of action. Within psychoanalytic thinking there has been a move to distinguish these two features as 'self' and 'person'.

> Self is a more delimited and specific term referring to the structure of a person's experience of himself. The self ... is a psychological structure through which self-experience acquires cohesion and continuity, and by virtue of which self-experience assumes its characteristic shape and enduring organisation. We have found it important to distinguish sharply between the concept of self as a psychological structure and the concept of the *person* as an experiencing subject and agent who initiates action. Whereas the self-as-structure falls squarely within the domain of psychoanalytic investigation, the ontology of the person-as-agent, in our view, lies beyond the scope of psychoanalytic enquiry.[52]

It was this issue of personhood that became the focal point of a number of American psychologists in the mid-twentieth century. Refusing to accept the view of man as a machine, they attempted a fully human alternative to the view of man that was prevalent within Western culture and reinstated fundamental questions regarding the nature of the human being and its development as legitimate questions for psychology. What became known as 'humanistic psychology' addressed itself to these concerns. However, it did so without any reference to the soul. Its primary focus was on the self and its actualisation.

Humanistic psychology

There is no one figure around which this effort was organised, but Abraham Maslow (1908–70), a professor of psychology, is generally acknowledged as being of central importance. Maslow challenged psychology for its neglect of the human and attempted a fully humanistic alternative to the mechanistic view of man prevalent in Western thought. He based his psychology on the assumption of an inner human nature, essentially a biological feature that is partly general to the species as a whole and partly individual and unique. He conceived of this inner nature or self as possessing a dynamic for growth and actualisation. Nevertheless, although fundamentally good, this inner nature is weak and easily frustrated, denied or suppressed. He believed that all human problems arose from stifling this true self and that denial or suppression of self was the major cause of illness and distress.

Maslow argued that human beings are more than their behaviour or physical bodies. They also have psychological and spiritual components. Each of these facets of the self has important needs that must be met for the individual to be healthy. The fully healthy person strives to fulfil these needs simultaneously and this culminates in self-actualisation. He considered health equivalent with self-actualisation, that is, the full expression of the self, culminating in transcendent or mystical experiences which he termed 'peak' experiences. This is an ideal state equivalent with perfect health. By contrast, if a person is not in touch with the real self and its needs, he or she will deny these needs and fail to meet them. Ill health, both mental and physical, is the result. The key to healthy functioning is therefore self-awareness — identifying personal needs and acting on them.

Like Freud, Maslow regarded self-denial as the major cause of psychological illness and distress. He claimed that Freud's greatest discovery is that the great cause of much psychological illness is the fear of knowledge of oneself — of emotions, impulses, memories, capacities, potentialities and of one's destiny. He held that this kind of fear is generally a defensive reaction to protect self-esteem and self-respect and that people tend to fear any knowledge that could cause self-dislike or give rise to feelings of inferiority, inadequacy, weakness or shame. In order to avoid such unpleasant truths they employ repression and similar defences. However, in denying the truth of him or herself the person also denies his or her best side, talents, finest impulses, highest potentialities and creativeness. Maslow argued that because of these fears the normal adjustment of the average common-sense person implies a continued rejection of self and the depths of human nature. The person effectively turns their back on themselves because they fear the consequences of doing otherwise. The result of being afraid of one's greatness is that most people are constrained to act in outmoded and ineffective ways. This generates what Maslow referred to as 'the psychopathology of the average' — the normal state of disease. For Maslow therefore what is generally viewed as being normal is unhealthy. He saw conformity to social roles and conventions as the fundamental source of psychological illness.

His psychology echoes that of Jung and ancient and oriental traditions and it found a receptive following during the 1960s in America which was experiencing a cultural reaction against the mechanistic scientific culture of the era. This counter-culture was fuelled by the growing belief that mechanistic, impersonal science would destroy the planet and humankind. Given the Cold War situation existing between the major world powers and the nuclear arms race, it seemed inevitable then that this destruction would come sooner or later. The Russian achievement in forging ahead of the West by putting the Sputnik satellite into space in 1958 merely served to intensify these anxieties. A further stimulus was the Vietnam War. This prompted wholesale reaction against the dominant culture by a great many Americans who saw their young men despatched as merely replaceable cogs in the American war machine to a pointless war from which they would not return or, if they did, they were disabled, traumatised or psychologically destroyed.

Maslow, however, was not opposed to science. He insisted that a truly scientific psychology must embrace a humanistic perspective, treating its subject matter as fully human and accommodating within its realm experience and subjectivity as well as objective behaviour. He therefore conceived of humanistic psychology as a unifying force that would synthesise the disparate fields of behaviourism and psychoanalysis and in so doing would integrate the subjective and objective, private and public aspects of human beings into a complete holistic psychology. Maslow claimed that humanistic psychology represented a 'third force' in psychology. He thereby used to good effect the Kabbalistic concept of the third force or middle pillar, that healthy force, similar to the principle of *Kundalini* in Indian thought, that results from a balancing of all the other forces within the body. He believed that inner human nature could and should be studied objectively through the application of the methods of science, and subjectively by way of psychotherapy.

Person-centred therapy

Although Maslow founded humanistic psychology as a distinctive approach to the study of human subjects and broke new ground in modern psychology, it was left to others to develop the approach in both theory and practice. In this regard Carl Rogers (1902–87) was perhaps its most influential pioneer. He too was a critic of the dominant culture and its mechanistic psychology. He pointed out that common sense and everyday experience indicate that man is more than a machine and that the understanding emerging from the physics of the time undermined the validity of a mechanistic view of the cosmos. He argued that human beings have free will and choice. They are not fixed like a machine but are dynamic, in a continual process of becoming. This theme underpins all his work.

Rogers' personality theory is located within his essentially positive ideology. It focuses on the importance of the true or authentic self. He considered the true nature of man to be benign or at worst neutral and that the aim of life is to actualise, or realise, full expression of this self. However, actualising the self is compromised by the requirements of others and society, and is rarely achieved. It largely remains an ideal, like perfect health, which is a desirable objective, even if its attainment is not possible for most people. Instead, because of the requirements of others and society, a person develops personality, which, in the manner of the Greek concept from which the term derives, builds up in layers and masks the authentic self. According to Rogers a person is healthy to the extent that his or her ideal authentic self and actual self are consistent or congruent. Such a person will feel at ease with herself because there is little or no tension between the true and the false self. Difficulties arise when the ideal and actual selves are incongruent and the person is inauthentic. Then the person does not feel at ease but feels uncomfortable because he or she is not true to the authentic self and because then tension arises between the two selves. This tension generates subjective feelings of anxiety that the person defends against in various ways and this in turn manifests physically in stress and stress-related disorders at both the psychological and physical levels. Conflict between the selves is therefore, in Rogers' terms, the basis of all dis-ease.

Rogers' theory went further than this. Having identified the structural features of the personality he also accounted for its development. He indicated that the authentic true self thrives when it is prized or valued by others. That is, when an individual is valued as him or herself he or she develops a sense of self-worth or self-esteem that promotes the expression of the true self. A child who is loved and valued for him or herself feels no need to compromise him or herself. Whereas a child who is not prized or valued or is not approved of will begin to act in particular ways to gain approval from others. This compromises the true self and the individual's own esteem for that self. Such a person's views tend to be 'if others don't love me, I must be unlovable.' The person thus begins to hide and conceal the true self and to be come inauthentic or unreal, leading to a split within his or her being.

However, the Rogerian self is not fixed or static but able to change and move in the direction of positive growth and development. A person can therefore become his or her true self. Rogers believes that the conditions for change exist within the person but can be facilitated by anyone as long as they provide three conditions: freedom from evaluation, genuine positive regard and empathy or listening. Rogers termed these 'conditions of worth'. In such circumstances, free from negative evaluation, a person has the freedom to explore his or her self and to express it; to perceive the self and its situation; to perceive choices and act on them. The basic principle therefore of Rogerian thinking is a commitment to individual freedom. For Rogers this self-actualisation is synonymous with health, wholeness or integration and he considered his therapy to be a process wherein this can be achieved.

Rogers concept of therapy accords with the origin of the Greek word *therapeia*, meaning attendance or service. Rogers emphasised that attending to a person is not doing anything to or for them but is simply about being. In his view simply being attentive, caring, open and genuine is therapeutic and brings about positive changes that move a person in the direction of wholeness and health. These qualities of being enable others to feel free to be themselves, to explore and express who and what they truly are. In this way the process of therapy is a getting behind the mask of personality — or socially constructed self or ego — to the true self or essence of the person underneath. He saw all human problems as ultimately arising from conflict between this essential or ideal self and the actual self, and the aim of therapy to promote congruence between them so as to heal the schism and bring about wholeness, or health. Rogers' fundamental philosophy can best be expressed by the maxim 'to thine own self be true.'

Rogers' contributions to psychology have been immeasurable. His theories not only underpin psychotherapy and the counselling movement, of which he is considered the founding father, but also humanistic or progressive education. He believed that education should facilitate the emergence and development of the true self and should therefore lead out potentials rather than a force in required facts and knowledge. This emphasis on human potential gave the name to the Human Potential Movement that is synonymous with humanistic psychology.

Gestalt therapy

Rogers' emphasis on self and its actualisation was shared by another highly influential figure, Frederick (Fritz) Perls (1893–1970), an Austrian psychiatrist, originally trained in psychoanalysis. Perls viewed the actualisation of self — the becoming of what one is — as an inborn goal of all human beings, plants and animals, and thus as a fundamental need of all living things. He argued that self-actualisation can only occur through integration of the various parts of the self because it is in this way that the self emerges as a unified figure against its environmental field. Only then, when the self is located in relation to others and the world, does it become possible for the individual to act and more importantly to take responsibility for such action, for this integrated self, like any unified energy field, is more able to utilise its potential. Such a process requires constant monitoring of the self and redefinition of its contact boundaries, because the features of the environment are dynamic and ever changing rather than static and fixed, as the demands of the self, others and external world alter. The satisfaction of these various needs, which is equivalent to psychological health, is something of a balancing act, maintained by a kind of psychological homeostasis, the fundamental requirement of which is awareness of the immediate situation. Hence the aware individual is able to perceive changes in existing self-environment patterns and to act to create new patterns, thereby restoring equilibrium between the self and its surroundings.

Perls attributed much of the difficulty in achieving this balance to society. He saw the problem as residing largely in the prescription of one central, enduring role to the individual who consequently is obliged to suppress, disown or project on to others and the environment all those aspects of the self that are inconsistent with maintenance of that role. This denial of self invariably results in a progressive fragmentation of the person and a difficulty in establishing boundaries between the self, others and the external world.

Perls viewed much psychological disturbance as resulting from this inability to perceive boundaries clearly, with the result that the person experiences the world encroaching upon them. Such a person is characterised by fear, anxiety, avoidance tendencies and elaborate systems of defence all aimed at avoiding this intrusion. Moreover, being unable to define personal boundaries, such a person manipulates the environment in numerous ways rather than utilising his or her personal potential. The person is therefore unable to satisfy his or her needs and remains in a state of psychological disequilibrium that might justifiably be thought of as 'unbalanced'.

The psychotherapy developed by Perls, Gestalt therapy, emphasises the ever-changing nature of all things and the illusory nature of the space–time concepts of Western thinking. Perls insisted that nothing exists or can possibly exist except the here and now and that everything is grounded in awareness of the ongoing process. He acknowledged that in this emphasis he was echoing the pre-Socratic, Heraclitan idea that everything is in flux. He also acknowledged the similarity of his thinking to that of Zen Buddhism, pointing out that the underlying principles of his therapy, and its focus on now and how, is similar to a Zen *koan*. His therapy aims to promote insight and thus integration, through focus on this *koan*. However, unlike Zen Buddhism, psychotherapy does not deal with people like Zen monks who in the pursuit of truth have made many sacrifices. Perls recognised this and he used many different methods by which integration might be achieved. In this respect his therapy is like Tibetan Buddhism, which employs strategies such as bodywork and visualisation. Perls believed that individuals could assimilate projected and disowned features of the self by role-playing, and many of the methods he used, with the aim of heightening perception, awareness and emotion, were of an essentially theatrical nature. In this respect Gestalt therapy is reminiscent of Greek theatre. Working with his clients 'centre stage' as it were, in front of an audience, Perls required them to play all the parts of the drama themselves, either by acting each role (including the 'props') in turn, or in the form of dialogues between these elements, whether animate or inanimate. For this purpose he developed his famous 'empty chair' method in which a person projects into a vacant chair any element of the drama in order to confront it. The 'occupant' of the chair might be an aspect of the self typically unexpressed in a given situation. It may be the repressed self or other aspects of the personality; real or imagined persons; creatures or objects; in fact, anything that the client or therapist wishes it to be. By bringing these features into the open and confronting them in this way, the person may be able to identify and integrate the diffuse parts of the self, distinguish them from other features of the environment and thus achieve a clear figure/ground discrimination or individual gestalt. In this way, Perls worked with clients on their unresolved conflicts, interpersonal relationships, thoughts and fantasies. He also used this method in working with dreams, which he regarded as 'existential messengers' because of their potential importance to individual self-awareness.

In his emphasis on dreams and his use of theatre and humour, Perls reflects not only the practices of the ancient Greeks but also shamanic practices in general. His approach also has much in common with Zen Buddhism and other oriental traditions. Like these traditions it is anti-intellectual in focusing on experiencing life rather than trying to understand it.

The psychological approach of Maslow, Rogers and Perls was very much in accord with the *Zeitgeist* of the 1960s and 1970s. The counter culture at the time did not merely involve protest against science and technology but also represented an active search for new meanings and answers in an era where traditional sources of authority such as religion had become obsolete. In its emphasis on human experience and subjectivity, and issues such as consciousness, emotion, values, personal freedom and responsibility, humanistic psychology could be said to reflect the popular psychology of the time. Its concerns were precisely those that Western psychology had so successfully avoided for the greater part of the twentieth century. Hence, its development was rapid. It thrived because in the cultivation of intellectual skills in the West, there had been an almost total neglect of teaching regarding the personal, personal experience and self-knowledge. Its popularity can therefore be seen as a critique of contemporary education in the West.

Psychotherapy as religion
In the wake of Maslow, Rogers and Perls, numerous 'self theorists' emerged in psychology and psychotherapies proliferated all with the aim of enabling people to find their true selves. There was a dramatic increase in the number of psychotherapies available and those who sought them. Recognition of the self as a modern substitute for soul, prompted redefinition of psychotherapy as 'the religion of the formally irreligious'.[53] This view of psychotherapy as, in many cases, *ersatz* religion is inconsistent with the institution of medical psychiatry. Nevertheless, many forms of psychotherapy were being developed and proclaimed with religious-like fervour and the validity of some, rather like belief in God, was an article of faith.

However, despite its perceived quasi-religious status, humanistic psychology does not address itself to spiritual issues as such. While for Maslow the capacity for mystical or 'peak experiences' was the defining quality of self-actualisation and evidence of man's ability to transcend present personal experience to some ultimate experience or reality, other pioneers of humanistic psychology ignored this dimension of subjective experience and effectively stripped self-actualisation of its spiritual component. Rogers neglected spiritual issues almost entirely in developing his person-centred approach, which was an oversight he admitted and regretted at the end of his life. It is not the case, therefore, as has been claimed,[54] that Rogers reminded psychologists of what it means to be a complete human being. His psychology remained incomplete. However, although not stated explicitly, it is difficult to avoid the conclusion that Rogers' authentic or true self, inner human nature, is other than the soul, and Rogers' concept of disease a consequence of conflict between the soul and the self. Viewed in this way his psychotherapy, in striving to heal the schism or incongruence between the two, is truly psychotherapy in the ancient sense of curing the soul. Moreover, the fundamental quality of being he advocated in therapists can be likened to that striven for in many spiritual disciplines such as *zazen* meditation.[55]

> This state, in which nothing definite is thought, planned, striven for, desired, or expected, which aims in no particular direction and yet knows itself capable alike of the possible and the impossible, so unswerving in its power — this state, which is at the bottom purposeless and egoless, was called by the master truly 'spiritual'. It is in fact charged with spiritual awareness and is therefore called 'right presence of mind'. This means that the mind or spirit is present everywhere because it is nowhere attached to any particular place. And it can remain present because, even when related to this or that object, it does not cling to it by reflection and thus lose its original mobility. Like water filling a pond, which is always ready to flow off again, it can work its inexhaustive power because it is free, and be open to everything because it is empty. This state is essentially a primordial state.[56]

Equally, while Zen-like principles are evident in the process of Gestalt therapy and were acknowledged as such by Perls, it is not directed to the soul. Nevertheless, in conceiving of the actualised self as an integrated force field enabling action, he was claiming functions traditionally attributed to the soul, and many of the methods he used in Gestalt therapy, such as drama, comedy, and role-play, were those traditionally used in healing the soul.

Similarities between humanistic psychology and Eastern psychologies

There are similarities between humanistic approaches and those of the Eastern psychologies, notably in the nature of the encounter between the therapist and the individual which, in the mutuality of the transaction, is more like that between master and disciple than that between doctor and patient or psychologist and client. There are also many similarities in the process, in the principles of insight and awareness facilitated and the methods used to achieve this such as focused attention and imagination.

To the extent that humanistic psychotherapy has principles and practices in common with Eastern traditions it can be considered religious. Buddhism, Taoism and Hinduism are characterised by their human attitude and have been identified as 'humanistic' religions in contrast to those, largely Western, religions with an authoritarian emphasis. The concerns of humanistic religion centre around innate human potential for transcendence for, insofar as they are theistic, God is viewed not as other or external but as residing within the individual. The person is therefore a manifestation of God and emphasis is upon the person realising his or her own nature, godliness or godhead. God is viewed as a symbol of human powers that the individual should strive to realise in life, not as a symbol of force and domination. The aim of such religion is to achieve the greatest strength, not the greatest powerlessness. Virtue is self-realisation, not obedience; faith is conviction based on personal experience rather than the propositions or dogma of others; and the prevailing mood is joy, rather than sorrow or guilt.

Humanistic psychotherapy clearly shares the themes and character of Eastern traditions. These elements resonated with other features of the 1960s and 70s when widespread experience with drugs and other consciousness-expanding methods such as meditation and yoga fostered interest in altered states of consciousness and transcendent experiences. There was growing fascination with the spiritual traditions of other cultures, especially the East. Ancient texts, such as the *Bhagavad Gita* were translated into English and astonishingly the

Bardo Thodol or *Tibetan Book of the Dead* and the *I Ching* became best-sellers in the United States. As more and more books presenting alternative and unfamiliar views of human nature and existence found their way on to the bookshelves, the practice of alternative disciplines flourished as more and more people explored Buddhism, Zen, Sufism, Yoga and various forms of meditation. By the mid-seventies five million Americans practised yoga and six million meditated regularly.[57] It became clear that the self-actualisation concept at the core of humanistic psychology was too limited and needed expanding to accommodate extraordinary and transcendent capacities. However, despite its apparent openness to experience of all kinds, there remained:

> ... a not-so-subtle resistance to incorporating certain approaches to the understanding of human life and human existence into the humanistic framework, that is, approaches that integrate aspects of ourselves that do not seem part of the more day-to-day conceptual, emotional, and languaged realities — the so-called transpersonal and/or spiritual dimensions.[58]

Certainly, humanistic psychology does not integrate understanding of human life and existence with the insights provided by quantum physics. The unbroken wholeness it describes points to loss of individuality of its constituent parts and this has a bearing on the question of personal identity at the core of humanistic psychology. Essentially, humanistic psychology rests on a model of the person as an individual that exists in isolation. In the light of the new physics such a model can be considered conceptually limited. Opponents of the counter culture also challenged the ideology of humanistic psychology, claiming that the fundamentally narcissistic model that follows from a psychology of the person produces an undesirably 'self-centred' culture. It was recognised that 'if we want to grow beyond that model we have to grow beyond the psychology on which it is based.'[59]

Furthermore, by the late 1970s the concept of self was being challenged within psychology. Definitions of and views about the self in psychological literature are many, various and problematic. It may be conceived as integral and continuous, multiple, changing and discontinuous, or integral and continuous, yet changing.[60] While over many decades 'self' theorists debated the nature of this entity, the emerging view within psychology was that there is no such entity, no self, no inherent human nature, because what is considered the self is socially constructed. The social constructionist view is that 'there is no universal transhistorical self, only local selves; no universal theory about the self, only local theories.'[61] The study of the self therefore cannot reveal self, only various cultural reflections of it. The conclusion of postmodern psychologists is that there is no single, separate, unified self, no universal human nature or abiding individual identity. There is no central personality in relation to which all varied behaviours might be seen as 'sides', aspects or features. 'We are, in other words, not absolutely anything.'[62] Accordingly, the subjectivity so avidly pursued by humanistic psychologists seems to lack a substantive self: 'something that would be a subject for the subjectivity, something that endures, but changes, something that exists, but is larger, more underlying ... than the psychological functions of id, ego, superego, or the psychological representations of self or other'.[63] Thus it seemed that psychologists were struggling to find the soul again.

This much had been anticipated by Maslow who in 1968 had written:

> I consider Humanistic, Third Force Psychology to be transitional, a preparation for a still 'higher' Fourth Psychology, transpersonal, transhuman, centred in the cosmos rather than in human needs and interest, going beyond humanness, identity, self-actualization, and the like ... These new developments may very well offer a tangible, usable, effective satisfaction of the 'frustrated idealism' of many quietly desperate people, especially young people. These psychologies give promise of developing into the life-philosophy, the religion-surrogate, the value-system, the life program that these people have been missing.[64]

Transpersonal psychology

It had been Maslow's hope that studies of peak experiences in which the person achieves a sense of heightened mental clarity and understanding, intense euphoria and an appreciation of the holistic, unitive, integrated nature of the universe and one's unity with it, would ultimately help to establish a truly scientific basis for spirituality.[65] He believed that human beings could live fairly consistently at this higher level of awareness and 'be on easy terms with the eternal and the infinite'. Although Maslow laid the foundations for a psychology that went beyond (*trans*) the personal, ego or self and considered spiritual development and experiences, the origins of transpersonal psychology are ancient. Vedanta, Yoga, Buddhism, Sufism, Taoism, Kabbalism, Native American traditions and Christian mysticism are all transpersonal in orientation and have spanned millennia. However, within psychology the term 'transpersonal' was first used by Carl Jung in 1917 as a synonym for the collective unconscious. Since then the term has been used in many different ways and has encompassed many themes. These have been synthesised into a definition of transpersonal psychology as 'the study of humanity's highest potential, and with the recognition, understanding and realization of unitive, spiritual and transcendent states of consciousness'.[66] Transpersonal psychology is concerned with scientific study of becoming, needs, ultimate values, unitive consciousness, peak experiences, ecstasy, mystical experiences, awe, bliss, wonder, ultimate meaning, transcendence, spiritual oneness, and cosmic awareness; that is, with the expansion of self-identity beyond the boundaries of ego, name and form.

> The history of Western psychology can be appreciated in the changes that have occurred in its directional focus. In this regard, psychoanalysis looks back, behaviourism looks at, humanism, looks forward and transpersonal psychology looks inwards (and thus beyond one's boundaries).[67]

Underpinning transpersonal psychology is the recognition that the universe has been known for millennia by deeply conscious human beings. These exceptional individuals have described all phenomena as creative illusory expressions of a primary unified field of pure consciousness that is held to be the fundamental source of all that exists in the phenomenal world, including human experience. They have claimed that humans can reach an awakened state of unity consciousness where the traditional concepts of space, time, isolated objects and cause and effect lose their meaning. The fundamental descriptions of reality passed down over thousands of years, most notably in the psychological traditions of the East, are strikingly similar to those provided by modern Western physicists and those that have emerged from explorations of consciousness. Transpersonal psychology reiterates the ancient and mystical view that there is more to being human than individual ego identity and personal awareness. It points to an extensive literature, ancient and modern that affirms the existence of human experience beyond the level of personal self awareness, experience in which identity is not confined to the individual mind or limited to the sense of self.

> Transpersonal psychology therefore calls us through and beyond our more familiar level of ego awareness to a critical examination of the very ground from which our behaviours, thoughts and emotions emerge as forms or manifestations. This shared reality has been conceptualised in many ways; philosophers and psychologists have spoken of unity, intuition, oneness, noumenal reality, collective unconscious, spiritual presence, mystic union, archetypal awareness.[68]

Transpersonal psychology holds that individuals can release themselves from the illusory restrictions imposed by the physical world and achieve a psychological state that recognises the universal consciousness underlying all of creation. In this state, the individual realises the true source of his or her identity and is freed of the boundaries and limitations of time, space and causality. It shares with the ancient traditions a commitment to turning inward towards one's deeper nature and this represents an involution or unfolding process that uncovers one's true source of being and the underlying unity of all existence.

Transpersonal psychotherapy 'makes that ancient wisdom concretely available to any who care to use it'.[69] Its aim is enlightenment, freedom, liberation, what is termed 'salvation' by Christians, *nirvana* by Buddhists and *samadhi* by Hindus. This is achieved by promoting transcendence of the conscious mind, enabling it to explore the unconscious and reveal a deeper (transpersonal) level of being referred to as the higher self, true or inner self, which is synonymous with the soul. The individual therefore has the possibility of going beyond personality and being in touch with the soul. A basic assumption of the transpersonal approach is that this deeper level cannot be encountered by intellectual analysis alone and so the interventions of therapists are less intellectual and more experiential than many other approaches.

Transpersonal psychotherapy is a process of awakening from a lesser to a greater identity.

> In transpersonal therapy, healing involves the realization of a greater identity that comes to light when we relinquish our unquestioned conceptions of self and world ... these conceptions of identity are the constructs of consciousness. According to the perennial philosophy, these constructs are not our true identity.[70]

Transpersonal psychotherapy has been likened[71] to a method of spiritual practice taught by one of India's greatest saints, Ramana Maharshi, to help his disciples realise the deep centre of their being. This involves meditation on the question 'Who am I?' and rejecting every answer provided by the discursive mind so as to probe deeper into the self. This takes the individual beyond the ego and socially adapted levels to more authentic layers of transpersonal being. The principle involved here is identical to that underlying transpersonal psychotherapy: by progressively relinquishing identification with ego the person can progress through the levels of the self and eventually transcend to true identity, the origin and source of all experience. The process is like peeling off the layers of an onion, letting go of all self-definitions and patterns of living that are impeding enhanced self-awareness and the emergence of a greater identity.

Important in this process is the crisis of awakening that occurs when the old identity gradually unravels and falls apart, and nothing appears immediately to replace it, resulting in feelings of anxiety, emptiness, darkness and chaos. This process, which has been described[72-4] as a crisis of death and rebirth, is comparable to the 'dark night of the soul' first described by the mystic St. John of the Cross. Just as this is recognised as a normal and important stage of the journey of spiritual development, in transpersonal psychotherapy a 'dark night' is considered a natural rite of passage inherent in psychotherapeutic change as a person awakens to any new identity. It is therefore a healing crisis rather than a pathological one.

In transpersonal psychotherapy, the therapist's role is to trust the psyche's natural healing process and to be supportive and accepting of the person throughout. The therapist has to have faith in the person's ability to give birth to a new identity, recognising that 'the inward experience of darkness, emptiness and death, this very void, is in actuality the womb out of which their greater identity ... eventually can be born.'[75]

Transpersonal psychologists recognise that the self often begins unfolding through images, dreams, fantasies and visions as these are the primary ways in which the soul expresses itself. Therapists facilitate this process by way of meditation, contemplative intuition, yoga, biofeedback, breathing techniques, inward focusing, visualisation, dreamwork and guided imagery. For transpersonal psychologists the truth lies within and any means to expand inner awareness can be included. They may therefore also use interventions including bodywork techniques, isolation and flotation tanks, journal keeping, hypnosis, prayer, chanting, drumming, movement therapy and energetic techniques. The work of transpersonal therapists is based on the idea that body, mind and spirit function as a harmonious unit and so their approach is holistic. They take into account all aspects of lifestyle, such as sleep patterns, diet, exercise, nutrition, leisure activities, body postures, movement and work.

Transpersonal psychology is thus an attempt to bring together the ideas of different eras, cultures and traditions into the framework, language and practice of modern psychology and to restore the 'soul' as the central focus of psychology. This is evident in the approach of influential contributors Roberto Assagioli and James Hillman.

Restoring the soul to psychology
The psychoanalytically trained Italian psychiatrist Roberto Assagioli viewed the unconscious mind as a source of wisdom and healing potential and he believed that people should be sufficiently in touch with the deep forces within their psyche to be able to use them, rather than be used by them. He conceived of symbols as 'containers' of meaning and therefore as transformers and conductors, or channels of

psychic energies, and used guided imagery, daydreams or symbols as a means of allowing his patients to mediate between conscious and unconscious material themselves. He viewed health as wholeness, requiring the integration of imagination, intuition and inspiration with rational, conscious processes. It is a psychosynthesis, bringing together different modes of consciousness. He developed a system of therapy bearing this name that draws heavily on the practices of oriental mysticism, using meditational and mystical techniques in the development of imagination and intuition, with the aim of integrating all aspects of the self.

Although influenced by Jung, Assagioli went further and distinguished between the collective unconscious and what he termed the higher or transpersonal self. Whereas the former can be considered as below or beneath consciousness, the latter can be conceived as above it, in a manner analogous to the underworld and the heavens of the shaman. The underworld of the collective unconscious is essentially the domain of the archetypal energies that may be differentiated and represented symbolically or imaginatively as gods or guides in various forms, whereas the heavens occupy an undifferentiated frequency domain beyond such conceptualisation which can only be experienced directly. Assagioli considered that psychoanalysis was unjustified in limiting its explorations to the 'underworld' of the unconscious and that the regions of middle and higher consciousness should likewise be explored.

A similar distinction between the world of spirits and the world of spirit is frequently encountered in religious and mystical traditions, notably those of the East that strive towards union with and direct experience of the Ultimate Reality or universal mind. These traditions emphasise that true seeing or direct perception of reality involves 'pure' consciousness, a nothingness or emptiness variously referred to as Brahman, the universal Tao and in Buddhism 'the clear light of the void', or undifferentiated uncoloured light that is encountered by looking inwards to the centre of one's being. These traditions all assert that this realm of consciousness is beyond all forms and appearances, even though all forms and appearances derive from it. Meditation or concentration on images and symbols is therefore a means to this end, which ultimately must be transcended. By differentiating the primitive, archaic contents of the collective unconscious from the 'superconscious', Assagioli was able to make subtle distinctions between the various kinds of psychic experience in a manner more fully consistent with ancient and oriental traditions, embracing mysticism and spirituality even more forcefully than Jung.

Since the 1970s James Hillman has been 're-visioning' psychology by calling for the return of the soul, which he considered its proper subject matter. He does not limit the soul to the individual or humanity but extends it to nature and the world at large. For Hillman each thing has a spark of soul at its core, and the idea that only people have souls alienates humankind from any encounter with the world. For Hillman psychology cannot be considered as a separate science; it must be concerned with the soul as this is at the core of all meaning. Psychology must therefore be considered a foundational, even a supreme, discipline because the psyche is prior to and must appear within every human undertaking. For Hillman, the ultimate aim of psychology is not to find answers and solutions to problems but to deepen experience of the problems themselves because the purpose of these eternal psychological problems is to provide the base to soul-making. This is because the soul that lies hidden behind human routines is most likely to emerge in chaotic pathological moments when beliefs, values and security begin to disintegrate. It is then that the essential and fullest view of the soul is possible.[76] The ultimate value of psychology therefore lies in deepening the meaning of the soul in a general sense. He considers psychotherapy to be fundamentally about soul-making. It constitutes a deep caring, love and appreciation of the soul and what it represents. 'In its widest sense it is the *anima mundi* that beckons us to regard it therapeutically in all of its manifestations.'[77] Accordingly psychotherapy must be practised on the world at large, not only on individuals. It should by concerned with healing the world. More specifically it is the 'imaginative possibility of our nature', a possibility that is realised primarily in dream, image and fantasy. These are the bearers of soul that is, for Hillman, synonymous with the unconscious.

The aim of therapy is soulfulness, leading the individual deeper into the unconscious. In this regard Hillman views psychopathology as the most valuable ally, as the primary vehicle through which soul-making is achieved. It is the royal road to deepening the soul because pathology is likely to exhibit the most salient structures of the unconscious. Accordingly pathological symptoms are the gateway to the soul. They are 'the first herald of an awakening psyche'.[78] By leading people into a dark night of the soul, psychopathology destroys their assumptions about themselves and the world and leads them back into the original chaos from which all passion, creativity and renewal are born.

The most comprehensive transpersonal theory to emerge in the twentieth century was advanced by Ken Wilber.[79] His theory unifies numerous approaches into a spectrum of psychological models and theories that reflects the range of human consciousness from the narrow focus of the individual ego or mind to that of cosmic consciousness, which Wilber terms 'Mind'. Wilber's spectrum psychology traces the development of personal identity through several levels of consciousness. It commences with the *ego level* at which the personal self, ego or mind is identified, and progresses in fine gradations through stages of *social awareness*, in which social and cultural influences are identified; *existential awareness* or self-awareness, in which dualism of mind and body, self and other are resolved; *transpersonal awareness* of the connectedness of the cosmos as a whole; and finally, the level of *Mind*, the mystical state of transcendence, where all dualities are resolved and all individuality merges into universal, undifferentiated oneness. As such it parallels human spiritual development as depicted by mystics and Eastern sages and the historical development of Western psychology. It draws together the traditional focus of concern of Eastern and Western cultures and their respective psychologies — mind and Mind, of which the former is but a part — in such a way that what were previously thought of as polar opposites can now be seen as aspects of one consciousness.

Within the framework set out by Wilber the stages of development addressed by Western psychology are identifiable as lower levels of consciousness. His model elucidates their relationship to higher mental states, including the psychic dimension relating to 'psi' phenomena, the powers of yogis and the highest spiritual states known as *samadhi* and *nirvana* in Hinduism and Buddhism respectively and *satori* in Zen. However, mainstream psychology still does not recognise this work and fails to understand the relationship of these higher states of consciousness to the 'normal' and 'abnormal' mental states with which it most frequently deals. It has difficulty integrating the information and techniques, which it is slowly learning, from such diverse fields as acupuncture and *Hatha* yoga, which deal with a subtle energy relatively unexplored by Western science but understood by yogis to be very much related to the evolution of higher states of consciousness.

> Our concepts aren't fundamental enough, for instance, to allow for a clear understanding of the interrelationships between the subtle energy flow of acupuncture and that of Western bioenergetics, or between the breath control exercises, body postures and moral and devotional practices of Eastern yoga and the mentally-oriented talk therapies of psychiatry. A deeper appreciation of spirituality would bring valuable understanding here.[80]

It can be argued that since the loss of the soul in the nineteenth century, Western civilisation has been progressing through its own dark night. With the demise of organised religions those persons who find themselves on the tortuous path of spiritual unfoldment often lack much-needed illumination and guidance. In the not-too-distant past many of them would have gained succour in the monastic life and within churches. Today they are, for the most part, obliged to undergo their spiritual journeys in the world at large and, for many, therapists have become their principal allies in the struggle for composure and peace of mind. It is to them that they turn in the hope of achieving enlightenment and the modern equivalent of salvation — mental health.[81] In acknowledging the spiritual dimensions of their problems, many people are admitting the soul in previously unthought ways. It is significant that there has been a return of soul in recent popular literature, suggesting some renewed interest in notions of soul and soul care in the West.

Although previously virtually non-existent within psychology, 'in the last few years, there has been a burgeoning use of the term soul in the title of articles, books, and presentations, but virtually no definition nor discussion of the term's meaning. Certainly in the recent history of psychological literature pertaining to the self, one is struck with the synonymous use of self and soul.'[82] Thus it would seem that the transition from soul to self may be undergoing a reversal, and that the soul may be becoming a more acceptable term.

> Today we are beginning to emerge from what is, in the long view, a relatively brief interregnum of radical positivism and its consort, psychological behaviourism. The emergence is certainly far from complete, and many academic citadels are still occupied by those who doggedly seek to produce a science in the model of an earlier century's notion of physics. Still the recognition that this is a truncated and distorting perspective is gaining ground steadily.[83]

Indeed, contemporary science is not only adding credence to the concept of the soul but it is providing descriptions of the soul and its functions that are remarkably similar to those passed down throughout history from ancient times.

6

SCIENTISTS OF THE SOUL

The insubstantial soul

According to ancient wisdom, the human soul is a tenuous, material substance; a subtle 'etheric' body that interpenetrates the dense physical body.

> The dense and etheric bodies are not normally separated during earth life; they normally function together, as the lower and higher strings of a single instrument when a chord is struck, but they also carry on separate though coordinated activities.[1]

Historically and biblically, Christianity, which until the nineteenth century underpinned scientific thinking in the Western world, also held a dualist notion of the human being as a unity of two distinct entities — body and soul. According to this view, the soul is a substantial unified reality that informs and causally interacts with its body and contains various mental states within it such as sensations, thoughts, beliefs, desires and acts of will. It survives death of the physical body, existing in an intermediate disembodied state upon death, before being reunited with a resurrected body.[2] This idea of the soul as 'thing-like', consisting of some tangible basic matter, substance or 'stuff', continued throughout history and survived into the early scientific era where it became problematic.

> What stuff is the soul made of? The question is as meaningless as asking what stuff citizenship or Wednesdays are made of. The soul is a holistic concept. It is not made of stuff at all.
>
> Where is the soul located? Nowhere. To talk of the soul as in a place is as misconceived as trying to locate the number seven, or Beethoven's fifth symphony. Such concepts are not in space at all.[3]

Accordingly, the soul was distinguished from body as 'immaterial' substance — as 'un-thinglike'- composed not of matter but 'mind stuff' such as thinking. The soul's insubstantial quality seemed to be necessary because the physical presence of souls is not generally seen or detected in any direct way, nor revealed during surgery. Nor does it comply with the deterministic and mechanical laws of physics as they apply to the world, and as most people understand them.[4] The insubstantial soul became an abstract notion, a concept that from a materialistic perspective 'is at best wrong and at worst incoherent'.[5] As such it was progressively dismissed as illusory and unreal.

However, abstract concepts, while not substantial, are not necessarily unreal or illusory. Nationality, ethnicity or religious affiliation cannot be weighed or measured, do not have a location inside a person's body, and yet they are meaningful and important, as anyone unfortunate enough to be persecuted because of them knows only too well. Abstract concepts such as Mondays, voices, haircuts and holes, do not involve 'things' in the sense of objects but relationships between and conditions of objects. However:

> Part of the reason that the self came to replace the soul as the proper subject of psychological study is the pervasive confusion surrounding what it means to say that the soul is an immaterial substance ... It is the loss of the idea of substance and its correct conceptualization that is the main culprit in this transition.[6]

In thinking about the human person the notion of a substantive soul was replaced by the concept of a structure or a system that is defined by its functions. The self is such a construct. In psychoanalytic thinking, for example, the self is seen as a form of psychic structure defined by its functions and so in the twentieth century the substantive soul was replaced by the idea of the self as a cluster of functions. At a stroke, functionalism solved most of the traditional problems associated with the soul simply by eliminating it. In the absence of the soul psychologists studied the nature, development and functioning of the self.[7]

Insubstantial science
Paradoxically, however, the discoveries of physicists during the

twentieth century led them to describe the universe in abstract rather than material terms. They revealed its substrate not as matter but as phenomena requiring explanations in terms of concepts like energy and immaterial, invisible, organising principles, or *fields*. The non-material nature of the universe — quantum reality — that was uncovered revealed the insubstantiality of substance. By describing the quantum vacuum as the underlying reality of all that is, physicists were restating the ancient view of reality as a living void comprising nothing but movement or dynamic patterns of activity. This principle of movement or energy is the vital force or life principle synonymous throughout history with the soul. It is the *anima mundi*, essence or soul of the universe; and at one and the same time the soul of the individual. Implicitly, therefore physicists reinstated the soul to the very centre of scientific concern. Moreover, their explorations of the quantum realm led them to redefine the 'stuff' of the universe as more like 'mind stuff', or consciousness. The quantum description of reality, proven experimentally to be the most accurate scientific description of the physical universe currently available, demands that it be considered one whole, indivisible and *conscious* entity. Indeed, it prompts the conclusion that the universe *is* consciousness.

> Essentially, the raw material of the universe is non-material. The 'stuff' of the universe is 'non-stuff', but it is not just non-stuff; it's thinking non-stuff.[8]

Physicist David Bohm[9] highlighted the striking similarity between consciousness and quantum processes and suggested that fundamentally they are essentially different aspects of the one overall order and may be understood in terms of the implicate order. Indeed, the idea that the mind and body are separately existent but connected by some sort of interaction is incompatible with the implicate order, according to which mind enfolds matter in general and therefore the body in particular, and similarly the body enfolds not only the mind, but in some sense, also the entire material universe.[10]

> So we are led to propose further that the most comprehensive, deeper and more inward actuality is neither mind nor body but rather a yet higher-dimensional actuality, which is their common ground and which is of a nature beyond both. Each of these is

only a relatively independent sub-totality which is the common ground and which is of a nature beyond both . . . and in which mind and body are ultimately one (rather as we find that the relative independence of the manifest order derives from the ground of the implicate order).[11]

This understanding is also found in Carl Jung's idea that psychic and physical energy are two aspects of one and the same reality, the world of matter appearing as a mirror image of the world of the psyche, and vice versa. He designated energy as physical when it is physically measurable, and as psychic when it becomes psychically or introspectively perceptible. Accordingly, 'the psyche should be capable of appearing in the form of mass in motion, and insofar as psychological interaction takes place, matter should possess a latent psychic aspect.'[12] A similar idea is found in Ayurveda: when the self interacts with itself subjectively it experiences mind and when it interacts with itself objectively it experiences body.[13]

As, according to Bohm, both mind and body are projections in a subtotality of a yet higher 'dimension', it is ultimately misleading and indeed wrong to suppose that each human being is an independent actuality that interacts with other human beings and with nature. Rather, they are all projections of a single totality.

> The easily accessible explicit content of consciousness is included within a much greater implicit (or implicate) background. This in turn evidently has to be contained in a yet greater background which may include not only neuro-physiological processes at levels of which we are not generally conscious but also a yet greater background of unknown (and indeed ultimately unknowable) depths of inwardness that may be analogous to the 'sea' of energy that fills the sensibly perceived 'empty space'.
>
> Whatever may be the nature of these inward depths of consciousness, they are the very ground, both of the explicit content and of that content which is usually called implicit. Although this ground may not appear in ordinary consciousness, it may nevertheless be present in a certain way. Just as the vast 'sea' of energy in space is present to our

perception as a *sense* of emptiness or nothingness, so the vast 'unconscious' background of explicit consciousness with all its implications is present in a similar way. That is to say, it may be *sensed* as an emptiness, a nothingness, within which the usual content of consciousness is only a vanishingly small set of facets.[14]

The very existence of a viable quantum model of consciousness 'takes consciousness out of the realm of the supernatural and makes it a proper subject for scientific enquiry'[15] As the distinguished astronomer and physicist Arthur Eddington observed:

> Recognizing that the physical world is entirely abstract and without 'actuality' apart from its linkage to consciousness, we restore consciousness to the fundamental position instead of representing it as an inessential complication occasionally found in the midst of inorganic nature at a late stage of evolutionary history.[16]

Bohm did precisely this. He considered matter, life, the cosmos and consciousness to be projections of a common ground: the ground of all that is. His theory provides a basis for speculating that the entire vacuum/universe is conscious, and 'a general theory of the vacuum is thus a theory of everything'.[17] Bohm's view of the universe as conscious and intelligent is strikingly similar to and fully consistent with the ancient Indian view of the 'void'. In Buddhist tradition the void is not nothingness or annihilation, it is the very source of life. Out of itself it creates everything.

> In speaking of this theory as taught in the Buddhism of China and Japan ... Hajime Nakamura, the Japanese Buddhist scholar, says 'Voidness ... is ... that which stands right in the middle between affirmation and negation, existence and nonexistence ... The void is all-inclusive; having no opposite, there is nothing which it excludes or opposes. It is a living void, because all forms come out of it, and whoever realizes the void is filled with life and power and the ... love of all things.'[18]

Bohm was not the only eminent physicist to hold such views. His theories about the unification of consciousness are part of a tradition within modern physics that includes some of the most highly acclaimed scientists of the modern era. Sir Arthur Eddington observed that the idea of a universal Mind would be a fairly plausible inference from the present state of scientific theory: 'at least it is in harmony with it.'[19] Erwin Schrödinger supported this view, stating 'I should say: the overall number of minds is just one.'[20] He acknowledged that the idea of collective consciousness, which he called One mind, found in ancient wisdom could be drawn from modern science. He considered that the Western world suffered from a global collective delusion in believing that consciousness or mind is localised in the body, that this idea is only symbolic, for practical use. Henry Margenau also subscribed to the idea of a Universal Mind.

'Their theories provide support for the idea of a genuinely nonlocal mind — mind that is not limited by space and time, mind that is not confined to brains or bodies, mind that is ultimately One instead of single and individual, and mind that is immortal'[21] — mind that has all the qualities traditionally associated with the soul. The views of these eminent scientists therefore run counter to the widely held view in the West that it is useless to speak of the soul because the soul does not exist.

> The theories of these physicists are so vastly important for us. They tell us that the verdict from science on 'something higher' is *not* final, that the opinion of great scientists is *not* unanimously negative, and that reasons can still be given from *within* science for the existence of the soul and its affinity with God. Even in an age of science in which God has frequently been pronounced dead, the recovery of the soul remains a project with bright hopes of succeeding.[22]

Hence recent conceptual development in the mind–brain sciences 'clear the way for ... a natural fusion of science and religion'.[23]

These developments in twentieth-century scientific thinking completely undermine the assumption within mainstream Western psychology and medicine that consciousness is a function or product of mind originating in the physical brain. Consciousness is being conceived as more fundamental than mind, as having created mind, brain and the entire cosmos. Hence, matter is an epiphenomenon of mind rather than the other way round. Such a shift in thinking is profoundly shocking to most people. 'It's not unlike realising that the sun does not revolve around the earth, the earth revolves around the sun and we've got it backwards. Rather than consciousness linked to spirituality as something that's out there in outer space, it's something that we can't ignore, it's primal. Consciousness creates reality. The data is in.'[24] Hence the idea that neuroscientists may eventually be able to fully map the brain and thereby account for consciousness is quite erroneous.

> Just as a person could totally understand a television set — could take it apart and put it together again — but understand nothing about electromagnetic radiation, we could study the brain as input–output: sensory input, behavior output. We make maps, but we should never confuse the map with the territory. I've stopped seeing the brain as the end of the line. It's a receiver, an amplifier, a little wet mini-receiver for collective reality.[25]

Even more shocking than the idea that 'consciousness is before the brain', in the sense that consciousness is the primary reality that actually creates mind and brain, is the notion that the brain may not be necessary to consciousness. Yet this is precisely the understanding that is emerging from the interdisciplinary science of psychoneuroimmunology (PNI) where it has been established that thought and emotion produce molecules known as peptides that have receptors throughout the entire body. Peptide chains within the body can effectively be considered as streams of thought, and greater understanding of the biochemistry of these processes leads to the conclusion that thinking or consciousness occurs throughout the body.

> One of the really shocking and exciting implications of the work [in this field of PNI] is the fact that the molecules of emotion are found not just in every system of the body but *running* every system of the body, connecting every system of the body to every

other system. This means that our body is really our subconscious mind ... The emotions are happening everywhere simultaneously and it really is about learning to think of ourselves in a totally new way. Not as a machine at all but as a field of information where things travel instantaneously everywhere.[26]

As peptides are the place where learning occurs there is memory wherever there are receptor sites. Intelligence and memory are therefore located throughout the body, as are some subconscious ways of acting. Hence 'trauma can be stored not just in little parts of our brain but deeply within our body, which may explain some of the very powerful aspects of the various kinds of body work.'[27] This awareness, and the recognition that thought and emotions can have a direct influence on physical functioning, just as physical functioning can exert influence on emotional and mental experiences, blurs any distinction between mind and body. Hence researchers in the field of PNI have introduced the term 'bodymind' to refer to the whole, fine homeostatic mechanism of information fields.

However, it is also being recognised that consciousness may not be confined to the bodymind, but extends beyond it. 'Consciousness may be projected to different places. It's like trying to describe what happens when three people have an incredible conversation together. It's almost as if there were a fourth or fifth person there; the whole is greater than the sum of its parts.'[28] Biologists are only reluctantly beginning, if at all, to realise that the mind is not physically dependent on the brain and body and that it will not be understood completely in terms of the brain's chemistry and anatomy.[29] Although the idea of a non-material field capable of causing physical changes to occur in the world is commonplace in physics it has not been warmly received in modern biology. 'It is as if the two disciplines were on fast moving trains, going in opposite directions and not noticing what is happening across the tracks.[30] Indeed, while physicists faced with compelling experimental evidence have been moving away from strictly mechanical and materialistic models of the universe to a view that sees mind as playing an integral role in all physical events, 'the life scientists, following the path of the last [nineteenth] century's physics, are trying to abolish mind altogether.'[31]

Unsurprisingly, therefore, a 'new science of life' proposed by the biochemist Rupert Sheldrake[32] which has at its core the idea that consciousness cuts across time and space and gives rise to non-local effects, has provoked great controversy. Sheldrake postulated the existence of morphogenetic fields — invisible organising fields — that act as a matrix or blueprint for both the form and behaviour of all living species, intelligently guiding and directing the evolutionary potential of all life forms. These morphogenetic fields are the energetic forces that guide cells to their particular destiny, assuring that they reach the correct differentiation and development for their specific purposes. 'An approximate analogy to this is when iron filings are placed on a magnet, they align with the magnetic field.'[33]

Sheldrake suggests that the morphogenetic fields not only govern the structure and differentiation of living organisms but also their behaviour and evolution. Morphogenetic fields also carry the organism's history. They are causative fields that propagate across space and time through a principle he termed *morphic resonance.* Accordingly, the behaviour and evolution of a species are not determined by laws but by acquired habits that if repeated often enough are incorporated into the template or matrix of the entire species. Thus, for example, if an animal finds a technique that helps survival and which is repeated, through morphic resonance it may become part of the behavioural repertoire of that species, acquired by others without direct genetic or geographical connection. Although difficult to establish, such habits become easier with repetition. 'Thus if rats learn a new trick in London, then rats everywhere should be able to learn the same thing quicker by tuning in to the experience of the previous rats. Likewise if chemists make a new compound, which has never existed before in the universe, it may be hard to get it to crystallise at first, but once this has been done, say in New York, it should become easier all round the world for this compound to crystallise in future.'[34] This idea accounts for what has become known as 'the hundredth monkey phenomenon'.[35] This refers to the remarkable case of Imo, one of a colony of *Macaca fuscata* isolated on the island of Koshima off the Japanese mainland intensively studied for many years. These monkeys were unable to eat raw sweet potatoes covered with sand and grit, until the young Imo carried the potatoes to a stream and washed them before feeding. 'In monkey terms this is a cultural revolution comparable almost to the invention of the wheel.'[36] Reversing the normal trend, Imo taught her mother and other monkeys to do this and slowly the new culture spread through the colony, with each new conversion observed by researchers. Within six years all the juveniles were washing dirty food, although the only adults over five to do so were those who had learned by direct imitation from their children. Then something extraordinary happened. The hundredth monkey learned this behaviour and in so doing 'apparently carried the number across some sort of threshold, pushing it though a kind of critical mass, because by that evening almost everyone in the colony was doing it. Not only that but the habit seems to have jumped natural barriers and to have appeared spontaneously, like glycerine crystals in sealed laboratory jars, in colonies on other islands and on the mainland in a troop at Takasakiyama.'[37]

Sheldrake's theory has already been subjected to a number of tests, some of which have been highly successful and lent support to the premise that nature, like an organism, may well have an inherent memory or habit, rather than being governed by eternal laws.[38] As such it resonates with ancient ideas concerning the soul and its implicit memory, known in some traditions as the *akashic record*, and described in modern times by Carl Jung as the collective unconscious. His ideas:

> ... like many of David Bohm's concepts of the enfolded implicate order, demand ... a reconsideration of our concepts of space–time constraints. It is very possible that our past is enfolded within the quantum potential or holographic field, and, therefore, would be much more likely to appear in the habits of nature than we are presently aware of.
>
> If we can see time as a continuous flux of projections into higher orders of the holographic universe and back again from a manifest universe to the holographic field, then the concept of past events affecting future events or future events affecting past events is not so far-fetched after all.[39]

Nevertheless, the theory remains highly controversial within science. It challenges conventional concepts of Darwinian evolution, casts doubt on the role that DNA plays in the formation and development of living species, overturns conventional concepts of time and space and does not involve any normal means of communication. Arguably, however, the controversial nature of the theory is less because it challenges the 'superstition of materialism'[40] — the mechanistic theory of nature, generally acknowledged by scientists as outmoded and inappropriate — but because it unashamedly seeks to restore the soul to the discourse of science, and to 'resacralize our relationship with nature'.[41]

Sheldrake argues that modern science presents a vision of nature that increasingly accords with that held throughout nearly all history, the view that nature is alive and everything is animated or ensouled. Yet as he points out, the desacralized, de-animated, soulless vision of the universe ushered in by Descartes, in which the animating principle or soul was withdrawn not only from the human body, but also from the whole of nature — which came to be regarded as an automatic machine with no spontaneous life and no purposes of its own — survives to this day, 'and is still the official philosophy which dominates the media, politics, education, and the whole ethos of development and economic progress',[42] although every tenet of this scientific modern view has been refuted or transcended by science itself. It has been supplanted by a new vision in which nature is seen once more as animated by immaterial internal organising principles in the form of *fields*, which even biologists are coming to recognise as crucial in the organisation of living things.

> A soul is a non-material and invisible organising principle, which provides something with internal purpose and motivation. Without soul then the whole of nature had to be thought of as being pushed from behind by causes rather than drawn by motivations to goals ahead ...
>
> Souls are motivated by attraction. The soul of the oak tree, according to Aristotle and to St Thomas Aquinas, was something which drew the oak tree towards its final form. Now, more than two centuries after this kind of vitalism has been expunged from science, it is again being smuggled back with the science of dynamics. The mathematical modelling of complex processes is now done in terms of where they are going to end up, rather

than in terms of how they are being pushed from behind. The final state is, significantly enough, called an 'attractor'.[43]

So far very little of the new scientific revolution as indicated by Sheldrake is generally realised. He acknowledges that resistance to accepting a new perspective ensures that at least 50 years elapse before any major scientific discovery penetrates public consciousness[44] and he anticipates that it will be about 2030 before his ideas become popular. If he is right it will be some time before it is generally recognised that modern scientists are identifying in terms of similar concepts such as energy and energy fields, albeit by different names, exactly the same soul principles that have been described throughout history.

Fields of energy

The traditional wisdom of the East tells us:

> Behind the visible garment of the universe, beyond the mirage of molecules, the *maya* — or illusion — of physicality, lies an inherently invisible, seamless matrix made up of nothingness. This invisible nothingness silently orchestrates, instructs, guides, governs, and compels nature to express itself with infinite creativity, infinite abundance, and unfaltering exactitude into a myriad of designs and patterns and forms.[45]

The Hindu called this field of infinite possibilities Brahman and the Chinese named it Tao, whereas contemporary physicists call it the unified field.

> The field is organizing everything in creation: the movement of galaxies, the movement of stars, the rotation of the earth, the cycles of the seasons, the biological rhythms of our bodies, birds migrating at the right season to the right place, fish returning to their spawning grounds, the biological rhythms of nature as found in flowers, vegetation, and animals. It is literally a field of infinite organizing power. It can do an infinite number of things all at the same time and then correlate them with each other. Even our human body is a field of infinite organizing power.[46]

Indeed traditionally everything is considered to have its own organising field or matrix which carries its blueprint or perfect pattern — its essence or soul. In different cultures these invisible patterns of subtle energy have been known by various names. Polynesians, such as the Kahunas of Hawaii, considered all phenomena, whether human bodies, thoughts, or material objects such as chairs, to have shadowy bodies or forms, referred to as *a-kas*, that remain after the gross physical form has been destroyed. These shadowy bodies interpenetrate the human body, being a mould of every cell and tissue in it. The Hindu refer to these shadowy 'spirits' without solid form as *devas*. Elsewhere they are known as angels, muses, fairies, elves, elementals and such like, but belief in the devic realm is universal. The tendency in all cultures has been to personify these energies or 'spirits', 'to clothe them'[47] in images in order to accept them more easily. These archetypes, found in the mythology of all peoples, are therefore a way of making sensible the subtle energetic influences that give coherence to the phenomenal world. Most commonly they are described in angelic images 'and the whole mythic tradition of the fall of the angels can be understood as a description of how the soul, from the realms of pure energy, incarnates and descends into the material paradox of human life.[48]

These spirits have traditionally been viewed as essential to the structural integrity of phenomena and therefore as fundamental to the health and well-being of living organisms. 'In any illness or disease, the perfect pattern envisaged and held by the relevant spirit is being obstructed and cannot fulfil itself.'[49] The expression of the matrix, blueprint or soul is therefore critical to the maintenance of health. The challenge for human beings is to allow the blueprint of their souls to be expressed in everyday life, in spite of the stimuli of life which often lead them to ignore or lose sight of the essential pattern of their being. The role of healers was to restore the energetic harmony between the soul's blueprint and its expression in everyday life — to put individuals back in touch with their soul or essential nature.

Traditionally, healers were seers or clairvoyants, mystics who could perceive these subtle energies directly. Typically they described a luminescence emanating from all matter, normally some five or six inches from the human body. This is commonly referred to as the *aura* and since antiquity there have been literary and pictorial descriptions of this phenomenon. It is sometimes represented as a luminous radiation around the entire body but more commonly as a kind of light around the head, or halo. In early Chinese and Japanese art a single, or occasionally a triple, halo is often shown around the head of the Buddha. In ancient Egyptian art, the aura is often shown as wings enfolding the body. Christ's raiment is described[50] as 'glistering', and typically Christ is depicted with a halo, as are the saints in Christian art, and angels are typically shown with both halos and wings. There is good reason, therefore, to believe that some ancient races were familiar with the idea of radiation from living creatures. In more recent times it was described by the poet Goethe, who suggested that the emanations from the human body should be studied.[51] His suggestion was later acted upon by the distinguished German chemist Baron Karl von Reichenbach who was fascinated by the experiments conducted by Franz Anton Mesmer in the late eighteenth century.

Franz Anton Mesmer (1734–1815), an Austrian doctor who practised in France, discovered that an ordinary magnet placed over any diseased part of the body would often effect a cure. He noted that during treatment with magnets muscle spasms often occurred and he theorised that some sort of ethereal fluid entered the patient's body. He realised that this force was magnetic in nature and could charge both animate and inanimate objects, but in order to differentiate it from magnetism produced by metals or minerals he initially termed it *animal magnetism*, and later *fluidum*. He claimed that recharging and rebalancing the body with fluidum was essential to healing as illness is a disharmony in the body's electromagnetic field. He considered the human body to be the strongest generator of magnetic energy and eventually concluded that it flowed from the hands of healers directly into the patient. By using their hands in sweeping passes over the body, in much the same way as a magnet is magnetised, healers could direct and regulate the flow of this energy in the patient's body and effect cure by realigning the magnetic field of the sick person. Accordingly he viewed the ancient technique of laying on hands as of paramount importance. As he was able to demonstrate striking cures, his concepts of animal magnetism and magnetic treatment, which became known as **mesmerism**, became very popular, especially among the poor who could not afford orthodox medical treatment.

There are indications that similar practices were used by healers in ancient Egypt, Greece and Rome;[52] in the middle ages by Paracelsus[53] who disseminated the idea that magnets possessed special healing powers and with their powers of polar attraction and repulsion could be used to influence the ethereal fluid he referred to as *illiaster*; and during the seventeenth century by the healer Valentine Greatraks.[54] Indeed in Mesmer's time healing by stroking and touch was common. The views of the sixth-century physician Galen were also still influential. He had claimed that an invisible essential fluid filled the universe, planets and all living creatures and that health consisted in a balance of the fluid essences of body, soul and the environment. What distinguished Mesmer from other healers of his time was his formulation of scientifically testable propositions that linked healing with the manifestations of 'a universally distributed and continuous fluid ... of an incomparably rarefied nature', with 'properties similar to those of a magnet'.[55] However, when Mesmer's claims were investigated by a Royal Commission in 1785 led by the US Commission to France, Benjamin Franklin, magnetometers failed to detect any magnetism and it was concluded that there was no substance to the claims, and Mesmer was discredited.

Interest in mesmerism continued, however, and when, in the mid-nineteenth-century, von Reichenbach (1788–1869) conducted experiments similar to those of Mesmer he accumulated a wealth of evidence indicating that there existed in nature a peculiar kind of energy which he named the 'odic force'. This exhibited many properties similar to those of the electromagnetic field that James Clerk Maxwell had described earlier that century and some unique features, notably that with the odic force like poles attract, rather than opposite poles as in electromagnetism. He found the odic force in magnets, crystals, light, heat and living cells and wherever chemical reactions occur. He discovered that this energy could be accumulated or conducted along wires and focused or distorted by a lens. He concluded that this was a vital energy since it could be transmitted by certain people to others for healing, pain relief or anaesthesia. His findings, published in 1844, created a considerable stir, but his claims were dismissed by scientists and doctors. 'Yet the great Humboldt said of his work: "the facts are undeniable: it now becomes the task of Science to explain them".'[56]

Scientists of the time did not rise to the challenge. Indeed they poured even more scorn on the claims of Albert Abrams (1863–1923), Director of Studies at Stanford University Medical School, who held that all matter emitted radiations; the human body could act as a receiver for them; and illness could be diagnosed and treated by way of them. He developed a diagnostic system based upon his findings and published many papers on it, claiming that in this way disease could be detected before it was clinically identifiable in any orthodox way. He began to experiment with the energy flow as a means of treatment and developed an 'oscilloclast' to treat patients by means of vibrations. On his death in 1924 his system was investigated by the Royal Society of Medicine in London. Although it was concluded that Dr Abrams' fundamental proposition 'had been proved to a high degree of probability', doctors of the era did not understand the relationship between energy and matter and it was decided that the system could not be taught in medical schools. His methods continued to be taught outside medicine, however, and were developed by George de la Warr, among others, who referred to the energy emissions as 'emanations'.

While the subtle energy fields around the human body have been evident to many healers throughout history, and used by them in the diagnosis and treatment of illness, they are invisible to most people. So, even in the modern era where the existence of invisible energies such as electricity, television and radio waves is accepted, the existence of subtle human energies is not.

> Energy fields are invisible structures around the body. They are invisible in the same way that television and radio waves are invisible. Their existence is made manifest by the presence of a receiver (the body), much in the same way that we need a TV or radio to detect television and radio waves. Unfortunately energy fields around the body are nothing like as simple as radio and TV waves.[57]

Until recently these subtle energy fields have eluded scientific measurement. This may be because they can only react with and be detected by living organisms, and so a detectable reaction only occurs when they find their counterpart in a living being. Certainly because these forces are not easily detected by physical instruments in the orthodox scientific world, they are generally deemed to have no physical reality and Western science has steadfastly denied their existence.

However, it is clear from the history of Western research into subtle energies during the twentieth century that scientific vision has been governed by the limitations of its tools. As these have become more sophisticated they have yielded more information about subtle energies and new theories about their influence and effects.

In 1911 Dr Walter Kilner of St Thomas' Hospital, London, published a dissertation, *The Human Atmosphere*, in which he claimed that a force field exists around the human body that can be charted and analysed. Consistent with various traditions that have described a radiant energy emitted from the body, he termed this 'the aura'. He observed that the aura is self-luminous, that is, it glows, but requires weak illumination for this to occur.[58] Kilner subsequently developed a special kind of glass, the Kilner screen, which, he claimed, enabled the aura to be seen objectively. This — and his prediction that in future it would be possible to photograph the aura and use it for more accurate diagnosis of all kinds of illness — was dismissed as fanciful. The views of F.S.C. Northrup of Yale University, who proposed the existence of dynamic fields around living organisms, were similarly rejected. So, too, was the claim of Yale Professor of Anatomy H.S. Burr that he had discovered an electrodynamic field or energy body which he termed the 'L[ife] field', possessed by all living beings. He spent over forty years investigating L fields, detecting them in humans, animals, trees, plants, seeds, eggs and plant moulds. In the 1930s he theorised that these L fields were responsible for the body's capacity to regenerate new cells that act and function in exactly the same way as those they replaced. He suggested that just as a jelly mould determines the shape of the jelly that will be produced within it, so the L field serves as a matrix or mould that preserves the shape or arrangement of the material it moulds, however often the material may be changed. Furthermore this 'invisible' and 'intangible' field can reveal the future shape or arrangement of the material it will mould. However, a distortion in the L field can give warning of an abnormality in the body, sometimes in advance of actual symptoms. Therefore a weakness in the L field of a living creature predisposes it to disease. Burr could tell how strong a plant would be by measuring its L field as a seed. He was able to detect cancer in animals and humans by measuring electrical potentials near to the skin and, through electrical measurements, assess the progress of the cancer.

Burr's discoveries were dismissed, although they lent credence to the centuries-old claim of healers that these energies can be detected through touch or sight and that they provide forewarning of illness. They also supported research conducted in Russia in the late nineteenth century by Yakub Yodko-Narkevitch. He had experimented with electrography or corona-discharge photography that does not require a camera. In this work, a high-voltage, high-frequency electric discharge passes between the object to be photographed and a conducting plate and, with the film between the two, an exposure is produced. In the course of his investigations, he found that a picture from a healthy person differs to one from a sick person, and that tired, excited, sleeping or awake individuals can be distinguished by the same means. Unfortunately, his publications and research tools were lost during the Russian revolution and electrography was rediscovered only by accident during the 1930s by another Russian researcher Semyon Kirlian.

Kirlian developed high-voltage photography that revealed streams of apparent energy flowing from the fingertips in a manner suggested by traditional aura theory. Subsequently other devices, such as the verograph, were developed that produced images similar to those obtained by Kirlian photography, and during the 1960s a lightless microphoto was developed that provided further objective evidence for the aura by capturing the fading life of a dying plant.

Over the course of many years of research Kirlian and his wife and co-researcher, Valentina, became convinced that these energy streams reflected the well-being or otherwise of an organism, and this view subsequently gained support from research on plants and humans. Working with a surgeon, Ruben Stepanov, the Kirlians found that electrography could be used to diagnose illnesses in human beings. They found that tissue from cancer patients produced many tiny white and grey spots on photographs, whereas non-cancerous tissue produced large well-defined spots.[59]

The Kirlians' work was developed further by Professor Vladimir Inyushin.[60] Unlike the Kirlians who attributed the energy they captured on film to the electrical state of the organism, he argued that it was caused by a biological plasma body. This, he claimed — as Burr had done previously — was a whole unified organism emitting its own electromagnetic fields, which are the basis of all biological fields. He considered *bioplasma*, as he called it, to be a fourth state of matter that could take on highly organised patterns and influence Kirlian images. As such, this may be equivalent to the etheric or astral body described by the ancients, generally referred to as the aura.[61]

Using Kirlian photography, Professor Viktor Adamenko has subsequently claimed to have found concentrations of bioplasma at hundreds of points on the human body corresponding to the acupuncture points of traditional Chinese medicine, and that these varied with different illnesses. However, he prefers to describe the phenomena not as bioplasma, whose existence in living things has yet to be proved, but as a 'corona', which he defines as the cold emission of electrons from the live object into the atmosphere. What is clear, he indicates, is that the Kirlian image is strongly influenced by electrical processes within the organism that are much more organised than is generally recognised.

Using Kirlian photography, Adamenko found that changes could be detected in the corona of a famous Russian healer during healing and that genuine healers could thus be distinguished from charlatans; it was also possible to discover healing ability in people who had never suspected they had any.[62]

Research with electrography convinced the Kirlians that their method provided evidence not only of a person's physiological state but also of mental states. Adamenko found that stress could be detected in mentally healthy people using Kirlian photography.[63] It could also be used as an effective tool in diagnosis of psychological illness.[64] Comparisons of Kirlian images from several hundred schizophrenics with controls have provided not only convincing evidence that Kirlian photography can be used in psychiatric diagnosis but also that it can be used to predict deterioration of clinical symptoms.[65]

Kirlian photography did not become known in the West until the mid-1960s and initially it met with scepticism. The suggestion that the observed phenomenon is simply the result of physiological variations at the surface of the skin was rebutted by Professor Thelma Moss of the Neuropsychiatric Institute of the University of California

School of Medicine, who was the first serious researcher of the phenomenon in the USA. She demonstrated that while there was no correlation between the observed corona and variations in skin temperature, or peripheral states of perspiration, there were apparent correlations with psychological states. Relaxation produced by meditation, hypnosis and acupuncture is characterised by brilliant coronas, while tension and emotional excitement result in a contracted corona with red blotches at the fingertips.

Further evidence that the phenomenon is not a physical variation of the photographed surface comes from the discovery that when a leaf has pieces removed or human fingers are amputated the corona discharge in each case shows as a whole image, albeit of poorer quality.[66] Physicist William Tiller of Stanford University has suggested that the energy apparently emitted from the fingertips is present prior to the formation of solid matter. This, he claims, may be another level of substance producing a hologram; a coherent energy pattern organising matter so that it produces a physical network in the manner of a hologram. Thus, if one part of the network is cut away, the forming hologram still remains. Adamenko observes that while a complete image can be reproduced from any part of a hologram, the smaller the piece of hologram, the worse will be the quality of the image. Since electrons can be considered waves as well as particles, he suggests that there is no reason why they could not form a holographic image just as well as light.

Electron-wave holography was first achieved in 1975 by physicists in the USA. As with light holography, it is necessary that the waves are in a highly ordered or coherent state, such as that produced by a laser.

> Could a living organism be so perfectly organised to emit coherent electrons in the intense electric field? If the answer is yes, then we shall see great developments of what is at present an embryo science: *quantum biophysics*. Kirlian photography will then be making a substantial contribution to the science of life.[67]

There is every reason to be optimistic about the future of Kirlian photography as a life-energy monitoring system. The German professor of biophysics, Fritz-Albert Popp, argues that living organisms are organised in precisely such a coherent way. Since the

1920s research has shown that virtually all living organisms emit exceedingly small amounts of light. The Russian scientist Alexander Gurwitsch first detected this radiation, which he termed 'mitogenic radiation', in onion roots.[68] However, other studies using physical methods failed to produce clear evidence for the existence of this very weak radiation and just before the Second World War the results were refuted. The phenomenon, known as 'ultra-weak biological light' was dismissed by many scientists as a by-product of metabolism, and interest in the subject declined in the following decades.[69]

Interest in the subject was revived with the development by Italian researchers of a sensitive photo-multiplier system.[70] Subsequent research on ultra-weak radiation in the 1960s was mainly carried out in Russia.[71] Pioneering studies were also carried out in the West[72-5] by researchers who independently developed methods for measuring the ultra-weak radiation in a variety of different cells by the use of highly sensitive equipment which allows for the maximal exploitation of the potential capabilities of a photo-multiplier tube. Systematic investigations using these instruments have revealed that every single cell emits detectable energy. Although emission of this light is very low in body cells it can be efficiently induced by ultraviolet light.

Much of the work on ultra-weak radiation in the West was conducted by Professor Fritz Albert Popp who coined the term 'biophotons' to refer to the ultraweak emissions by cells.[76] These biophotons have remarkable properties that cannot be explained in terms of random metabolic errors. Popp proposes that the light is released from a coherent electromagnetic field which accounts for biological organisation and biocommunication. Many significant correlations exist between features such as cell division, death and major shifts in metabolism, which may indicate that the light is a sensitive global expression of biological regulatory processes. Furthermore, there are strong grounds for believing that rapid communication takes place by way of electromagnetic fields. Studies of light emission have provided evidence for long-range communication between cells and have shown such communication to be defective in cancer cells.[77] This research suggests that there is a fundamental sense in which all organisms are 'beings of light'.[78]

An organism may be likened to a candle flame. The structure of the flame is only maintained by the dissipation of energy in the process of burning. It is a very simple example of what Prigogine calls a 'dissipative structure'. Likewise an organism only maintains its structure by the constant dissipation of metabolic energy. The instant this is cut off it starts to fall apart. The organism should therefore be thought of as a process or a 'happening' rather than an object.[79]

Evidence for coherent states (known as Bose–Einstein condensates) in living tissue is now abundant. Scientists working independently of Popp in Japan have discovered the same effects and believe them to be clearly associated with vital activities and biological processes.

As a possible means of detecting electromagnetic fields, there is growing interest in Kirlian photography in the West, where it has been used successfully to identify patients with cancer.[80, 81] However, although there have been some successes in a number of applied fields many scientists simply have not taken Kirlian photography seriously. Attitudes are slowly changing, however, and the full potential of this method is being explored in high-quality research.[82]

Other attempts have been made to measure patterns or currents of electromagnetic energy in and around the body. New York orthopaedic surgeon Dr Robert Becker has shown that the human electromagnetic field relates directly to the functioning of the body, and its patterns and strength vary with physiological and psychological changes.[83, 84]

This research established the relationship between regeneration and electrical currents in living things. The flow of electrons through the perineural cells of the nervous system (those cells containing bundles of nerve fibres surrounded by an extensive layer of connective tissue) and the resultant magnetic field are the factors that effect an organism's ability to sense and evaluate damage occurring anywhere in the body. This electromagnetic flow also provides cells with the appropriate electrical environment to either sustain health within an uninjured cell or stimulate healing in a damaged one. It has been suggested[85] that this same perineural structure is the passageway healers use when channelling energy into a subject during healing.

Scientific research has also focused on the chakras as possible patterns or currents of electromagnetic energy in and around the body. The first modern description of chakra energies was by Sir Isaac Newton in 1729 in his second paper on light and colours. In this he spoke of electromagnetic light as a 'subtle, vibrating, electric and elastic medium that was excitable *and* exhibited phenomena such as repulsion, attraction, sensation and motion.' He anticipated in many ways the electromagnetic field theories of Michael Faraday and James Clerk Maxwell a century later that paved the way for quantum physics.

Scientific measurement of the chakras in the twentieth century was pioneered by Japanese professor Hiroshi Motoyama who since the 1960s has developed various physiological devices for measuring subtle energy fields. He devised an apparatus (AMI) that measures the flow of energy within each of the acupuncture meridians in order to ascertain the functional condition of meridians and their corresponding internal organs. The instrument measures the initial skin current and steady-state current in response to DC voltage applied externally at the terminal points of meridians. Experiments on some 2000 subjects strongly suggest that the relative magnitude of such skin currents reflect the functional conditions of Ki energy in the meridians. Motoyama has also developed a Chakra Instrument to detect minute changes in energy emitted by the body. It measures the electromagnetic fields around the body and can show subtle changes in these when chakras are naturally active or activated by some other means.[86, 87] On the basis of experimental studies using these devices, Motoyama has concluded that despite differences in terminology the energy systems underpinning traditional Chinese and Indian medicine are fundamentally the same and are consistent with the age-old observations of clairvoyants and mystics.

Bioelectrical theories are now used being used to explain the sensitivity of clairvoyants and intuitives who perceive chakra and aura energies and use them in diagnosis and treatment, and of doctors who diagnose illness through the energy field they perceive around their patients or the energy vortices connected with the endocrine system.[88] Some experiments have reported a correlation between the measured electromagnetic fields of the body and the aura perceived by clairvoyants, and have supported the claim that healers can detect electrodynamic or energy patterns through touch or sight. Studies at the University of California at Los Angeles by Drs Valerie Hunt and Andrija Puharich[89] have shown a direct correlation between the frequency and wave patterns of alternating electrical currents on the body surface and the specific colours perceived by the clairvoyants. The research conducted by Dr Hunt discovered energy emanations from the body surface beyond frequencies previously found to emanate from biochemical systems. It provided the first objective electronic evidence of frequency, amplitude and time which validates the subjective observation of colour emissions from the aura described for centuries by clairvoyants. Three different data resolutions by wave form, Fourier frequency analysis and Sonogram frequency representation all produced the same results, measuring frequencies and energy patterns from each chakra location that directly corresponded with the aura reader's descriptions of each chakra and the total aura. Dr Hunt was able to measure seven harmonics or varying frequency bands of colour, vibration and colour of each chakra. Her study highlighted the importance of balance and harmony by showing that when all the chakras are aligned and functioning appropriately healthy process occurs. When their energies are not aligned or balanced ill health results. These results lend support to the teaching of all spiritual disciplines throughout history that see the purpose of life as to express the harmonics of the soul in everyday life[90] and emphasise the importance of maintaining balance in life or balanced living. Other conclusions may be drawn from this study:

> From the extensive detailed study of energy field emissions from the body meticulously recorded and processed, strong conclusions are warranted. The energy field described as aura has dynamic changes that coincide with emotional states, imagery, interpersonal relations and the state of resiliency and plasticity of the connective tissue of the physical body. A skilled aura reader can accurately describe the color and dynamic interplay of this electromagnetic energy radiating from the chakras and forming the auric field.[91]

Further studies of electromagnetic fields[92] have suggested that healers world-wide exhibit the same brain wave pattern of 7.8–8 Hz during healing, irrespective of where or when the healing occurs. These patterns correspond with the fluctuations of the earth's magnetic field between 7.8 and 8 Hz which are called Schumann waves. Indeed during healing the healers' brain waves synchronise with the earth's Schumann waves. This process, known as 'field coupling', has been studied by Dr John Zimmerman,[93] whose findings suggest that healers 'ground' themselves by synchronising with the Schumann waves and that, by linking with the earth's magnetic field in this way, they may be tapping this energy source for healing.

Bioelectrical investigations and theories not only appear to have great promise for explaining phenomena such as healing but also for understanding specific treatments such as acupuncture. The determination of the existence of acupuncture points by electrical means began in the 1950s. Dr Rheinhold Voll first measured acupuncture points using a standard circuit to measure resistance. Dozens of studies have subsequently confirmed that there is a significant difference between the electrical activity of true and non-points, and concluded that acupuncture points represent at least an area of high conductivity (electrical permeability) relative to nearby tissues.

Research also suggests that meridians can be identified with measurements of electrical impedance and conductance. In fact the objective existence of the meridian system is argued for most strongly by the electrical specificity of acupuncture points.[94] Various studies have found that, by applying a direct current over the body surface, points on the skin of higher electrical conductance can be identified; these correspond with the meridians.[95] In general, the research appears to acknowledge the bioelectrical identity of both acupuncture points and channels as specified in traditional acupuncture. This has led to a bioelectric theory of action which postulates that acupuncture points and channels are electromagnetic in nature; that acupuncture treatments induce alterations in the electromagnetic properties of channels and local tissues; and that electromagnetic fields significantly influence biological matter and physiological functions. The available evidence indicates that acupuncture points and their connecting channels are definable electrically. Relevant research has focused on electromyogram readings that correlate with subjective reporting of propagated sensations along the channels in both healthy subjects and patients with neuromuscular disorders.

Accordingly a theory of acupuncture action has been developed based on the concept of the organismic energy field.[96] This hypothesis, known as the *standing wave superposition hypothesis*, implies that acupuncture has the capacity to induce changes in the standing wave pattern of the person, and that shifts in electromagnetic fields created by such interference can produce changes in biological response that may promote healing. The theory is attractive because it accommodates many of the features of acupuncture, including its holographic nature, that is, the way in which the entire body is represented in parts such as the ears, hand and feet. It also explains the anomalous skin resistance points and their interconnectedness.

The last few decades of the twentieth century saw the emergence of a new science of bioelectromagnetics, which studies the interaction of electromagnetic (EM) fields, and life. It 'has already opened the door towards another way of seeing life, from the viewpoint of a nonlinear dynamic system that collectively interacts within a sea of EM fields'.[97] From this perspective, 'life turns out to be electromagnetic through and through.'[98] There are a growing number of electromagnetic applications in medicine, whereby a large variety of externally applied electric, magnetic and electromagnetic fields of low intensities are used to diagnose and/or treat disease.[99]

> Energy fields offer a tantalizing opportunity for early diagnosis and the selection of appropriate treatment in a way that some of us have not even begun to grasp. We are slowly groping our way to a more objective way of looking at these fields and thereby experimenting with them. In my view this must be one of the most exciting areas of potential development for biology in general and medicine in particular.
>
> Already the measurement and healing of energy fields has generated the fast growing field of energy medicine, sometimes called vibrational or non-local medicine. This has enabled enormous progress to be made with a whole range of chronic diseases which so far have been untreatable. We are clearly on the brink of several breakthroughs in this area of medicine which will herald an era of highly focussed causally directed medicine.[100]

Physicist Danah Zohar has suggested that the coherent electromagnetic field identified by Popp provides the physical basis for consciousness. She indicates that one of the many implications of this discovery is that it lends support to the view that rudimentary consciousness may exist in all living systems. 'Indeed there is no reason in principle to deny that *any* structure, biological or otherwise, which contained a Bose–Einstein condensate mightn't possess the capacity for consciousness.'[101] She goes on to indicate that in the quantum model of consciousness she is suggesting, the vibrating molecules in the neurone cell walls, or photons associated with them which give rise to a Bose–Einstein condensate account only for the ground state of awareness, the 'blackboard' on which perceptions, experience, thoughts and feelings are 'written'. The 'writing' itself could be supplied from a wide range of sources such as the genetic code, memory, synaptic activity in the brain, and all the phylogenetic echoes resonating within the nervous system.

> Each of these would appear individually or in some combination as excitations of the underlying condensate, as patterns within it like waves on the sea, or bubbles on the surface of a pot of boiling stew. And it would be these patterns, the mathematics of which are actually the mathematics of a hologram, which we recognise as the familiar contents of consciousness. Interestingly too Descartes believed that perceptions were excitations of our underlying soul.[102]

Certainly, the aura or human energy field emerges as twentieth-century science's candidate for the soul. Kirlian photography and related research suggests that it is the matrix for life — the 'negative space–time-frame body', as William Tiller has termed it. As such, it conforms with Plato's view of the soul as the perfect form of the body, its archetype. The aura has also been claimed to be the 'missing link' between biology, physical medicine and psychotherapy — the 'place' where all emotions, thoughts, memories and behaviour patterns are located.[103] It quite literally embodies every function attributed to the soul throughout history, and places human spiritual concerns firmly within the remit of scientific endeavour. Accordingly, the term 'spiritual', which traditionally has been used to connote the relationship between the person and the universe, can now be reformulated as the person's relationship to the universal energy field or quantum reality — the unified field, or realm of infinite possibilities. The 'soul', which has always been a more self-referential term, can be conceived as the organismic energy field, or life field, a subset of that all-embracing unified field; and the body as a function of this field. These fields need to be understood not simply as physical fields but as fields of intelligence and information, or consciousness. Certainly it would now seem that 'Science has actually advanced to the point where formerly religious questions can be seriously tackled.'[104]

The science of mysticism

This being the case, does redefinition of the soul in terms of organismic energy or life fields shed light on the mystical universe?

> The 'perverse' upside-down physics of the shamanic universe — in which time is stretched, space is solid, matter is transparent, and conventional manifestations of energy are replaced by invisible subtle forces — cannot be grasped by our customary mode of perception. Nevertheless, all tribal societies as well as our ancestors — and cultures of both the Old world and our present world — did at some time subscribe to the idea of such a universe. Our modern Western culture forms the only exception to this general rule. Its determined scientific exploration has confined itself to what is observable within three-dimensional space. In other words, it has concentrated itself exclusively on a reality accessible to a system of logic based on purely sensory perceptions.[105]

Certainly, the peoples of Eastern cultures have less difficulty than Westerners in accepting the world as a kind of magic show in which what is seen is both substantial and insubstantial, true and not true, taken for what it essentially is not. As a result they have fewer difficulties in accepting the insights of modern physics, which for the most part still play little part in the everyday lives and thinking of people in the West. Viewed from the perspective of quantum physics, the apparent weirdness of the shamanic universe becomes comprehensible. From such a perspective, shamans and sages throughout history emerge as 'the scientists of consciousness in the spiritual world'.[106]

Many notions of magic central to shamanism are consistent with modern scientific thinking:

• Other living and non-living forms possess a second body, a 'soul body' of a spiritual, immaterial nature.

• The cause of illness resides in the soul body and healing must focus on harmonising it.

• The realm in which the soul lives is embodied in the qualities and capabilities of the soul.

• Since all material forms not only possess a soul body but at the same time are bearers of the spiritual essence, they are connected — the soul and the ensouled universe are a whole.

• By altering the structure of consciousness people can access the soul body and thereby the realm in which it resides, the non-material cosmic reservoir of energy.[107]

When each of these ideas is examined it can be seen that there is firm scientific evidence to suggest the existence of an immaterial 'soul body' or energy field that carries the essential blueprint for life. This corresponds with the idea of the soul carrying the essential archetype, the perfect form of the body, and the pattern for perfect fulfilment. There is also evidence from research to support the age-old view that health consists of an energetic harmony between the soul's blueprint and its expression in everyday life. Valerie Hunt's study suggests that the human energy system is designed to function in a particular way. When all its energies are balanced health occurs and when imbalanced, ill health is reported. Her study also demonstrates that greater coherence of the energy field occurs as a result of healing.[108]

Contemporary physics makes sense of the shaman's belief in the vitality of all that exists, the relatedness of all beings and phenomena at every level and a universe pervaded by a creative essence that not only transcends normal existence but gives it inner cohesion. In the realm of quantum reality, as in magic, 'everything is interrelated, nothing exists in isolation. Here rules the principle of *pars pro toto* [every partial aspect contains and resonates with the whole]. This level of consciousness, like a gigantic telephone exchange, affords access to all levels of awareness.'[109]

The science of ecstasy

But does modern scientific thinking admit the idea of leaving the body, (the literal meaning of 'ecstasy') and undertaking journeys of the soul, which is probably one of the oldest underlying principles of shamanism and magic? This notion is found wherever there is belief in the soul. Kalweit insists that it is more than simply an idea but an actual experience that the shaman wilfully induces and that occurs spontaneously in many Western people as out of body experience (OBE) or near death experience (NDE). Indeed, it is known that the shaman usually first becomes aware of the nature of the universe as a result of a near death experience. Mystical awareness, prophetic insight, ecstasy and self-knowledge are commonly reported by those who have undergone NDEs. These experiences appear to be universal.

The universality of experience reported in tribal cultures, occult and esoteric traditions and by those who have undergone OBEs and NDEs suggest that it is not a spiritual invention but a living experience no less real than experiences people have in the material world. It is generally reported that after consciousness leaves the body it remains connected to it in a characteristic manner, as if by a delicate rope, thread or cord. Most people observe themselves from a vantage point outside the body. They may experience 360-degree vision, may see through solid objects and have greatly enhanced distance vision. Many have a comprehensive view of happenings and events, access to extensive information and a feeling of omniscience. This knowing is instantaneous. So is travel; they can move about the universe 'in a flash'.

People who describe such experiences are not psychologically deranged. Research has established that they are for the most part ordinary persons, of above-average education and intelligence, below-average religious involvement and very high psychological well-being.[110] OBEs are surprisingly common. They are experienced by one in every ten to twenty people and occur most frequently during sleep, or unconsciousness following anaesthesia or a blow to the head, and during stress.[111] They can also occur spontaneously during any kind of activity. Psychologist Alan Gauld describes motorcyclists riding at speed who have suddenly found themselves floating above their machines looking down on their bodies, and airline pilots who have found themselves apparently outside their aircraft struggling to get in. He points out that not all OBEs occur spontaneously, but those who induce them describe experiences which are similar in all respects to spontaneous occurrences. People undergoing OBEs experience themselves as still embodied but in a body whose shape, extension, character and spatial location are easily altered at will. These experiences are vivid and resemble everyday waking experiences rather than dreams. Moreover, some cases of OBE are reciprocal. That is, the person is objectively seen at a spot distant from the physical body to which he or she has projected him or herself.

Gauld highlights the similarity of OBEs and NDEs and the fact that NDEs are much more common than has previously been thought. The medical definition of death is where an individual has sustained irreversible cessation of circulation and respiratory functions or irreversible cessation of all functions of the brain, including the brainstem. Brain death means that no part of the brain functions. The person cannot breathe without a respirator. In common vegetative state only part of the brain is destroyed. The person is capable of stereotypical reflex functions such as breathing, sleeping and digesting food, but is considered incapable of thought or even any awareness of the world. A person can remain in this state for years. Behaviour in vegetative coma is generally assumed to be meaningless.

Scientists and doctors have long recognised that people who have died and been resuscitated, or who have been in coma, report strange visions and experiences, but explanation of these has been hotly disputed. The most commonly held view is that people close to death are vulnerable to delusions and repeat what they have previously seen and heard. However, a study at the University of Virginia by Dr Bruce Greyson[112] has established that NDEs are not related to delusion or mental illness but are part of the way the body copes with intolerable stress. His study contributes to growing evidence that NDEs are not a symptom of psychiatric disorder and that those who experience them should not be treated as mentally ill. Greyson found in a study of 134 people who had been close to death that 72 per cent had experienced some form of dissociation of their thoughts and feelings from their bodies, or out of body experience. Younger people and women were more likely to have these experiences, which were mostly accompanied by feelings of peace and joy, although 'hellish' experiences can occur.

Arnold Mindell, a psychotherapist who has spent twenty-five years working with people in coma, also disputes common assumptions about them.[113] He insists that 'there are powerful, dramatic and meaningful events trying to unfold themselves in comatose states,'[114] and that the use of terms such as 'ill', 'psychotic', 'deranged', 'comatose' or 'drugged' can be considered an aggressive act that cuts people off from their experience. 'We need to know that these terms are consensus reality terms for internal and unknown processes. They are our way of dealing with what we do not know.'[115] He insists that comatose people are not simply brain-damaged 'vegetables' who need oxygen, suffering from limbic lobe syndrome triggered by endorphins or like substances. Nor are they merely machines whose central nervous systems, stimulated by excessive physical states, produce haphazard hallucinations and visions. Rather, they are human beings in an altered state of conscious that may be an important and meaningful experience for them. He considers coma a trance state, one of many states of consciousness in an ongoing process, and has shown that the comatose person is able to communicate with others and can often make conscious, rational decisions, thus adding a new dimension to ethical and legal debates about near-death conditions. He indicates that when they have processed the experience, some people in coma actually choose to return to ordinary consciousness and live, and 'when a trance is fully processed it always gives rise to more life, not less.'[116]

> In fact, people in comas resemble mythical heroes. Storytellers the world over have always enchanted us with tales of the shaman, the king and the hero, figures who journey through the outermost gates of reality seeking information in the unknown reaches of existence to return with a divine message for the rest of us.

Up to now only shamans have been able to leave this reality, to alter states of consciousness through dance, drugs and dreaming to return with messages for all of us. Now it seems that comatose people are attempting the same sort of shamanistic feat. The more we learn about these feats the more we shall learn about living completely and bringing together the various worlds we encounter.[117]

Undoubtedly the experiences described by those who have undergone OBEs or NDEs are identical with traditional shamanic descriptions of the Beyond — the primordial domain of the life substance or soul, which is considered to be the world of the dead. However, as Jung pointed out, this world of the dead is not 'dead'. In most cosmologies the Beyond is structured in the same way as the terrestrial realm, and the feelings and actions of the souls in that realm are in no way different from those of the living. The funerary rites of the ancient Egyptians and Tibetans and the medieval *ars moriendi* are based on the assumption that the departed soul is present; they represent attempts to give final instructions to them, to make the surviving consciousness aware that it constitutes the world of the Beyond. 'The Beyond consists of all those properties particular to our consciousness, once it is completely independent of the body.'[118]

Kalweit suggests that some indication of the way in which consciousness is experienced outside the body can be gained from studies of sensory deprivation. When they are insulated from light, sound or temperature variations, people experience magical and paranormal sensations such as those described by those who have had OBEs. In these experiments subjects lose touch with their senses and are unable to use sensory cues to distinguish their body boundary from its surrounding environment. This body/other or figure/ground discrimination is known to be the first stage in the development of a sense of self, self-identity or self-concept. When a person loses the sense of the body, he or she loses the sense of individuality in which self-concept or identity is rooted and becomes immersed in the environment. Contact with ordinary reality, as such, is lost. Kalweit observes that anyone can gain access to expanded consciousness if the sense of identity is dissolved or dismantled as a result of accident, near death experience, a long fast, prolonged rhythmic dancing, shock, pain, extreme stress, or some other blockage of the normal neurological mechanism. They can also do so through deep relaxation, meditation and any other means in which they lose the sense of an individual self rooted in the body. All spiritual traditions aim at surrendering the sense of self or ego in order to experience cosmic unity. Indeed 'In every human being there is the possibility of consciousness separating from the body and penetrating the nonphysical world of the spirit.'[119]

> Since ordinary consciousness with which we are concerned in ordinary life is before all things rooted on the little local self, and is in fact self-consciousness in the little local sense, it follows that to pass out of that is to die to the ordinary self and the ordinary world.
>
> It is to die in the ordinary sense, but in another sense it is to wake up and find that the 'I', one's real, most intimate self, pervades the universe and all other things — that the mountains and the sea and the stars are part of one's own body and that one's soul is in touch with the souls of all creatures ... So great, so splendid is this experience that it may be said that all minor questions and doubts fall away in the face of it. And certain it is that in thousands and thousands of cases the fact of it having come even once to a man has completely revolutionized his subsequent life and outlook on the world.[120]

This view is supported in studies of NDEs. They confirm the impression conveyed by OBEs and shamanic experience that what lies beyond normal waking consciousness is a realm that cannot be adequately described in ordinary language, or understood in terms of logic, cause and effect and the space–time concepts of ordinary Western thinking. These experiences also lend support to the animistic idea that the human mind 'whether in its before or after death state is essentially and irreparably bound up with some kind of extended *quasi*-physical vehicle, which is not normally perceptible to the senses of human beings in their present life.'[121] It is clear from them that mind and brain are not the same.

The case of Janet related in the introduction to this book is a case in point. She returned to a body declared brain dead with knowledge and information of the past, the future and other places that were subsequently shown to be correct. There can be little doubt that she travelled beyond her body with full consciousness, and cannot now explain to herself how this could have been possible. Nor has it been explained to her.

In another case[122] a woman undergoing rare, extremely specialised and risky brain surgery with her eyes and ears completely sealed, experienced herself viewing her operation from above and behind the surgeons. She was subsequently able to describe in minute detail the intricate procedures she witnessed and the specialised equipment used. Given the rarity of the operation it is highly unlikely that she could ever have seen either before. One explanation offered by commentators on her case — that during the operation she nearly died and her soul departing from the body witnessed the procedures — was dismissed without consideration by her doctors. They conceded that she had 'died' during the operation and attributed her sensory experience to a hallucination or false perception caused by physiological processes in the dying brain. No explanation was offered as to how a 'false' perception could have given rise to such valid and accurate information. To hallucinate is, literally from the Latin *allucinari*, to wander in the mind, so the 'explanation' proffered is little more than a description of what occurred. The question not addressed is how this was achieved.

The case of Sarah[123] is still more intriguing. Sarah's heart stopped beating during the final stages of surgery to remove her gall bladder. She was successfully resuscitated and subsequently amazed the surgical team by describing the surgery schedule posted on the corridor outside the operating theatre, the colour of the sheets on the operating table, the hairstyle of the head scrub nurse, the names of the surgeons in the doctors' lounge waiting for her operation to be concluded, and the mismatching socks worn by the anaesthetist — details she knew despite having been fully anaesthetised throughout the surgery and cardiac arrest, and despite having been blind since birth. However, although the critical care nurse acknowledged that after anaesthesia patients often know full details of procedures and test results, none of the medical team would discuss her experience with her.

It is not necessary to die or nearly die in order to obtain

information normally beyond sensory awareness. Remote viewing refers to awareness of locations, events and objects unable to be perceived by the known senses, typically owing to distance. The conclusion presented by the US House of Representatives Committee on Science and Technology in 1981 was that 'recent experiments in remote viewing and other studies in parapsychology suggest that there is an 'interconnectedness' of the human mind with other minds and with matter ... The implications of these experiments is that the human mind may be able to obtain information independent of geography and time.'[124]

Remote viewing is achieved by directing or projecting the imagination to locations beyond normal sensory awareness. Most people are aware that they can travel in their mind by using their imagination. They often choose their holiday destinations in precisely this way, by imagining Barbados or Barcelona, but most do not 'imagine' that by so doing they can obtain valid and reliable information about these places. Yet this is precisely how Albert Einstein acquired the knowledge on which his epoch-making theories of relativity are based. His insights were based not on laboratory research, as might commonly be supposed, but on *Gedanken* or thought experiments in which he imagined himself travelling in space at the speed of light. He was subsequently able to translate the insights he derived from such 'flights of fantasy' into the language of mathematics and so communicate them to other scientists. The 'magic' worked by Einstein was precisely that described by shamans throughout the ages as a 'soul journey' into the Beyond. Einstein journeyed into the 'heavens', but he might equally have travelled to the underworld. It seems that the reason most people do not do likewise is simply because they do not imagine that they can. The images of dreams, fantasies, reverie and daydreaming are widely seen as vehicles of the soul; the means by which the soul expresses itself in everyday life. 'Your challenge as a human being caught in all the stimuli of life is to allow the blueprint of your soul to come into daily experience.'[125] However, most people ignore the pattern of their souls. The imagination is discouraged in favour of the rationality, reason, analysis and logic of ordinary consciousness.

The idea that ordinary consciousness acts as 'a reducing valve'[126] limiting perception in a way described by the Hindu as 'not-seeing', or *avidja*, has been put forward by many Western scientists. Psychologists and neuroscientists realise that reality is not what the eyes perceive, but is an interpretation made by the brain. The neuroscientist Karl Pribram indicates that the brain may act as a lens that transforms mathematically the blur of primary reality into hard reality. Without these mathematics humans would probably know a world organised in the frequency domain; a world without space and time such as that described by mystics throughout history and by modern physics. The physicist David Bohm also lent support to the mystical idea that what is essential is invisible to the eye. He suggested that humans learn to see the world in certain ways and so do not necessarily notice the primary order of the universe because they are habituated to the explicate order of manifest reality which is emphasised in thought and language, both of which are predominantly linear and sequential. Indeed, Western culture as a whole is habituated to the rational, logical, linear and sequential and to descriptions of a manifest explicate reality. Accordingly, the way the world is perceived and experienced is predominantly a mental construct with little reference to what actually is. Thus, consciousness is historically and geographically conditioned and represents only a small part of total consciousness.

The psychologist William James claimed that there is a continuum of consciousness against which our individuality builds barriers and as a result of this habitual tendency human beings use only a small part of their potential powers. Consequently, like the Buddha, he considered humans beings only half-awake and with a greatly restricted range of perception. 'I have no doubt whatever that most people live, whether physically, intellectually or morally, in a very restricted circle of their potential being. They make use of a very small portion of their possible consciousness and their souls' resources in general, much like a man who, out of his whole bodily organism, should get into the habit of using and moving only his little finger ... We all have reservoirs of life to draw upon, of which we do not dream.'[127] Given that ordinary consciousness is partial, an appropriate life task, as suggested by Jung, is to create more and more consciousness, 'to kindle a light in the darkness of mere being'.

Enlightenment is the aim of most traditional spiritual beliefs, especially in the East. These systems of belief all maintain that enlightenment can only be achieved when the blinkers imposed by the ordinary ego are transcended or circumvented in some way. Attainment of this egoless state is normally depicted as a studied path of spiritual development. It can occur haphazardly in many different ways. The physicist Danah Zohar has described the experience of losing her ego boundaries during pregnancy.

> During the pregnancy with my first child, and for some months after her birth, I experienced what for me was a strange new way of being. In many ways I lost the sense of myself as an individual, while at the same time gaining a sense of myself as part of some larger and ongoing process.
>
> At first the boundaries of my body extended inwards to embrace and become one with the new life growing inside me. I felt complete and self-contained, a microcosm within which *all* life was enfolded. Later, the boundaries extended outward to include the baby's own infant form. My body and my self existed to be a source of life and nurture, my rhythms were those of another, my senses became one with hers, and through her, with those of others round me.
>
> During those months, 'I' seemed a very vague thing, something on which I could not focus or get a grip, and yet I experienced myself as extending in all directions, backwards into 'before time' and forwards into 'all time', inwards towards all possibility and outwards towards all existence.[128]

She observes that Sigmund Freud would have called this an 'oceanic feeling', a term that resonates with the Hindu idea of the universal soul as an ocean. Such an experience is not confined to the 'earth mother', an image that in itself embodies the principles of the universal soul, but is also possible during sexual union and other states of bliss where the divine in each person is glimpsed.

> If it was once feared that one had to make a choice between intellect and emotion in answering the call of the Divine, then surely we may lay this fear to rest. If we choose to hearken exclusively to the soulless messages of science that have predominated up to now, for fear of compromising our reason,

then this choice can only be described as self-indulgence — for within science today we see the unmistakable emergence of a a new latitude for the human spirit which simply did not exist in the recent past. As the eminent physicist Werner Heisenberg was said, '"consciousness" and "spirit" can be related in a new way to the scientific conception of our time.'

In the end we can choose to continue to believe that we are local, isolated, doomed creatures confined to time and the body and set apart from all other human beings. Or we may elect to open our eyes to our immortal, omnipresent nature and the One Mind of which we are each part.[129]

This choice confronts both psychology and medicine as they enter the twenty-first century. If, however, they wish to retain any credibility as 'life' sciences they will not be able to stand against the progress of scientific knowledge and will need to accommodate the soul. To do so they will need to merge so as to address not only the whole person but also 'the whole of things' and reflect this change of perspective in all their procedures and practices.

The following chapters examine the principles that twenty-first century 'psychological' medicine will have to address as regards the therapeutic relationship, diagnosis and treatment.

THE THERAPEUTIC RELATIONSHIP: BEING A SOUL-MATE

What is 'psychological medicine'? If asked to define the term most doctors would probably identify it with psychiatry, while psychologists would describe it in various ways as clinical psychology, medical psychology, psychotherapy, behavioural medicine, behaviour therapy, psychoneuroimmunology or health psychology, depending on their theoretical orientation. Members of the general public might find the question difficult to answer because until relatively recently the modern disciplines of psychology and medicine have been largely divorced in both theory and practice, and many people are unclear about the distinctions between psychiatry and psychology. Furthermore, the term 'psychological medicine' is not included in dictionaries of psychology or medicine. Yet it has been used within both disciplines since 1872 when it appeared as the title of a classic textbook written by Daniel Hack Tuke. His use of the term was based on an analogy with organic medicine. He considered there to be diseases of the mind that affect intellectual and emotional functioning, just as diseases of the body affect physical functioning. Accordingly, psychological medicine is the appropriate term for that branch of medicine concerned with the diagnosis and treatment of mental diseases. Its use continued for several decades but was gradually overtaken by the term 'psychiatry'. One of the last textbooks to appear with this title was published in 1945.[1] However, 'Psychological medicine seems a very appropriate description for the aspect of medicine concerned with psychological factors in the predisposition, precipitation, perpetuation and prevention of disease. This term allows for a wide range of topical discussion, favours no particular theoretical position, and puts psychological medicine on an equal footing with chemical, botanical, nutritional, homeopathic, surgical, physical and other medicine that are used by the entire spectrum of practitioners and physicians.'[2] Hence it has been 'reincarnated' as mind–body or psychosomatic medicine, that is, the application of psychology to problems that are presented primarily as somatic disorders.[3]

However, the term 'psychological medicine' derives from the Latin *medicina*, the art of healing, and the Greek words *psyche*, soul, and *logos*, usually translated as 'study' or 'knowledge'. Literally, therefore, 'psychological medicine' means applying knowledge of the soul in the art of healing. From this perspective, psychological medicine becomes a very ancient discipline rather than a modern subset of either psychology or medicine because it embodies the principles that form the basis of the healing arts in every culture since the earliest times. These principles are fully consistent with the latest developments in scientific understanding, which point to the limitations of the biophysical or biomedical model on which orthodox healing approaches in the West have been based for the last two hundred years. This model, which focuses almost exclusively on the body, is quite aberrant in the history of medicine, and is simply inadequate to deal with the true nature and complexity of living beings.

> This leaves a vast area that is badly taught, poorly understood and indeed almost ignored by modern Western medicine — the mind, the soul and the spirit. So badly have most doctors been trained in these area that they can't even recognise the malfunction of the mind, soul or spirit when it stares them in the face, and if they did, most of them wouldn't be adequately trained to cope with it.[4]

Western medical 'science' is based on a totally outmoded scientific model of the universe which is no longer tenable, a model that was fundamentally flawed from the outset, but which is now inappropriate to the world we live in. The scientific vision of nature is undergoing a radical change that is proceeding on all levels and resulting in an understanding of the world totally new in the West. While the physical sciences have recognised this and attempted from the early years of the twentieth century to revise their model, medicine has ignored these developments almost totally. Mistaking it for science, medicine remains 'steeped in the superstition of materialism'.[5] This superstition is that the world is made up of physical objects in space and time and, if there is such a thing as thought or consciousness, it is the epiphenomenon of matter and occurs because of biochemical reactions within the body. The consequences are considerable, and clearly evident in a widely acknowledged crisis within Western medicine.

The need for a new medical model

Simply stated, 'medicine isn't right and we know it.'[6] Evidence to support this claim may be found in prestigious medical journals and research reports. These reveal that there is no direct relation between changes in disease patterns and the 'progress' of medicine and that the environment is the primary determinant of the general health status of any population. 'People are healthier today not because they receive all this well-publicised better treatment when ill, but simply because they tend not to become ill in the first place.'[7] Therefore the effectiveness of doctors is largely illusory. So too is the role of drugs in combating infection. Two-thirds of people receiving drugs in treatment suffer side-effects, in many cases more serious than the problem being treated and in the USA more people die annually from adverse drug effects than on the roads.[8] Results of the world's first study on hospital safety in 1995 show that one in six people are hospitalised because some medical treatment has gone wrong, and there is a 16 per cent chance of dying or suffering injury while there. Since half the risk is caused by doctors or hospital error, there is an 8 per cent chance of being killed by hospital staff. In the USA, where some 40,000 people are shot dead each year, a person is three times more likely to be killed by a doctor than a gun.[9] Some 1.17 million Britons are hospitalised each year as a result of doctor error or a bad reaction to a drug. This is equivalent to the entire population of a city the size of Birmingham.[10] These are just a few of the statistics that suggest medicine itself has become a major health threat, with levels of dysfunction, disability and morbidity resulting from its technical interventions rivalling those as a result of traffic- and work-related incidents and even war.[11]

The expression of discontent is not confined to medical journals. Almost everyone knows of those who have suffered desperately from treatment methods, incorrect diagnosis or treatment, whose records or test results have been lost, or who have been told 'ten different truths by ten different doctors'.[12] Such experiences have led many people to lose confidence in medicine and to question its progress and its emphasis which is predominantly on 'plumbing'.[13]

Many nurses are disillusioned with current approaches to health. Although they are trained to assess and respond to the person at every level, in practice within the existing system this holistic approach is denied. This, and the fixed attitudes in medicine, are major causes of staff wastage in nursing.[14] The failure of many doctors to respond to patients as human beings also accounts for much of the drift to 'alternative medicine', whose proliferation is clear testimony to dissatisfaction with orthodox medicine. An increasingly well-informed general public is becoming progressively disappointed with the failure of scientific medicine to live up to its promise and fulfil popular expectations. 'Advice like "it's your age" or "you'll have to learn to put up with it" are beginning to wear a bit thin and many people are searching desperately for alternatives that will hold the promise of improved health.'[15] The number of alternative medicine consultations is increasing dramatically in all developed countries. Surveys suggest that the major reasons for this are orthodox medicine's neglect of psychosocial factors such as the doctor–patient relationship and the failure to satisfy other personal needs, and the emphasis of alternative approaches on treating the whole person. The more personal and holistic approach of non-orthodox medicine is preferred by women in the USA[16] where most female patients surveyed use some form of unorthodox medicine at some time in their lives. Indeed in the USA the projected growth of alternative medicine into the twenty-first century predicts an 88 per cent increase in supply of alternative medicine by 2010 compared with a growth in the supply of physicians by 16 per cent.[17]

The implication of this is that if orthodox medicine retains its status as the form of medicine authorised by the state in most western countries, it will continue to be 'orthodox' in the narrow political sense but may no longer be 'orthodox' in the cultural sense of being the form in which the public at large has the most confidence and regards as the most legitimate.[18]

HRH The Prince of Wales voiced the views of many when in his address to the British Medical Association in 1982 he observed that, for all its successes, medicine, like another imposing edifice, the Tower of Pisa, is slightly off-balance. He claimed that one of the most unfortunate consequences of this unhealthy imbalance — which he attributed to a move away from traditional methods of psychological healing towards biomedical therapeutics — is that the patient's emotional, mental and spiritual needs are lost sight of.

Indeed this 'loss of vision' is the fundamental problem underpinning the current crisis in Western medicine, rather than economic recession, government under-funding, government policies, widening economic division, mass unemployment and failure to tackle smoking, alcohol use and poor nutrition — all recent explanations for the failure of modern medicine. The fundamental crisis in modern medicine, and one that urgently needs to be addressed is not finance, politics or organisation but perception — the way in which the universe and man's place in it are viewed. Western medicine has built its notions of health and disease around a particular view of the universe. The world-view underpinning orthodox medicine generally remains unquestioned. It is assumed to be correct and the only view possible in the light of modern discoveries and knowledge. This idea has become a set of blinkers, preventing many people in the medical establishment from seeing that the world-view that emerged in the physical sciences in the West in the twentieth century is radically different from those on which its medicine is based.

An inability to see the whole picture emerging from the physical sciences also maintains the strong divisions that traditionally segregate orthodox medicine from 'alternatives', physics from metaphysics, biology from cosmology and science from religion.

The new knowledge emerging in such fields as physics and biology ·is, however, moving towards the recognition of a common ground or centre in which it is increasingly apparent that all systems (whether of a physical or metaphysical nature) come together and meet each other. It is at this centre or meeting point that we encounter the blueprint or matrix for the life of the human organism which provides the potential formula for our new model.

This blueprint emanating from the universal mind is identifiable in each and every one of us, and is unique for each individual human life. Our understanding of its formulation has significant implications for the future of medicine as it may provide doctors and practitioners with a broader insight in the diagnosis of the underlying causes of illness and disease. At the same time it offers physical and metaphysical medicine the potential to heal illness and disease and within the blueprint by healing the patient's mind and the physical body and giving direction to that patient for their own evolution within the universal order. The course of this setting and unfolding is affected by the interplay of numerous energetic forces which, in acting through the various subtle bodies as well as the physical body, combine together to form the whole individual. The continued good health of the individual organism as a whole depends upon the maintenance of a harmonious balance between these different energetic forces within the blueprint of life of each individual — and this harmonious balance has the potential to be sustained or regulated through the energetic elements of allopathic and complementary medicine ...

Medical practice has shown that it is also possible to heal humans and animals through the corrective influence of the mind and its projected thoughts. For us to explore this potential for healing within the universal order the traditional medical or biophysical model of man as an individual mechanism needs to be replaced by a new model that incorporates these additional universal dimensions.[19]

Principles of a new medical model

What are the principles of a new model of healing that incorporates the universal dimensions being addressed at the cutting edge of contemporary science? These principles have always been at the forefront of traditional psychologies and religions. The first principle, as it applies to this model and to all creation, is that of unity or oneness. The universe, from the Latin *universus*, all together, is a whole in which there are no separate parts, in which everything is connected or related. **Relationship** is fundamental to the universe and therefore to healing, which literally means 'making whole'. Literally, and traditionally, health means wholeness, and incorporates being at every level: physical, psychological (mental and emotional), ecological and spiritual. It concerns the ways in which an individual relates within itself, to others, the environment and the universe. These are the fundamental concerns addressed by shamanism, which underpins all traditional forms of healing throughout the world. In traditional medicine illness is considered a disruption, a breach in relationship at any level, and healing is viewed as restoring relationship or harmony, joining together (from the Latin *harmonus* meaning joint) that which has come apart, making a connection. The healer recognises the whole of things and does not consider disease an isolated phenomenon. This principle is embodied in the Hippocratic doctrine:

> There is one common flow, one common breathing; all things are in sympathy.

As a consequence the unified field is self-organising. It does not refer to anything outside because there is nothing it does not include. This self-organising principle is evident throughout nature. The human body is a self-organising field.

> There are six trillion reactions occurring in the human body every second, and every one of them is correlated with every single other reaction; every single other biochemical event knows what other biochemical event is occurring in the body. A human body can think thoughts, play a piano, sing a song, digest food, eliminate toxins, kill germs, monitor the movement of stars, and make a new baby all at the same time, and correlate each of these activities with every other activity. So, inherent in the field itself is infinite organising power.[20]

Traditional medicine recognises the life force inherent in all living things as nature's healing power, referred to by Hippocrates as the *vix medicatrix naturae*, and that fundamentally all healing is self-healing; something an organism does to and for itself. Although a physician may suture a wound or splint a bone fracture, these procedures do not in themselves bring about healing. They merely assist the body's own self-healing by creating the most favourable conditions for such a process. In traditional medicine the healer is considered simply a servant of nature whose role is that of helping nature heal itself: restoring the balance disturbed by disease but not interfering with nature. Hence the healer is a therapist — literally (from the Greek *therapeia*, attendance) an attendant to the healing process. Hence, fundamental to the new model of medicine is the understanding that 'Treatment is not pills. It is the way we treat people. The way we attend to them.'[21] Treatment is about relating to others in ways that facilitate the healing process.

The therapeutic relationship

Probably the most despised aspect of contemporary Western medicine is the 'five-minute consultation', the maximum period of time a patient can ordinarily expect to spend with a practitioner in general practice. The attention the patient receives from the doctor may be cursory. The doctor often pays more attention to written case notes or computer records, and delegates collection of fluid samples, measuring of blood pressure and such like to nursing assistants. Often the doctor's only task is to administer a hastily written and often illegible prescription for drugs or other preparations, explanations about which may be left to the dispensing pharmacist. This procedure does not conform to what most people think of as 'attention'. Nor does it conform to the literal meaning of the term that derives from the Latin *attendere* meaning to reach out. Attention, quite literally, is an attempt at relationship, a reaching out towards something; if the shift towards complementary medicine in the developed world shows anything at all, it is that more and more people are choosing to seek attention in practices other than those of orthodox medicine. Concerns about communication with doctors, or more usually the lack of it, are among the chief reasons given for seeking alternative treatment.[22]

Most of the alternative approaches to treatment commence with a lengthy history-taking of the patient as a whole person. This focuses not only on symptoms of illness but on details of personal history, lifestyle, attitudes, preferences and such like. It is both objective and subjective in that it takes into account the individual's perception and interpretation of his or her symptoms and individual features. The encounter between the practitioner and the patient is an intimate interaction for both — it 'remains personal within the frame of impersonal professional treatment'.[23] The practitioner is therefore a therapeutic partner in the healing process rather than remaining 'external' to it. In homeopathy, for example, the homeopath 'is not merely a passive observer protected behind a wall of objectivity. Each patient engages the homeopath in a deep and meaningful way ... When homeopathy is practiced with this degree of involvement it stimulates growth in the homeopath just as it does for the patient.'[24] The reciprocal action of relation between therapist and client was also considered fundamental by Jung, who insisted that 'the doctor is effective only when he himself is affected ... When the doctor wears his personality like a coat of armour he has no effect.'[25] This understanding underpins all traditional forms of healing, such as Tibetan medicine:

> The feeling tone of the healing experience is extremely important, perhaps more important than the specifics of medical practice. A certain caring and trust has to be present and mutually experienced.[26]

In order to reach out or attend so as to connect with another there must be nothing in the way. Normally, there is a good deal in the way — ego, or self, and all the baggage that implies. Ego tends to demand attention for itself. The therapist who wants to make a good impression, be liked by patients or clients and appear knowledgeable, who worries about inadequacy or failure and is concerned with his or her own affairs, is attending to him or her self and cannot possibly give full attention to another person. Hence ego acts as armour, as a barrier between people. Most Western people are very attached to ego and wish to strengthen rather than diminish it. They do so through the power and responsibility invested in social roles that confer status, standing, identity and respect. Some roles are more powerful and prestigious than others, and one of the most powerful and respected roles in Western culture is that of physician. Many are attracted to the role for this reason and most of those in the role are very attached to it, and all it implies, and tend to act in ways they see as consistent with it. Hence, Western medical practitioners tend to be heavily armoured. They typically adopt a 'professional manner' whenever they are in the presence of patients or clients, having been carefully trained to do so.

The problem is that the professional role, the *persona* — literally, from the Latin for mask — can act as a barrier to any real contact. Hence the 'helping' role of the medical practitioner is often a major impediment to actual help. It can not only prove unhelpful but can be downright dangerous, even deadly in some circumstances. It has been observed[27] that some hospital nurses may be so concerned with giving the impression that they have a 'good bedside manner' that they consequently do not listen to what patients are trying to tell them. In some cases, despite all the apparent attention given to patients by plumping up their pillows and telling them that they are in good hands, they failed to attend to what the patient was trying to communicate. As a result, cases were found where the nurses did not discover allergies to penicillin or other drugs, which when subsequently administered proved almost or actually fatal.

Attending to others is not about *doing* anything; it is about *being*. In order to attend effectively to another, a person must be able, temporarily at least, to suspend his or her ego and enter into an ego-less state — a state of authentic being, so that the ego does not act as a barrier to contact and allows the other person to be the focus of the encounter. This state can be likened to a meditative or Zen state,[28] a state of consciousness altered from the usual state of preoccupation with oneself and one's world. The ego-less state of the therapist, like that of the master in Eastern and magical traditions, can be likened to a mirror that reflects but does not hold reality, and so reveals it in a non-selective way.

This principle of mirroring or reflection is central to Carl Rogers' ideas about therapy. He indicated that, provided the therapist can put aside or suspend his or her ego, the other person will effectively be facing themselves, encouraged to talk as if to a mirror and, in so doing, will be confronting features of themselves, possibly for the first time. Rogers' therapy focused on mirroring the verbal communication of the person and, as the Chinese sage Lao Tzu observed, 'such listening as this enfolds us in silence in which we begin to hear what we are meant to be'. However, it is also possible to mirror facial expression, postures and gestures, beliefs or physiology. Rogers claimed that confronted with such sustained reflection, persons attend more to themselves and come to see themselves more clearly. Their awareness progresses from the general to the specific; from the superficial to the deep; from thoughts to feelings; and from the abstract to the concrete — a similar progression as that resulting from meditational practices that traditionally aim to develop 'soulfulness' and insight. These new insights can then be used for personal growth and change.

Rogers claimed that when persons see themselves and their situation more clearly they are able to make choices, find solutions, take responsibility for their actions and increase their freedom. Similarly, in Buddhist meditation, by focusing on the gaps or spaces between thoughts, going beyond the illusion of self — the realm of infinite possibilities, ultimate freedom, is accessed.

> Freedom is inherent in the unified field, and when we contact that field then freedom comes to us. It is freedom that comes from the experiential knowledge of one's real nature. And our real nature is that we are the joyful, silent witness, the nonattached, immortal spirit that animates all manifestation. And to have the experience of that silent witness is to just Be.
>
> This is real freedom — the ability to enjoy the choices we make in every successive moment of the present. It is the ability to spontaneously put our attention on those choices that bring joy to us and also to others.[29]

Hence Roger's therapeutic relationship, like meditation, provides 'space' for creative action and change. The catalytic role of the therapist is to remind the person of his or her freedom.

Somewhat paradoxically, therefore — given Carl Rogers' 'self theory' and what many see as 'self-centred' therapy — achieving an ego-less state of being is the essence of the therapeutic relationship he described and advocated, and at the very core of the humanistic therapies he inspired. His thinking was based on the premise that self-actualisation, which is synonymous with wholeness or integration, is the aim of therapy. Consistent with traditional healers who considered expression of the soul or essential blueprint as life's purpose, Rogers' ideal of health was actualisation of the authentic or ideal self, as opposed to the actual self or ego which is the product of social conditioning. He believed that the actualising tendency in every individual awaits only the proper conditions to be realised. He insisted that while the potential for actualisation resides within the individual, the conditions for its facilitation lie in a relationship which is emotionally warm, free from evaluation and allows freedom for the person to be fully him- or herself. He claimed that these 'conditions of worth' must be a feature of therapeutic relationships if they are to be effective.

The type of therapeutic relationship Rogers sought to provide has several important qualities. The first is authenticity or genuineness. The therapist must be him- or herself and not present any façade or defensive front, openly being the feelings and attitudes that are flowing in the moment and willing to express them where appropriate. There is harmony or congruence between what the therapist is at any point in time and what he or she appears to be. If the therapist is experiencing one thing in the relationship but endeavours to be something else then this condition is not met. Rogers claimed that the less the therapist hides and presents a façade, the more accurately he or she can listen to what another person is trying to communicate and the more likely it is that the person will feel empathically understood. By being congruent, the therapist is offering the opportunity for a genuine encounter with the other person because in being him- or herself the therapist allows the other person to be him- or herself also. In other words, when the therapist is able to 'bare his soul' and be fully authentic in a relationship he or she acts as a catalyst enabling another person to do the same. This ability to 'be and let be' means that the therapist does not 'do' therapy, but lives it:

> He does not seek to make interpretations, he does not evaluate and judge; he allows what is to be, so that it can reveal itself in the essence of its being and then proceeds to elucidate what he understands.[30]

Being and letting be means that the therapist accepts the other person unconditionally, just as he or she is, irrespective of his or her circumstances or condition, behaviour, attitudes and feelings. Rogers emphasised that attending to a person is not about doing anything to or for them but is simply about *being*. In his view, simply being attentive, caring, open and genuine is therapeutic and brings about positive changes that move other people in the direction of wholeness and health. Rogers claimed that within such a relationship significant changes are possible because there is implicit freedom for individuals to explore their true selves. These changes include greater acceptance and awareness of feelings they have lost touch with, living life according to their personal values rather than those of others, and trusting the spontaneous aspects of themselves.

It is often wrongly supposed that the principles of the therapeutic relationship set out by Carl Rogers apply only in the field of psychotherapy. However, what he described is the common human bond, generally known as rapport.

> Rapport is the ability to enter someone else's world, to make him feel that you understand him, that you have a strong common bond. It's the ability to go fully from your map of the world to his map of the world. It's the essence of good communication.[31]

It is essentially a relationship of trust — a relationship in which 'people feel as though they've found their soul-mate, someone who really understands who can read their deepest thoughts, who is just like them'.[32] and of responsiveness. People respond positively to those with whom they have rapport and this connection is undoubtedly very powerful. This is nowhere more evident than with people in coma. Arnold Mindell[33] points out that *connecting* with comatose persons is all-important. By communicating congruently — speaking in the rhythm of their breathing and touching them so that the verbal message matches the non-verbal message, it is possible to establish rapport. He suggests that the individual's breathing rate matches the experiences he or she is having and so speaking and touching the person at the same rate is communicating on his or her wavelength or frequency. Many people in persistent vegetative comatose states will respond to these attempts at relating by giving minimal cues such as changes of breathing rates or eye and mouth motion indicating that contact has been established. He claims not to have met any person in coma who has not responded to this kind of encouraging, interested and gentle interaction. He indicates that after the comatose person begins to respond the process involves relating to his or her experiences in the modality in which they are expressed. Listening to and mirroring breathing patterns and sounds is important because they can convey much information. As Mindell observes, the process is similar to ordinary forms of psychotherapy and allows the signals descriptive of the state to unfold. It is a form of refined communication. An intimate relationship in which the therapist helps a person in this state to work on and communicate with themslves. 'We are teaching the person to reflect, meditate, and value altered-state experiences in order that they may become self-healing and elucidative. Thus the lessons we learn from working with comas will be applicable in all of our relationships.'[34] Rogers observed that within such relationships healthy biological changes may occur. Support for this claim comes from studies of healing.

Healing

'Healing' is the term most commonly used to refer to contact healing by the laying-on of hands. It is almost certainly the most widespread therapy in the world, the most ancient, and possibly the most misunderstood. As a result it is not widely accepted by modern medicine, although there is more supporting evidence for its efficacy than for most of the complementary therapies combined.[35, 36] There is documentary and pictorial evidence for its use in Western civilisations since the times of the ancient Egyptians and Greeks, but nowhere is it more evident than in the scriptures of the early Christian Church.

Christ appeared to teach of a spiritual realm in which healing energies work more powerfully than man ever dreamed, and in this respect his teachings were fully consistent with those of ancient traditions of both the East and West. He directed his disciples to heal with this knowledge. There can be little doubt that Christ's original mission was to establish a healing ministry.[37] Healing the body played an enormous role in the early Christian period, as the Acts of the Apostles reveal. Numerous acts of healing by Christ are documented, as are those of his followers, Peter, John, Ananias and Paul.[38] The laying-on of hands therefore became an established religious practice. Indeed, as a result of its purges on witches and other 'lay' healers whose practices were condemned as 'the work of the devil', the Church held a monopoly on healing from the Middle Ages onwards. In Britain until 1951 lay healers were under threat of prosecution under the Witchcraft Act, which carried a death penalty, and in the USA they were subject to legal prohibition of anyone without a recognised qualification manipulating another's body. As a result, the practice of healing in both countries tended to be confined within churches, outside of which it has flourished only since relaxation of these laws.

Healers in Britain have been able to treat patients in hospitals since 1959, but only in 1977 did the General Medical Council change its policy and allow doctors to suggest or agree to patients seeing healers. Negative attitudes towards healing no doubt owe much to the legacy of the Church and its opposition to witchcraft, but a good deal results from misunderstanding of what healing involves. Its religious connotations have to a great extent meant that healing is widely thought to be synonymous with faith healing, and its effects the results of suggestion.

Belief and suggestion have an undisputed role in all healing, including orthodox medical treatment and cure as is amply demonstrated by the *placebo effect*, but these factors do not account adequately for the effects of the laying-on of hands. Faith, belief or suggestion are merely an auxiliary to actual healing,[39] and if this were not so, the healing of children, the mentally ill, those with learning difficulties, animals and those unaware of receiving this form of treatment could not occur. Yet it does. 'There is solid experimental work and enough careful evaluation of reported claims to make this clear.'[40]

Experiments using plants and animals as experimental subjects eliminate the possibility that the effects of healing are attributable to the patient's beliefs. A series of double-blind experiments established that a noted healer, Oskar Estebany, was able to prevent the development of thyroid goitres in mice, and injured mice healed much faster than controls when he held his hands over them.[41] He was also able to significantly affect plants and fungi in this way.[42, 43]

Other experiments[44, 45] revealed that Estebany was able to increase enzyme reactions over time, and that the longer he held a test-tube of enzymes the more rapid the reaction. Similar effects have been noted in response to high-intensity electromagnetic fields. Indeed it was found that Estebany's hands, although not emanating any measurable 'energy', affected the digestive enzyme Trypsin in a way that was comparable to the effects of an electromagnetic field measuring 8–13,000 gauss (normally human beings live in an electromagnetic field of 0.5 gauss). Irrespective of the type of enzyme investigated the change noted after exposure to the healer's hands was always in a direction of greater health of the cells and greater energy balance. Other noted healers, such as Olga and Ambrose Worrall, could cause damaged enzymes to reintegrate and return to normal structure and function, and enhance plant growth. The latter effect was subsequently confirmed in other experiments.[46] Other studies of Olga Worrall[47] used a cloud chamber, an electron detection device developed by nuclear physicists to make visible the path of high-energy particles. The experimental procedure involved Mrs Worrall placing her hands around the apparatus in an attempt to determine whether they might exert any influence on its uniform vapour pattern. They were found to produce a wave pattern in the vapour that seemed to move vertically from her palms, and altered course when she changed the position of her hands — an effect not found in any non-healer control subjects. Furthermore, she could affect the cloud chamber from a distance of 600 miles, when it was found that the aftermath of the energy turbulence in the chamber took about eight minutes to subside.

Studies of healers have shown that they can affect living tissue *in situ*. Following treatment by Estebany, the haemoglobin levels of patients exceeded pre-treatment levels,[48] and other healers could also accelerate repair in living organisms.[49] Furthermore, after receiving training from Estebany, nurses could also produce statistically significant effects.[50]

The British healer Matthew Manning was found in various studies to be able to prolong by up to four times the life of red blood cells in a weak salt solution in which they would normally burst. (The probability of this occurring by chance is 100,000:1). He was also able to influence cancer cells in sealed containers. Indeed, of 140 controlled trials of healing on enzymes, cells *in vitro*, yeasts, bacteria, plants, animals and humans, 61 per cent demonstrated highly significant effects and another 16 per cent showed marginally significant effects.[51]

Manning's brain wave patterns during healing have been found to show a large increase in low *theta* and *delta* range frequencies, a pattern which has been termed a 'ramp function' because of its appearance on EEG records. This pattern, suggestive of very deep sleep, has been found to originate in the limbic system of the brain, and Canadian studies have shown that it is transferred to people receiving healing from him. Moreover, when held by him, the hands of those receiving healing show a highly unusual Kirlian image with a brilliant white corona. Other healers have also been shown to produce greater corona emanations during healing.[52, 53]

The EEG patterns of healers while healing are similar to those of clairvoyants and yogis[54] and the brain wave patterns of those receiving healing alter simultaneously with those of the healer, suggesting energetic resonance between them. 'The diverse range of experimental data on the biological effects of healing is supportive of the hypothesis that a real energetic influence is exerted by healers on sick organisms.'[55] Furthermore, this would appear to be exerted while healers are in a highly relaxed state.

Most healers believe that they are originators or transmitters of energy they attribute to various sources. Some healers experience this energy physically as a pattern of activity within their hands and body, and heal by trying to transmit it to another person by way of the hands. The attempt to heal by 'doing' something to or for a person in this way has been distinguished as quite different from and less important than healing where the healer attempts to do nothing other than experience a feeling of being 'at one' with the person to be healed.[56] However, this is a false distinction because a universal feature common to all healing, irrespective of idiosyncratic rituals, is that all healers do one thing similarly; they shift consciousness and become one with the person to be healed, albeit momentarily. This is not achieved by concentration, but on the contrary, by mental abandonment or relaxation. The resulting state of being united or in harmony with another is similar to Rogers' concept of empathy in which the person attends or reaches out towards another without barriers. Accordingly 'true healing is a partnership between healer and patient. The removal of the personality barrier results in a condition known as contact or rapport.'[57] Hence despite appearances to the contrary, the contact achieved by the laying-on of hands is not physical but psychological.

A seminal study of healing by the psychologist Lawrence LeShan confirmed that healers do not 'act' in the sense of doing anything. Rather, they enter a state of consciousness in which they simply and literally perceive themselves and the person to be healed as one entity within a metaphysical system which LeShan terms 'the clairvoyant reality'. Within this frame of reference, reality is clearly perceived as a timeless and unified whole in which there are no boundaries and nothing is separated from anything else. All things flow into each other and are part of a larger whole where neither time nor space can prevent exchange of information and energy. LeShan suggests that when healers alter their consciousness to this clairvoyant mode with the person to be healed as its focus, they are able to mobilise the self-repair system of that person, even at a distance, simply by bringing them to mind.

> Remember, attention brings the particle into existence out of a probability amplitude, out of a field of all possibilities. Attention is the very mechanics of precipitating a space–time event in the field of all possibilities. So when we put our attention on that particular quality of the field, it brings it not only into our awareness, but into our life in its material expression.[58]

In this mode the healer does not attempt to 'do' anything to the person but simply 'is' at one with them.

> When the healer — for a moment — absolutely knows this to be true, that he and the healee are one, the healee sometimes responds with a mobilization of his self-repair and recuperative abilities.[59]

LeShan proposes that when the healer attends with love, which is equivalent with Rogers' concept of unconditional positive regard, this is in some way transmitted to the healee, who knows it also. The healee is then in a different existential position, part of a unity or whole, and more complete. This, LeShan observes, constitutes healing, and under these conditions positive biological changes may occur. The world-renowned British healer Harry Edwards has described the relationship between healer and healee as establishing an interplay of energy that is frequently experienced by one, other or both parties and accelerates the patient's self-healing. In physical terms this may be thought of as a state of attunement or harmony in which the healer 'gets on the same wavelength' as the other person, enabling healing to occur through the principle of resonance. In psychological terms it is the removal of personality barriers that allows this to occur.

> The boundaries between one and another may be temporarily removed so completely that, for the time being, the two personalities become merged into one. Now the action which takes place between healer and patient depends on this principle.[60]

Accordingly, it is the relationship between the healer and the healee that is healthy in the sense that it is integrative, or wholesome. Nevertheless, LeShan considers that the changes that occur in the healee's body as a result of this union are confined to the kind of result the body can normally achieve on its own under optimal conditions, and that the healer cannot influence these energies in any way. The healer is therefore constrained to 'be' rather than to 'do'.

As the contact between healer and healee is essentially a psychological relationship between them, it follows that physically laying on hands is not a requirement of the process. Indeed, in most cases hands are laid on the body only when the psychological relationship has been established and is only done to reinforce the psychic contact already established. Healing can be achieved without any physical intervention of any kind. That this is in fact the case is suggested by the phenomenon of absent or distant healing, in which the healer makes psychic contact with a person at a distance, without even being in their presence.

LeShan considered that everyone has the ability to heal, and that it can be trained. In 1970 he established a five-day training programme and found that of some 400 people who took part in the course over a ten-year period, 80–90 per cent learned to alter their consciousness to the clairvoyant mode and achieve positive biological changes in others. LeShan's results support Edwards' claims who observed that, despite appearances to the contrary, any ritual of 'doing' is unnecessary in healing and may even be an impediment because, ultimately, healing is a state of mind or quality of being. However, having trained himself and others to heal in this way, LeShan admitted having 'not the faintest idea as to why it gets results or what is happening', despite having claimed that the frame of reference he calls the clairvoyant reality is common to mystics, mediums and physicists. These categories of person would all probably agree that what they share is an ability to perceive and thereby access the field of infinite possibilities, the unified or quantum field, and within that creative realm to bring about changes.

> If the student has grasped all that has been said on the subject of spirit and matter, he will see that in mental treatment time and space count for nothing because the whole action takes place on a plane where these conditions do not obtain; and it is therefore quite immaterial whether the patient be in the immediate presence of the healer or in a distant country.[61]

It is not what a therapist does that is important, but what he or she is. The effective therapist can be likened to a magnet, a metallic substance within which there is a characteristic organisation of domains or regions in which all the atoms have their magnetic moments aligned in the same direction, as a result of which it attracts and magnetises other metals. A magnet, therefore, does not 'do' magnetism — it *is* magnetic: the very nature of its being effects changes in other substances. Rogers' notion of congruence can be compared with magnetism in that it implies an internal organisation or harmony. The greater the degree of harmony within the individual the greater is his or her ability to facilitate this in others. Effective therapists therefore elicit and reinforce authenticity in others by manifesting it themselves. The harmony in such therapists arises essentially because they are at one with their true nature, aligned within themselves to their essence or soul. They may also align consciously or unconsciously with the universe, grounding themselves in that fundamental reality. By so doing they become more forceful. According to unified field theory, the more integrated and unified a physical field the more force it exerts. It therefore 'appears quite incontravertible that in any interaction between two persons, especially when one is more congruent and the other is less congruent, that some 'directive' influence will occur, however unconscious or unintentional'.[62] Studies[63] have shown that when therapists are open others respond in like manner. Hence a resonance or sympathetic relationship occurs.

Establishing rapport

The principles of the therapeutic relationship as identified by Rogers, LeShan and Edwards in which the therapist does nothing other than simply be open and spontaneous is quite alien to the West. It is not that the nature of the therapeutic relationship is not understood in the West, where it has been subjected to considerable scholarly investigation. It is rather that Western medical practitioners, for the most part, choose to ignore it or to rely on the rather overused excuse that they simply do not have time to engage in such relationships with their patients. There are several reasons for this, all rooted in Western psychology. One is the mistaken idea that time is something one has rather than makes; that treating people is a race against time; and that it is better to treat more people 'at a time' than to treat fewer people effectively. It is not *time* people need but attention, not the quantity or 'amount' but the quality that matters. These ideas arise because the majority of Western practitioners have been conditioned not to simply 'be' but to do, which means performance is usually measured against time, and they are obsessively concerned with means, ends, objectives, outcomes, performance and achievement. There is a considerable dread of passivity among therapists,[64] who are frequently attracted to techniques that make them feel they are doing something to make their patients well. The authority, power and prestige conferred by such techniques have considerable appeal, with the additional attraction that they can be learned. Yet herein lies the danger; in becoming technically efficient, all too often they have become inefficient in human qualities such as awareness that cannot be achieved technically. Technical behaviour may impress patients but to the extent that it is a manipulation of them, rather than an open spontaneous response, it often produces vigorous defences rather than rapport. This is no less true of attempts to 'do' things to put people at ease such as effecting certain postures or mannerisms.

However, patients are also conditioned to doing rather than being. Most people in Western culture, conditioned to doing and 'always being on the go' simply do not know what it means to rest and may become more tense and anxious if they are required to. Yet rest can be viewed simply as another way of providing a person with much-needed space in which change can occur. This may provide an opportunity to regroup energies, allowing the person to be revitalised. A period of rest or non-doing may allow the person to get in touch with him- or herself again. When a person stops listening, however temporarily, to what others expect of them, they may be able to hear their own inner voice and its wisdom. The person may learn from that inner self the correct course of action and be able to cultivate it as a guide or ally to self-healing and growth. This understanding is that of both the shaman and the psychotherapist. However, it may not be that of the 'patient'.

The expectation in the West that something has to be done to or for patients in order to make them well is another reason why rest cures tend to be ineffective. Patients expect, and often demand, medical practitioners to do something for them, even if this is little more than to please them by giving them a prescription for inappropriate medicines, as is the case where antibiotics are prescribed for viral infections they cannot treat. This insistence on the doctor doing something to help is currently a major problem in Western medicine; it is responsible for the development of super bugs resistant to antibiotics and the proliferation of pointless surgical procedures such as most hysterectomies. Nevertheless, the doctor pleasing the patient can in itself be the most powerful medicine of all.

The power of the placebo

The word *placebo*, Latin for 'I shall please', refers to a medicine or procedure with no intrinsic therapeutic value, which is applied more to please and placate the patient than any other reason. It is highly probable that many remedies of traditional medicine considered highly effective by patients and revered by physicians such as crocodile blood, asses' hooves and putrid meat were placebos, and throughout history medical practitioners have quite deliberately exploited the power of placebos. Within Western medicine 'placebo' is a pejorative term implying quackery and pseudoscience. The 'doctor who resides within'[65] has been dismissed as a nuisance factor that contaminates the effects of 'real' treatments rather than nature's own pharmacy at work. For this reason, placebos — fake substances — are used in control studies when drugs are tested to find out exactly how much effect is the action of the drug or whether the drug's effectiveness is really the patient's imagination. Although it has long been acknowledged that the prescription paper rather than what is written on it is often the vital ingredient in recovery, it is only relatively recently that placebos have been systematically investigated. They have been demonstrated to be as or more effective that real medicines in the treatment of pain and a variety of diseases ranging from hay fever to rheumatoid arthritis, which implicate the autonomic, endocrine, and immune systems. It is now recognised that the placebo can have more profound effects on organic illness — including 'incurable' malignancies — than conventional drugs. Studies suggest that a 55 per cent placebo reaction is involved in the administration of every medication and therapeutic procedure.[66] This response is likely to vary according to circumstances and physiological make up of the individual but the relationship between the therapist and patient is undoubtedly a highly significant factor. This is because the placebo, rather than being a pill or a procedure, is a process which begins with the patient's confidence or trust in the therapist and then extends through to the full functioning of his or her own immunological and healing system.[67] A person can be given exactly the same inert preparation and, depending on the label given to it by the doctor, can convert it into a beta blocker, stimulant, anxiolytic, antidepressant or anti-cancer drug. Given such a substance and told that it is a painkiller, a person will produce painkilling effects that cannot be reversed by a narcotic antagonist and so, in effect, is producing substances more powerful than morphine. The same inert substance, when used to treat ulcers, may be converted into an H2 receptor blocker, a specific molecule that has to interfere with hydrochloric acid binding to the receptor. When given to treat high blood pressure, the same substance may be converted into a specific molecule — a beta blocker — that could not be more different. A patient given such a substance as an anti-cancer treatment may find that his or her hair falls out and the gums begin to bleed. What this means is that in each case a person converts a belief into a very specific molecule, that is, a very different biochemical reality, which in turn produces a very different physiological result.[68] So-called 'miracle cures' can be effected in this way.

However, what were formerly considered miracles must be considered today's science. The understanding emerging from PNI is that the way a person interprets events determines his or her physiology. For example, if a person enjoys a ride on a roller coaster his or her body produces Interleukin 2, and interferons, substances that stimulate the immune system. Whereas if the ride creates panic, the body produces cortisol and adrenalin which destroy the immune system. Similarly every thought, feeling, emotion or desire a person has is transformed into peptides, 'messenger molecules from inner space',[69] located throughout the body. Accordingly, the cells, not only of the immune system but of the entire body, can be considered to be 'eavesdropping' on every thought, emotion, feeling and desire, transforming these fluctuations in energy into molecular, biochemical and ultimately physiological and physical effects. So, if a patient believes what a physician tells them about their condition, treatment or survival, there is a high probability that this will be realised. Stated another way, what the physician relates to the patient, intentionally or otherwise, and how, is related to what occurs subsequently in the patient's body.

A case in point is a patient of the cardiologist Bernard Lown. While on his rounds with medical students Dr Lown pointed out that this patient's heart had 'a wholesome very good third-sound gallop', which in medical terminology means that it was badly damaged. Indeed, the patient was critically ill and with little hope or recovery. Yet, on hearing what he took to mean that his heart was as strong as a horse, he recovered.[70] In another extraordinary case, a contemporary American doctor performed a de-hexing ceremony in an attempt to reverse a shaman's deadly spell. The dying patient recovered, suggesting that his belief in the medicine of the 'orthodox' physician was greater than in that of the shaman.[71]

Undoubtedly the doctor is the most powerful placebo of all. The chances of successful treatment seem to be directly proportional to the quality of the doctor–patient relationship, that is, the extent to which the patient believes that the doctor's interventions can and will be effective. The placebo will not work in all circumstances. The healer's attitude to the patient, his or her ability to convince the patient that he or she is not being taken lightly, and his or her success in gaining the patient's full confidence, are all vital factors, not only in maximising the usefulness of the placebo, but also of the treatment of disease in general. It is doubtful whether the placebo or any other treatment would prove effective without the patient's will to live, that is, without a positive attitude to life.

The importance of positive attitude is highlighted by the recently acknowledged negative placebo or *nocebo* effect whereby treatment known to be effective does not work because the patient does not expect it to. This phenomenon is well illustrated in the case of Mr Wright who achieved a remarkable remission in his cancer in response to the newly introduced and much acclaimed 'wonder drug' *Krebiozen* only to succumb quickly to the disease when the drug was derided as ineffective.[72] Mr Wright's case shows that negative prognoses will be translated into that reality.

> [Medical] staff should realize that the way they inform their patient has the effect of a hypnotic induction and could be murderous. There are many ways to tell a patient that the treatment is not successful and the prognosis is poor. But to tell a patient 'You will die soon' is a form of murder.[73]

For this reason doctors are now advised against giving negative expectancies in the form of prognoses to patients. Doctors have to be very careful about what they say.

What the placebo effect shows is not only that 'the word is made flesh', as indicated in the Bible, but that people can and do relinquish their personal power to the words of doctors. 'Cancer' is one such word and it is a nocebo; most people in Western society perceive it as a virtual death sentence. So too are medical statistics. They can be regarded as collective nocebos. For example, medical statistics may reveal that for a specific cancer mortality is likely to be 90 per cent within six months. The doctor has no idea when a patient with this cancer walks into his or her office whether he or she falls into the 90 per cent who will soon be dead, or the 10 per cent who won't. By giving the 90 per cent statistic the doctor is reinforcing the former belief, when in fact the patient could easily be within the 10 per cent unlikely to die in that time. By giving them this information the doctor is probably initiating a self-fulfilling prophecy. So, by not employing these statistics, the figures would probably change because they induce, quite simply, a collective nocebo response.[74]

It may well be that any effective treatment is a ritual that culminates in some patients believing that the treatment will work and creating the physiology consistent with this belief. Such a view is consistent with the observation that 'human suffering responds to the spoken word rendered by compassionate persons cast in the role of healer,'[75] and with studies in the field of PNI which suggest that the immune system learns how to respond. Expectancy or belief is known to influence blood levels of the hormones cortisol and prolactin which are important in activating the immune system.[76] Positive and negative expectancies have opposite effects, respectively enhancing or depressing the immune system. Expectancy is a major factor in stress.

Relating to the world

Stress is a state of physiological activation characterised by increases in heart rate, blood pressure, pulse rate, muscle tension, elevated blood levels of sugars, fats, cholesterol and homones such as cortisol and adrenaline. Prolonged stress or recurrent stress, where the body remains in a continually reactive state, results in the wear and tear of various bodily organs and inevitably takes its toll on health. It may result in cardiovascular problems, stroke, heart disease, kidney failure, gastro-intestinal disorders, diabetes and much else. Stress is now thought to contribute to 80 per cent of all illness.

The neurological changes resulting from stress have been demonstrated to affect immune function both directly and indirectly. Direct effects are possible because lymphocytes bear receptors on their surfaces, for many neurohormones and transmitters and lymphocytes are exposed to neurochemicals in lymphoid organs and in peripheral blood. More indirect mechanisms for neural-immune interactions may involve changes in lymphocyte tracking resulting from changes in sympathetic vascular tone.

There is a wealth of evidence from human and animal studies that acute stress, whether physical or emotional, can produce immuno-suppression and that chronic stress may cause significant dysfunction of the immune response leading to increased susceptibility to disease.[77] Research in the field of PNI has only relatively recently shed light on the mechanisms by which stress and emotional states can have such profound effects on immunity. It has become increasingly evident that factors such as expectancy or belief and coping style are instrumental in determining the impact of stress on the autonomic nervous system and susceptibility to disease. Confronted with similar circumstances individuals may act so as to minimise or maximise the threat it poses. This idea is conveyed in the Chinese word for 'crisis', which is composed of two characters that separately mean 'danger' and 'opportunity'. Implicitly, therefore, every crisis presents these two features, and the individual response to it depends on which view of it is favoured. If a person sees the situation as dangerous or threatening they will experience stress, whereas if they see it as a challenge, an opportunity to learn, grow and develop they will not. These differences in appraisal or interpretation can result in enormous differences in how people respond to potentially stressful events and the amount of stress they experience. 'We can be transformed from victims to heroes depending on how we respond to crisis.'[78] What this means in effect is that stress is an option rather than an inevitability that arises mainly from the individual's attitude towards and interpretation of events. Stress is not 'out there' in the world but is determined by how people interpret and relate to the events and circumstances of their world. 'People construct circumstances for themselves which they then react to with stress: that is, they are not being stressed by external events beyond their control but are stressing themselves.'[79] In other words, 'as we think, so we experience.'[80]

Studies of cancer patients[81] have suggested that attitude is vitally important in determining the outcome of the illness. Those with spontaneous remission of cancer have been found to be positive in attitude and a clear correlation has been found between mental attitude and length of survival.[82]

However, people are largely unaware that their attitude to life may determine its length and their experience of it, and many are unaware of what their attitudes are. Some people may be unaware that they are stressed because they repress their feelings and keep them under control. Repression as a coping style has attracted considerable attention, particularly the association between a repressive coping style and the onset of cancer. One theory is that because people with a repressive coping style display inattention to internal cues of distress they may also fail to detect significant bodily feedback. Some support for this idea comes from the finding that repressive cancer patients report fewer and less severe side-effects of treatment,[83] yet they are no different from other patients in terms of disease and treatment status. What this suggests is that people with this coping style have a poor level of internal communication and that the way in which they relate to themselves is limited. Such people are out of touch to a great extent with their feelings and their bodies. Therefore the ways in which people relate to themselves and their world emerge as highly significant factors in health and illness.

Studies of the placebo effect, stress and coping style also provide clear proof that there is no separation between mind and body, and their relationship has to be considered of primary importance in healing. In the light of this new evidence about the way the mind–body system functions as a whole, 'attempts to treat most mental diseases as though they were completely free of physical causes and attempts to treat most bodily disease as though the mind were in no way involved must be considered archaic.'[84] Furthermore, the bodymind complex cannot be regarded independently of its context. These elements are interrelated aspects of one whole and their relationships needs to be fully understood and addressed in order to promote healing. This understanding was fundamental to traditional systems of healing where relationships within the person and between the person and the environment were regarded as being of primary importance.

A growing body of research is highlighting the importance of the therapeutic relationship. From considerable research on the connection between psychological and physiological factors, a picture is emerging of the specific ways in which emotions, experiences and attitudes can create physiological change, and how complex psychological factors govern the functioning of the immune system. 'There has been enough replication involving controlled studies to point to a presiding fact, namely, the physician has a prime resource at his disposal in the form of the patient's own apothecary.'[85] These findings, increasingly featured in respected medical journals, have led to more widespread recognition of the need for a biopsychosocial or holistic approach to health which incorporates full utilisation of both medical science and the human healing system, and combines the high technology and symptom suppression techniques of biomedicine with an understanding of psychological and social factors in health and illness. There is, of course, nothing new in this model. It is precisely that established by Hippocrates over 2000 years ago and which originated in the magico-religious practices of the ancient world. What is new is that for the first time in Western scientific medicine there is acknowledgement of the need to examine, understand and restore to their proper place in health care the principles and practices of the psychology of healing, or psychological medicine.

The challenge for Western psychological medicine in the twenty-first century is to be able to identify with precision the mechanisms by which the body's own pharmacy can be targeted at specific organs and disease conditions to bring about cure and to develop understanding of the therapeutic relationship in facilitating these processes within the person. However, this challenge is far from being met. While research in psychology and PNI continue to add to knowledge about psychotherapeutics, much of this remains unknown within medicine. It is not reflected in medical training which at present is guided by the belief that disease is an almost exclusively physical phenomenon that arises in bodies separated from each other and from their psychosocial context, and is to be treated impersonally. Furthermore, as technological medicine advances, it is difficult to avoid the conclusion that 'the more we learn about the technical craft of saving physical life, the less we seem to care about the human art of caring about the person.'[86]

Pain, for example, is one of the most common symptoms that doctors have to deal with. It is a complex biopsychosocial phenomenon, extensively researched within psychology, yet it is treated almost exclusively as a physical condition. There is teaching on pain in only four of the twenty-one medical schools in Britain and even where it is taught it is covered in an average of 3.5 hours of a five-year medical degree course.[87] Similarly, there is little or no training given in psychological and social aspects of health and illness. The general disregard of mental and social factors in health has been likened to the attitude prevalent in the 1800s when surgeons ridiculed the concept of sepsis and the germ theory of disease and 'persisted in operating in unclean surroundings, sometimes defiantly sharpening their scalpels on the soles of their shoes to show their contempt for the putative power of invisible germs'.[88] Similarly, it is claimed[89] that the current ignorance of and insensitivity to the 'invisible' symbolic messages in human interactions between doctor and patient limit the effectiveness of contemporary medicine. Arguably a more fundamental limitation on the effectiveness of medicine is the failure of many doctors to listen to the spoken messages of their patients, much less the subtext of these subcommunications, or to give them information about their condition and treatment. Recognition of this fact led Glasgow University to announce in 1987 its intention of following the universities of Manchester and Leicester in examining all future medical students in their ability to communicate with and relate to patients. However, most medical schools do not give any teaching in these skills. The understanding that the therapeutic relationship is the context in which all aspects of therapy — assessment, diagnosis, treatment, rehabilitation — take place, is thus ignored in medical training. Yet in the wake of the conviction of the British general practitioner Dr Harold Shipman for mass murder in February 2000, the greatest concern expressed by doctors and medical commentators was that this verdict might undermine the relationship of trust between doctor and patient and destroy 'this very valuable faith which patients need to have in their GP, and which is the basis of our medicine'.[90]

8

DIVINING THE SOUL: DIAGNOSIS

Twentieth-century physics has revealed that energy and information exist everywhere in nature. 'In fact, at the level of the quantum field, there is nothing other than energy and information. The quantum field is just another name for the field of pure consciousness or pure potentiality.'[1] Furthermore, everything in the universe is related — part of the whole. This has tremendous implications for medical diagnosis (which derives from the Greek *gignoskein* meaning to perceive or know). The changed view of the universe dictates a different way of viewing organisms, bodies, health and disease. 'The separateness of bodies, and absolute distinctions between health and disease cannot be maintained in a context of quantum wholeness.'[2] The underlying unbroken wholeness of all manifestations of the entire universe has to be acknowledged, and the principles of relatedness, oneness and unity have to be addressed rather than their fragmentation and isolation. Translated into practice these new conceptions of reality require bodies, health and disease to be viewed as dynamic processes rather than discrete entities, and understood in terms of patterns of relationships within the organism and its environment rather than in terms of separate parts. Heath and illness need to be viewed in relation to the wholeness or integration of these processes, rather than in terms of symptoms or the lack of them.

These principles are embodied in traditional systems of medicine, all of which examine the life situation of the patient and consider, in Hippocratic manner, 'the whole of things' spiritual, emotional, physical and ecological. Ayurveda takes into account the patient's constitutional type, individual susceptibilities, seasonal and climatic variations and other ecological factors. Diagnosis is not simple given that Siddha, the Tamil language version of Ayurveda, recognises 4492 different sicknesses. Traditional Chinese medicine views the person as inextricably part of the environment, and diagnosis relies heavily on environmental factors. It also considers internal factors such as emotion. Whereas orthodox Western medicine relies primarily on quantitative data, traditional systems of medicine consider the patient's subjective experience, including dreams, daydreams and fantasies and intuition as the primary data in diagnosis.

Intuitive diagnosis

Traditional systems of medicine also emphasise the importance of the practitioners' intuition. In Ayurveda diagnosis of a person's constitutional type is achieved in part by the observation of the individual's attitudes and behaviour, but more fundamentally it relies on the practitioners' intuition.

> When an Ayurvedic doctor looks at you he sees signs of the three *doshas* everywhere, but he cannot literally see the *doshas* themselves. They govern the physical processes in your body without being physical themselves. We have called them 'metabolic principles', a term which is quite abstract. Yet the *doshas* are concrete enough to be moved around, increased and decreased; they can get 'stuck' in tissues and displaced to parts of the body where they don't belong — so they are on the borderline of being physical. Lying as they do in the gap between mind and body, they resemble nothing that exists in our Western scientific framework. *Vata, Pitta* and *Kapha* only come into clear focus once you begin to view yourself within an Ayurvedic perspective.[3]

Intuition derives from the Latin *intueri* meaning to gaze upon and it refers to knowledge or intelligence gained by insight rather than reasoning. Intuitive diagnosis, whereby a person obtains reliable information about another's state of health and uses this as a basis for treatment, is as old as medicine itself. It is fundamental to shamanism and to Hippocratic medicine. Indeed 'most physicians arrive at a diagnosis through their use of intuition,'[4] and some physicians regard the use of intuition as essential in medical practice.

> Intuition in medicine is crucial ... More than half of medical practice requires decisions which have little or no technological basis. There are no absolute rights or wrongs; there are only decisions of the head and heart, of wisdom and compassion ... The good physicians is able to combine ... intuition and common sense.[5]

However, throughout the history of medicine there have been many individuals with exceptional intuitive ability. Perhaps one of the most influential of modern times is the twentieth-century physician Edward Bach (1886–1936), whose intuitively derived flower remedies are increasingly used and researched throughout the world.

The first formal study of medical intuitives was conducted in the nineteenth century by Dr John Elliotson, professor of medicine at University College Hospital, London. He discovered that patients who were mesmerised could properly diagnose medical cases whose illnesses had confounded medical experts. However, his discovery was dismissed by his medical colleagues as nonsense and so he resigned to pursue his interests in mesmerism in private practice. James Esdaile, the British physician who did much to promote mesmerism in the nineteenth century, published a book on mesmeric-induced intuition in 1850, but this was also ignored.

No further attempt was made to investigate the subject scientifically until the late twentieth century, when medical intuitives such as Edgar Cayce, Olga Worrall, Jack Schwarz, Rosalind Bruyere and Carolyn Myss were studied. Norman Shealy, himself a highly intuitive American neurosurgeon, conducted research on several intuitives during the 1970s and claimed to have found 'a significant rate of accuracy as determined by computerised evaluation'.[6] On the basis of his studies he concludes that intuitive diagnosis is not only possible but also highly successful.[7] One of the most outstanding intuitives he studied was the internist Dr Robert Leichtman, who was 96 per cent accurate in his evaluation of patients compared with 80 per cent accuracy among physicians generally. Shealy observed that many doctors who acknowledge that there is a strong element of intuition in all medical diagnoses might be more persuaded by the claims made in respect of Dr Leichtman than those made by intuitives with no medical training. However, Leichtman demonstrated his accuracy using only photographs, the patients' names and birth dates.

Unlike Leichtman, most outstanding intuitive diagnosticians studied have no medical training. The terminology they use in diagnosis and the description of diseases and their causes often bear little or no relation to the terms and concepts used in orthodox medicine. Nevertheless, the therapeutics they prescribe are appropriate and effective despite their lack of medical knowledge. The most famous and intensively researched intuitive diagnostician of all time, Edgar Cayce, made some 15,000 diagnoses and therapeutic recommendations. The latter involved conventional and unconventional medications. Many of the more unorthodox remedies, not recognised or understood by Western medicine at the time, have since been found to be effective.[8]

Like Cayce, the medical intuitive Carolyn Myss has no medical training yet she is able to intuit the nature and precise location of physical disease in a person's body, and is claimed by Shealy to be 93 per cent accurate in her diagnosis. Although Shealy provides insufficient detail to enable independent evaluation of his findings, the most compelling evidence for the accuracy of Myss' diagnoses is that Shealy has successfully conducted neurosurgery based upon it, and has sufficient confidence to do so. Nevertheless, despite considerable evidence for the accuracy of intuitive diagnosticians, the view within medicine is that the studies are inconclusive and there is need for more rigorous investigation.[9]

Intuiting the soul

Orthodox Western medicine that relies on diagnosis based largely on quantitative 'factual' information obtained from objective tests has a fundamental problem in accepting as valid and reliable diagnosis that appears to have no rational, objective basis. Edgar Cayce and Edward Bach both explained illness in terms of the soul and soul principles. According to Cayce the body and mind come into being for the purpose of manifesting the soul in the material realm, and that all health and illness need to be understood in the context of these three aspects. He regarded attitudes and emotions as having critical importance in determining health and illness, describing emotions as 'electronics' that act as vibratory communication between the body, mind and soul. Similarly, for Edward Bach, disease is caused by conflict between the soul and the personality which manifests in a distortion of the wavelength in the 'soul' or energy field around the body resulting in negative 'soul states' like worry, anxiety and impatience, for example. Bach claimed that these negative states deplete the individual's vitality and result in the body losing its natural resistance to infection and illness.

Robert Leichtman also views the person in terms of body, mind and emotions but emphasises that the consciousness behind these is a:

> ... center of life essence that creates the three vehicles of the personality, animates them and maintains the health according to its own ideals, plans and purposes. This life center can be called the soul, the inner being, the higher self, the superconscious or the human spirit.[10]

For Leichtman, the purpose of the body is to express the light of the soul, which is pure consciousness. The soul is the origin of health because it contains all the ideal patterns of health for mind, emotions and body. The purpose of the mind is to be a channel through which the soul can condense its wisdom and intent and enlighten the life of the personality. The measure of the healthy mind is therefore clarity of thought; the extent to which the mind is responsive to inspiration of the soul and aware of its connections and purposes. Ultimately, therefore health lies in the integrity or oneness of the whole.

These principles are acknowledged by most intuitive diagnosticians. However, like Jack Schwarz and Rosalind Bruyere, Carolyn Myss describes her experience[11] of working with intuitive diagnosis as corresponding to the teachings of Eastern spiritual traditions. These emphasise the human being as a system of energy as opposed to the Christian tradition that emphasises humanity's experience in the physical world.

> The Eastern tradition speaks of the 'energy' of the human being, and their language includes terms that are specific to what I need to describe. Of particular value from the East is the

> description that we are a combination of mental, emotional, psychological and spiritual currents of energy that come together to form the physical body, and that our bodies have energy centers called 'chakras'.[12]

Eastern traditions describe all material phenomena, including the human body, as different forms of energy that emerge from the field of pure energy. Twentieth-century physics also describes matter as no more than 'a state of information'.[13] The process of energy manifesting as form is essentially that of being in-form-ation. 'Information is implicate-order awareness arising from some universal awareness (to us incomprehensible) that manifests "in forms".'[14] It is not material 'but may utilize materiality and have material effects. It "in-forms", that is, directs into form an awareness of formal intentionality, to something able to receive that awareness and respond to it.'[15] Even when energy has taken form this process is maintained because all things being dynamic fields of energy rather than static objects. The human body, for example, completely renews itself every year. Hence it is always in-form-ation, in a process or becoming.

> As far as our ordinary personal awareness is concerned, many of these programs and ends are largely unconscious. We cannot directly perceive the awareness and patterning intention of a leaf. Neither do we directly experience our immune reactions, our organism's rejection of self-pattern-foreign elements, or the objection of our organism to a particular food item until our stomach has chosen (regardless of and even contrary to our conscious volition) to reject it or until, perhaps days later, our skin responds to the information with protesting hives. On the other hand, through what we call 'altered states of consciousness' (ASC) — such as those reached through meditation, hypnotic trance, or by means of some mythical imagery — our conscious selves have been able to tune into direct experiential awareness of the fields that our customary consciousness cannot reach and the existence of which Western science has consequently chosen to deny.[16]

Intuitives apprehend this energy in-form-ation as information or knowledge and so are able to intuit what will manifest in the body long before it does so. They are able to do this because, having once attuned themselves to a specific energy field, they sense its vibrations in their own energy field through the principle of resonance. Moreover, this sensitivity is not specific to intuitives.

> We have a nervous system that is capable of becoming *aware* of the energy and informational content of that localized field that gives rise to our physical body. We *experience* this field subjectively as our own thoughts, feelings, emotions, desires, memories, instincts, drives, and beliefs. This same field is expressed objectively as the physical body — and through the physical body, we experience this field as the world. But it's all the same stuff. That is why the ancient seers exclaimed 'I am that, you are that, all this is that, and that's all there is.'
>
> Your body is not separate from the body of the universe, because at the quantum mechanical levels there are no well-defined edges. You are like a wiggle, a wave, a fluctuation, a convolution, a whirlpool, a localized disturbance in the larger quantum field. The larger quantum field — the universe — is your extended body.[17]

This means that the human nervous system is capable of becoming aware of the information and energy of its own quantum field or soul, and the universal field beyond, the energetic or non-material spiritual realm, in which is located the quantum fields of all other organisms. Intuitive diagnosticians differ from others only insofar as they have developed their awareness of these energy fields. Their ability in this respect is simply more refined than that of the ordinary person and so they are able to make more subtle distinctions in terms of their feelings. Carolyn Myss describes this as projecting her emotional energy towards a person and feeling emotional responses that convey information about that person's spiritual, psychological and emotional state.[18] John Pierrakos,[19] a doctor with this sensitivity, explains that emotion is a whole-organism pulsation. The feeling of well-being, for example, is consciousness of energy streaming freely.

The explanation offered by these two highly intuitive diagnosticians is consistent with the theory recently advanced by neurologist Antonio Damasio[20] that human consciousness evolved from the development of emotion. This proposition challenges the hierarchy established in Western thinking, which locates feelings in the body and reason in the brain, dismisses emotion as irrational and primitive, and considers even study of emotion unreasonable. Its basic premise is that awareness of emotion — *feeling* the feeling — is the significant step in the development of human consciousness. The process of feeling alerts the organism to the problem that the emotion is concerned with. Thus emotional responses involve both the body and the brain rather than only the body. Not only does recognising feelings for what they are — sensory processes — have tremendous survival value, but it enormously enriches the capacity of human beings to respond imaginatively and effectively in novel situations. Although Damasio's ideas are breaking new ground in contemporary Western scientific thinking, they are not original. The ancient view is that organisms are moved — e-motionally and motivationally — by energy, a moving and intelligent life force that is the essence or soul of all phenomena. This idea found expression in modern times in the theories of Wilhelm Reich, who based his approach to treatment on the understanding that emotional intelligence is found everywhere in the body, because human beings respond as a whole to the events and circumstances of their lives. This conclusion is also that drawn from discoveries in the field of PNI.

Nevertheless, the idea of emotions or feelings as information-gathering or sensory processes is not commonplace. Under ordinary circumstances most people can only perceive the energy plane of the physical body with their senses, whereas intuitives can attune or align themselves emotionally with the energy flow of another and become sensitive to it. However, the ordinary person can develop this sensitivity. It can be trained. Indeed, in most traditional forms of healing, medical training is training of intuition. Although not trained as such in orthodox Western medicine, it has been established that many physicians have the ability to diagnose illness through the energy field they detect around the patient or energy vortices they perceive as being connected with the body's endocrine system.[21]

Various physical sensations can be distinguished by feel as the hands and fingertips are passed through the energy field or aura of another person some two to three inches above the surface of the body. These sensations of heat, cold, tingling, pins and needles, pulsation, pressure or electric shock can provide reliable information about pain and other symptoms of disease, as has been recognised by healers and masseurs throughout history. They indicate areas in which the vibration is noticeably different from what it should be and hence the presence of bodily dysfunction. With appropriate feedback from others, this sensitivity can be developed and used diagnostically. It has wide application in healing of all kinds as the aura reveals a person's health, character, emotional disposition and tendencies, abilities, attitudes, past problems and spiritual development. Accordingly, within psychological medicine as it is being conceived here, diagnosis does not focus only on the signs and symptoms of disease evident in the physical body but also on apprehending signs and symptoms of soul disturbance at the energetic level before they manifest within the body.

Divining information

The emotional sensitivity of medical intuitives amounts to a heightened awareness of feelings mostly experienced as subtle vibrations. As such it is a resonance with the energies or emotions of another organism. Some of the frequencies detected by intuitives can be registered by technical devices, such as EEGs. A more complete picture of the energy fields surrounding the body is provided by Kirlian photography, which shows promise as a tool in the diagnosis of both physical illness and psychopathology. Various other techniques have been developed in attempts to make objective what is essentially a subjective awareness of energy information. Divining is perceiving or understanding by intuition or insight. It is the basis of divination, which is the art or practice of discerning future events or the unknown. Its essentially spiritual character is suggested by its origins in the Latin *divinus* meaning God. In ancient Greece divination occurred at sacred oracles such as Delphi. In the civilisations of the ancient world it was one of the functions of priest-healers, who used rods, sticks or pendulums as divining instruments, to detect subtle energies, and they are depicted on both Egyptian and Mayan reliefs. Pendulums are among the objects recovered from many Egyptian burial sites. Divining, also known as dowsing, has been used throughout the centuries not only to diagnose illness but to locate water, minerals and lines of force deep within the earth, and more recently to sex newly born chicks and detect submarines.[22] The Chinese have used divination or *feng shui* for many centuries to determine good location of their houses and public buildings and to create harmonious living and working environments.

Although practised throughout medieval Europe, the earliest references to dowsing in the English language were by Robert Fludd in 1638. At the end of the nineteenth century the term 'radiesthesia' which means sensitivity to radiations, was applied to the practice in the belief that the phenomena observed in the act of dowsing — movements of the dowsing instrument — result from some kind of radiation.[23] Radiesthesia has also been described as radiation perception and defined as the innate ability to detect vibrations or waves of force emanating from objects in the physical universe and from levels of consciousness that lie beyond the range of physical sense perception.[24]

> These waves or radiations can be detected by any person who is sufficiently sensitive to record their impression, or who is prepared to take time to develop the sensitivity. It is a fact that some people are sensitive enough simply to use their hands to pick up the energy fields of various objects, but most practitioners use a pendulum which amplifies the neuro-muscular response to provide a clear set of signals. These signals provide data relevant to the search for what the radiesthetist is carrying out which may be for water, oil or mineral prospection, missing objects or persons. In the medical field a simple example would be the identification of the correct medicine for a patient.[25]

Although ostensibly a physical method, dowsing or radiesthesia ultimately depends on the sensitivity of the practitioner to subtle radiations of varying vibrational frequencies. The dowsing instrument, whether a rod, stick, pendulum or more complex device, merely serves to indicate what the human 'instrument' initially detects. Therefore while a person may be unaware of subtle energies they are nevertheless processed by the nervous system and expressed through unconscious neurological and motor pathways. Tiny muscle movements register these influences and produce visible movement in the dowsing instrument.

Radiesthesia first gained popularity in Europe at the end of the nineteenth century largely because of two French priests, the Abbés Mermet and Bouley. The Abbé Mermet could find with unerring accuracy whatever he was looking for. He could pinpoint a water source in countries many thousands of miles away, and describe its depth, the geological strata overlaying it, its potability, temperature and rate of flow. When describing a missing person he could tell of their movements from the time they were lost. His ability to diagnose disease was equally dramatic and he used radiesthesia to determine the homeopathic or herbal remedies appropriate in treatment. In so doing he was a pioneer of what is now known as phytotherapy.

The Abbé Mermet observed that the body of a person is basically no different from the body of the earth. Each has cavities and streams of fluid flowing beneath its surface and so just as it is possible to detect what lies under the earth it is possible to establish whether disease has invaded a body, and to do so at the site or from a distance.

Dowsing became popular in Britain in the 1930s and in 1933 the British Society of Dowsers was founded to study the field in general. By 1939, a Medical Society for the Study of Radiesthesia had been established by Dr Guyon Richards and other physicians, and medical radiesthesia became widely used in detecting hidden causes of disease that could not be identified by standard clinical tests, and to find treatments that would eliminate the disease. Psionic medicine, developed by Dr George Lawrence, represents a modern development in the application of radiesthesia to health.[26] The concept on which psionic diagnosis is based is that health is a balanced, harmonious state of energy patterns and any imbalance indicates ill health. Gross and chronic imbalance is disease and this can be detected by dowsing specimens of blood, saliva or hair from a person.

Applied kinesiology, developed by American chiropractor George Goodheart in the 1960s, is based on similar principles. It uses manual muscle testing to provide muscular feedback on responses to given stimulation, evaluate body function through muscle–meridian connections and indicate appropriate treatment. A kinesiology muscle test involves the practitioner placing a person's limb in a certain position in order to isolate and contract the muscle being tested. Light pressure is applied in the direction that would extend the muscle. On the practitioner's instruction to 'hold' the person tries to match the applied pressure. The muscle will either lock in place or give way. This is not a test of muscle strength but of neurological function. This, it is claimed, can be used to test the individual's response to any stimulus, whether a remedy, food, emotional word or phrase; to locate dysfunction in the body; and assess imbalances in the energy field that may undermine future health. The explanation offered for this is that if a given stimulus produces stress, the resulting neurological responses can be detected by way of imperceptible muscle movements. Although the reproducibility and reliability of muscle testing remains the subject of considerable debate, applied kinesiology is widely used in diagnosis by many practitioners of complementary therapies.

Dowsing by pendulum is also widely used diagnostically in complementary therapies. A pendulum held over a chakra will usually begin to move within a few seconds in response to the amount and direction of energy flowing through it. Clockwise movement of the pendulum indicates a chakra that is functioning effectively. The feelings and processes it governs are therefore balanced and healthy. Anti-clockwise movement indicates that energy is not flowing through the chakra, with the result that the feelings and functions it governs are not balanced and are probably experienced negatively by the person. Between these two extremes various other movements may be described by the pendulum, all of which have diagnostic validity.[27]

Radionics is also based on sensing the energy field around living systems. It originated in the work of the neurologist Dr Albert Abrams, Director of Studies at Stanford University Medical School. He pioneered diagnosis by percussion within orthodox medicine. He found that tapping various parts of the body produces resonating sounds, and hollow sounds where disease is present. His investigations led him to conclude that this involves some kind of energy and he developed a box containing resistors to measure disease reactions in ohms. Abrams wrote many papers on his new diagnostic system, claiming that it enabled disease to be detected before it was clinically identifiable in any orthodox way. This attracted the interest of doctors throughout the world and many travelled to California to learn about it. However, the medical orthodoxy was hostile to Abrams' system, despite the fact that the practice of percussion has a very long history in traditional medicine and is demonstrably effective as a diagnostic technique. Indeed, an investigation by the Royal Society for Medicine in London in 1924 found that Abram's fundamental proposition had been proven to a high degree of probability, but being unable to understand the relationship between energy and matter, decided against it being taught in medical schools. Most radionics practitioners today are therefore not medically qualified.

George de la Warr developed the theory and practice of radionics after Abrams' death and it was subsequently further developed and refined by a number of pioneers. Radionics is based on the principle that physical organs, diseases and remedies have their own characteristic frequency or vibration that can be expressed in numerical values known as 'rates' and calculated by radionics instruments developed for this purpose. Using these instruments the chiropractor Dr Ruth Drown identified a series of rates that in effect constitute the vibrational pattern of known diseases. In making a diagnosis, the radionics practitioner uses the 'radiesthetic faculty' involved in dowsing, detecting disease in much the same way that the dowser detects the location of oil, water or mineral deposits, that is, by asking a series of mentally posed questions and thereby obtaining information about the health of a patient to which his or her conscious, thinking mind has no direct access.

Radionics systems that indicate this sensitivity more accurately than dowsing devices such as rods, sticks and pendulums have been developed and tested in the USA and Europe for several decades. These have been termed 'psychotronic technologies'[28] because of the central role of the operator's consciousness in obtaining information from the device. The operator sensitises him- or herself to various subtle energies through a process of attunement.

> The psychic process of tuning in ... occurs at the level of our higher frequency vehicles of expression. In most individuals this energy linkup takes place at an unconscious level. The unconscious mind acts as a passageway through which higher frequency levels of consciousness may interact with the physical body. Higher psychic impressions are translated into various forms of the body's neurological circuitry. If the psychic

information reaches conscious awareness, it does so through the expressive mechanism of the cerebral cortex. Unconscious intuitive information may filter through the right cerebral hemisphere and then be transferred to the left hemisphere where it is analysed and expressed verbally. While psychic information may not always reach conscious awareness it is still processed by the nervous system and expressed through unconscious pathways of neurological and motor activity.[29]

Whereas in dowsing, tiny unconscious muscle movements are expressed via the pendulum or other device, in radionics the medium of expression is the radionics instrument. Typically, the radionics procedure involves a biological specimen — a drop of blood or a lock of hair — referred to as the 'witness'. This is placed in the well of the radionics instrument, a device consisting of a black box with a number of tuneable dials on the front, each numerically calibrated, and usually attached to variable resistors or potentiometers inside the box. These are also connected by wires to a circular metallic well and to a rubber pad which forms the interface between the operator and the device. While mentally tuning in to the patient, the radionics operator then lightly strokes a finger across the rubber pad and while doing so slowly turns one of the dials. A positive response is registered when the operator feels a sticking sensation in the finger as the pad is stroked. This is considered to be a sympathetic resonance reaction that occurs between the energy frequency of the patient and the subtle energy field of the operator. The dial is left tuned to the setting that induced the resonance response. The procedure is repeated with a series of dials, each of which represents a digit in sequence that when combined produces a multi-digit number or rate. This reflects the energetic frequency characteristics of the patient being remotely tested by the radionics device. By comparing the patient's rate with the known vibrational frequencies associated with particular illnesses the practitioner is able to make a presumptive diagnosis of the patient's pathological condition.

A similar frequency matching procedure is carried out in homeopathic diagnosis, except that homeopathy matches the frequency of a remedy to a symptom complex, whereas radionics measures the patient's primary energetic frequency disturbance.

Although this frequency matching procedure conforms to the principles of biological resonance, to most orthodox physicians the process may appear nonsensical. Nevertheless, it is also consistent with the principles of holography central to modern scientific thinking. The witness is considered to reflect the total energetic structure of the entire organism and continues to do so because of resonance with the person from which it came, remaining in equilibrium with its source regardless of distance.

Diagnosing the whole from its parts

The holographic principle that diagnosis can be effected by way of any given part of the organism because information about the whole is contained within each of its parts underpins many traditional systems of medicine.

Iridology is based on observations of the iris of the eye. Traditionally the eyes have been called the mirror of the soul and it has long been thought that they indicate the condition of the whole body. Observation of the eye is as old as medicine itself. It is referred to in the works of Hippocrates and other early Greek physicians, and is a key element in traditional oriental diagnosis. In 1670 Meyens discussed signs in the iris and their relation to disease in his *Chiromatica Medica*.[30] In 1881 a Hungarian doctor, Ignatz von Peczely published his findings on iris diagnosis. He claimed that markings on the iris are related to organic disease and that by localising these markings disease can be related to a specific organ. Later that century Pastor Felks made further advances in mapping the iris. Correspondences between the various parts of the iris and the organs of the body have since been fully charted and developments in modern technology allow images of the iris to be photographed and projected for analysis. However, although widely used in oriental diagnosis, iridology has gained little acceptance in orthodox Western medicine.

Tongue diagnosis is a feature of *Bo-Shin*, the Chinese art of seeing or diagnosis by observation, based on the principle that information about the entire constitution is reflected in the structure of parts of the body such as the eyes, head and face, and the spine. This is more accepted within Western medicine, where it is recognised that deficiencies of B vitamins can be indicated by scarring, colouring or coating of the tongue and cracks and fissures in its surface.

Traditional Chinese medicine also involves diagnosis by touch, *Setsu-Shin*. In Chinese medicine there are 12 major bodily organs each with a pulse. According to a theory drafted by the physician Pien Ch'io in 6–5 BC, the state of energy flow along meridians associated with each organ can be assessed at the pulses, six on each arm, which can be felt just above the wrist. Energy imbalance and the state of various systems of the body are indicated by the pulses and can be estimated before any signs or symptoms become apparent. According to this theory the meridians have terminals or 'well points' located next to the bottom corners of the fingernails and toenails. Energy level at these points is said to reflect accurately the condition of the entire meridian. Meridian functioning can also be assessed by pressing the well point and noting the colour. When on light pressure the skin appears white or cold, *chi* energy is held to be deficient. *Chi* is normal when the skin is warm and red in response to pressure, excessive when pressure results in pain, and deficient when pain only develops with deep pressure. The half moons of the nails also show the state of the associated meridian. If no moon is apparent this is an indication of deficient energy flow, and excessively small nails suggest long-term deficiency of *chi* in the corresponding meridians. A nail showing normal pink colour indicates a healthy meridian. Vertical wrinkles in certain nails are an indication of deficient blood supply and consequent deficient meridian flow, whereas ridges or bumps reflect deficient blood supply through the entire body, as do excessively white or pale nails. Another way of checking meridian functioning is by noting the way the fingers form when contracted into a fist and opened out again. Fingers feeling or appearing weak reflect weakness in the associated meridians. Deficiency of *chi* is also reflected in peeling skin at well points and excessive flow in rashes.[31]

Acupressure and shiatsu involve diagnosis by pressure, as does reflexology. Reflexology probably has ancient origins. Hand and foot pressure is known to have been used therapeutically for over 5000 years in China and India and by Native Americans. It appears to be based on energy principles similar to oriental medicine. Modern reflexology is attributed to an American ear, nose and throat specialist, William Fitzgerald. He found that gentle pressure applied to specific areas of the hands and feet produces partial anaesthesia in areas of the ears, nose and throat, and claimed to have used this method of anaesthesia in minor operations. He mapped out the correspondence between these organs and parts of the hands and feet and since then various schools of reflexology have developed. These are all based on the common assumption that every part of the body is connected by energy channels or pathways, known as reflex zones, that terminate on the soles of the feet, palms of the hands, ears, tongue and head. These pathways, equivalent to the meridians of Chinese medicine, relate to all areas of the body through ten zones that divide the body longitudinally on either side of the medial line. These divisions are conceptual rather than actual, as the energy is considered to flow in a continuum. Tension or imbalance in any part of the reflex zone will affect the entire zone and give rise to malfunction in the organs it influences. Whenever an organ is dysfunctional the corresponding reflex in the feet or hands will be very tender on pressure.

In the traditional systems of medicine of China and Tibet the voice is also used for diagnosis. According to *Bun-Shin*, the Chinese art of hearing, the way in which individuals use their energies is revealed by their voice quality and so their general health can be assessed by listening to them speak. Vocal features are classified as *yin* or *yang*. *Yin* energy is expressed in low, slow, soft, wet, unclear, flat, loose and irregular speech, whereas *yang* energy characteristically sounds high, fast, loud, sharp, dry, clear, penetrating, tense and regular.

The resonance of the voice indicates the possible location of energy stagnation in the body because according to Chinese medical tradition different sounds resonate in different parts of the body. By establishing which sounds are vibrating and which are not, a practitioner gains insight into a person's physical condition.

Typically voice quality is noted during *Mon-Shin*, the art of questioning, when the patient's own views and opinions regarding his or her condition are sought. This process provides insight into the person's character or personality. In Chinese medicine no distinction is made between physical and psychological problems. A person's emotional state and attitudes are indicative of deeper physical symptoms because the major bodily organs are governed by certain emotions. In health the heart and small intestines, lungs and large intestines, spleen and stomach, kidney and bladder, liver and gall bladder are governed respectively by happiness, positiveness, trust, courage and peacefulness. While in illness, these organs are ruled by hysteria, depression, suspicion, fear and anger. The practitioner determines the weakness or strength of these organs by assessing the mixture and predominance of the emotions the individual expresses. Hence character or personality is an important factor in diagnosis.

In traditional oriental medicine, the mind is believed to reflect the overall health of the person as reliably as the body. Accordingly energy imbalances can be revealed in dreams by the predominance or absence of a particular element or correspondences of that element. Dreams are therefore scrutinised for signs such as images of fire, burning, coolness, dryness and so on. Mental images have been used in diagnosis throughout the world since the earliest times. Shamans invoked powerful images in themselves and others as a means of discovering unconscious clues to the onset of illness, emotional and mental factors that might have contributed to its development. This use of visual images to divine or see what others could not was termed 'using the strong eye'. Dream imagery was used diagnostically by the ancient Egyptians and Greeks. Diagnosis also took place in the state of consciousness just prior to sleep when what are now known as hypnogogic images occur. Many cures were attributed to insights derived from this procedure.[32]

In Hippocratic medicine, images, especially those of dreams, were thought to reveal clinically important information and to foster the development of malignancy once established. Galen anticipated modern research findings by indicating that images of sadness, fear and terror produce discrete physiological effects. During the Middle Ages witches, in the manner of shamans, undertook flights of fantasy within the unconscious for the purpose of divining information relevant to illness.

Imaginative methods of diagnosis flourished long after the witches. 'The methods of the shamans and the wise women — healing in non-ordinary reality and invoking visions of spirit guides — has been a part of Christianity since its inception. Only the names have changed.'[33] Churches dedicated to the healing patron saints Cosmas and Damian used the method of incubation sleep, modelled on the *incubatio* or divine sleep cures of the ancient Greeks. In these the sick received diagnostic information and cures from revered healers whose images appeared during the twilight state between sleep and wakefulness. The practice continues within the Christian Church, as does its reputation for effecting exceptional cures.

Carl Jung described the images of dreams as messengers of the soul and like Freud he regarded them as providing highly important diagnostic information. Both men also used waking images of fantasy and daydreams as a means of uncovering unconscious problems, as did numerous psychotherapists influenced by them. Roberto Assagioli viewed images as transformers or conductors of psychic energy, containers of meaning. He considered every element of images as representing at one level or another a personality trait, albeit a distorted, misplaced or projected one.

During the 1960s humanistic psychologists focused attention on imaginative methods. Fritz Perls demonstrated that images, especially those of dreams, were a rich source of information about an individual and developed a wide range of methods by which images can be accessed and explored. Influenced by him, many therapists have used guided imagery diagnostically. Imaginative exercises such as visualising journeying through the body; taking imaginary inventories of the body; engaging in imaginary dialogue with internal parts of the body, creating and interacting with an imaginary inner guide, and dying in one's imagination have all been used in order to gain insight into physical problems and attitudes.

Jung advocated art as a way of revealing hidden features of the self and Freud viewed art diagnostically as evidence of a patient's pathology. Undoubtedly everything that a person creates has an autobiographical aspect in that these products are expressions of imaginal experience and as such can be regarded as self-portraits of psychic life. Art of various kinds can therefore provide useful information, especially about issues normally hidden or avoided. Art has proved diagnostically very effective in working with children.[34] As a child's fantasy process is usually the same as the life process it is possible to look into inner realms by way of fantasy and so find out what is going on within a child's life from his or her perspective. Fantasy is also a means for a child to expressing things which he or she has difficulty admitting and expressing in reality. However, the diagnostic value of art is not confined to children or to psychological problems. It has been applied effectively in the fields of physical medicine.

During the 1970s the American oncologist Carl Simonton used imaginative methods, including art, in the treatment of cancer. He recognised that as emotional and mental factors, including stress, play a significant role in susceptibility to and recovery from all disease the first step in getting well is to understand how these factors have contributed to illness, and to find ways of influencing them in support of treatment. He believed that visualisation might help cancer patients confront their fears and help them gain a sense of control over their illness. Simonton also hoped that visual images produced by patients during fantasy and in artwork might also provide a means of accessing and exploring unhealthy beliefs hidden in the patients' unconscious mind and so yield valuable insights into their condition. He taught his patients a simple form of relaxation and encouraged them to visualise their illness and the form of treatment they were receiving in any way they appeared to them. Having done so they were asked to imagine their cancer shrinking or otherwise responding in a positive way to treatment. Patients were encouraged to imagine pain in the same way rather than trying to suppress it, and they were encouraged to draw their cancer and pain and to use these drawings as a basis for exploring these issues with those who were treating them.

This method was found not only to provide invaluable diagnostic information regarding patients, beliefs, attitudes, fears and expectations but also to produce remarkable results. Of 159 patients with a diagnosis of a medically incurable malignancy treated over a four-year period, none of whom were expected to live more than a year, 22.2 per cent were reported to have made a full recovery. The disease regressed in a further 17 per cent of patients and stabilised in 27 per cent. Further tumour growth was reported in 31 per cent of patients but average survival time increased by a factor of 150–200 per cent. Those who eventually succumbed to malignancy maintained higher than usual levels of activity and achieved a significant improvement in their quality of life.[35]

These results suggest that by changing the fundamental beliefs or expectancies about their malignancies as revealed through imaginative methods patients could bring about significant changes in their physical condition. This supports the evidence regarding placebo effect and findings in the field of PNI which suggest that the interpretations people consistently create become physiology, and highlights the importance of correctly diagnosing beliefs, attitudes and other mental states. As Carolyn Myss[36] has observed, identifying the physical presence of illness is only the first step in the diagnostic process. Of equal importance, or perhaps even more significant, is helping a person understand how and why an illness has developed. This is the complex part of any intuitive diagnosis because it involves identifying a person's emotional, psychological and spiritual stresses.[37]

Recognition of the importance of imaginative methods in revealing inner states and subjective experiences such as pain and anxiety associated with medical procedures has led to their increasing use in diagnosis within orthodox Western medicine. Moreover, such methods are also being increasingly applied as therapy in many health care settings. The pioneers of these methods in modern Western medical practice, who believe that techniques that have served the world so well in medicine since the beginning of recorded history should not be discarded but improved on, have been described as shaman/scientists trying to bridge the gulf between the different worlds of magic and medical science, mind and body.[38] Such a term is misleading, however, because for the most part modern medical practitioners who adopt these methods ignore the soul, not realising that they are methods of divining the soul, which shamans traditionally consider the most important factor in disease, health and healing.

In order to accommodate the soul in contemporary medicine and so bring about a true psychological medicine, a change of approach is needed.

> We have to learn to accept and acknowledge a phenomenology in which information is contained and exchanged by various personal or transpersonal fields, each with their own 'code' systems induced and 'transduced' into other field and code systems, one of which happens to be our conscious mind.[39]

This involves recognising that:

> ... information is encoded in different ways on the organic as well as the inorganic planes. The cellular, biologic level as well as instinctual and psychologic or soul level. Hence information

is present not only in the functioning of our bodies and conscious minds but also in dream, myth and art. The understanding of its code systems is, however, not necessarily accessible to that fractional awareness that is our rational ego-consciousness.[40]

Hence successful diagnosis — divining the encoded information — may need to embrace methods conventionally considered irrational and absurd. Moreover, treatment may need to directed to the level at which this information is encoded.

9

TREATING THE SOUL

For the past two hundred years Western medicine has focused almost exclusively on treating the body. Mental disorders have been viewed largely as a product of brain dysfunction and treated within the medical specialism of psychiatry. The body has generally been regarded as functioning independently of mind and where the mind has been acknowledged as a component in illness such conditions have typically been dismissed as 'merely' psychosomatic, that is, as unreal or insubstantial: illusory. The very word 'psychosomatic' is pejorative.

The emphasis on treating the body has inevitably meant that much medicine is concerned with treating physical symptoms that have manifested there, rather than healing the ultimate cause of illness, the disease itself. These concerns of modern Western medicine are quite aberrant in the history of medicine which, throughout the world since the earliest times, has viewed all sickness as symptomatic of some fundamental dis-ease or disturbance, as sickness of the soul; and mind as a major factor in its onset and development. Accordingly, treatment has been directed to establishing the underlying problem and the contributory psychological factors, where possible influencing the disease factors before they manifest in the form of symptoms within the body. Hence traditional forms of healing can be considered systems of preventative medicine in that the role of the physician is to prevent disease and pre-disease conditions. This is reflected in the Chinese proverb 'the superior doctor prevents illness; the mediocre doctor imminent illness; the inferior doctor treats actual illness.'

Information medicine
Much traditional medicine has to be considered as information medicine because its primary concern is arresting diseases that are in-

form-ation, rather than actually formed or manifest in the body. Until very recently this idea has been quite alien to Western medicine which has directed its attention to identifying *substances* that can give rise to illness and discovering those that will counteract it. The notion that the causes of illness, much less its treatment, could be insubstantive was unthinkable. Yet this is precisely the notion that is supported by modern science: when viewed at the level of cells and molecules the body is ultimately comprised of no-*thing* but energy and information. Such a view underpins all ancient wisdom. As the Sufi poet Rumi observed, 'we come spinning out of nothingness, scattering stars like dust.' Although modern physics supports the concept of information medicine, it is nevertheless very difficult for most conventionally trained doctors to accept that treatments amounting to *nothing* in themselves can be effective.

> Thus, herein lies the first and most important difficulty that orthodox medical science has with alternative approaches. So many of them do not base their rationale on any theory with natural laws as we now understand them. It is simply not possible, to take one simple example, for orthodox scientists to accept that a medicine so dilute that it may contain not so much as one molecule of the remedy in a given dose can have any pharmacological action.[1]

This view expressed in a British Medical Association report on alternative medicine published in 1986 represents that of the governing body of medicine in the United Kingdom. Yet it misrepresents two very important issues:

- the 'natural laws' as they are *now* known are those revealed by modern physics, not the materialistic, mechanistic principles on which orthodox Western medicine is based, and are fully consistent with the principles on which all complementary medicine is based[2]

- the principles of homeopathy (the treatment being referred to), which does not claim any pharmacological action in its remedies. Indeed it is attempts to explain the action of homeopathic remedies which have led to the concept of 'information medicine'.

Homeopathy

Homeopathy was developed in the nineteenth century by the German physician Samuel Hahnemann (1755–1843). It was his view that there are certain basic vibrational patterns of disease, which he termed 'miasms', that originate in the energy fields or auras of living organisms. They may be inherited genetically, or acquired by resonance, the principle whereby energies vibrating with a certain frequency and amplitude reverberate with similar energies in the environment. The former, in the genetic code, and the latter in the form of bacterial or viral attack, toxic pollution in water, food or the environment, can lie dormant for many years and flare up at times of weakness when they influence all the energies of the organism. Then the organism reacts to this disease or imbalance in its energies by attempting to restore balance and in so doing produces the symptoms and signs the patient feels and the doctor observes. Unlike the orthodox physician, Hahnemann considered these not to be illness *per se*, rather the body's reactions to the original state of imbalance. They are the body's defence mechanisms. As such they are an indicator of the extent of the imbalance and how profoundly the organism is affected by it and can be used to determine appropriate treatment for restoring balance. Implicit in Hahnemann's system is the understanding that imbalances occurring in the body are symptomatic of energy imbalances occurring at more subtle levels. These imbalances first manifest at a higher vibrational level than that of the physical or material body — in the psychological or emotional energy fields — the soul plane — and energy imbalances successfully treated at this level do not manifest as symptoms at the physical level.

The treatments Hahnemann developed aimed to restore the balance of subtle energy fields of the body by matching various natural remedies of different vibrational characters or soul qualities with the disharmonies of the body, thereby restoring harmony and inducing health. They utilise the principle of resonance, applying remedies which subject the organism to a periodic disturbance of the same frequency of the body, at which frequency the body displays an enhanced oscillation or vibration. By using a natural substance that in its raw state can produce similar effects to those of the illness, homeopathy (literally meaning 'similar suffering') employs the principle of treating 'like with like'. Hahnemann discovered the importance of this principle while studying the toxicology of cinchona or Peruvian bark from which quinine, used in the treatment of malaria, is extracted. He noted the similarity between quinine poisoning and malaria and realised that it could be the basis of the drug's healing effects. He subsequently discovered that any medicine can cure the particular kind of disease whose symptoms most resemble the effects it produces when taken by healthy individuals. The idea that like cures like, often rendered in Latin as *similia similibus curentur*, is also used in orthodox medicine, notably in vaccines and in the treatment of cancer with cytotoxic drugs and radiation that are in themselves carcinogenic. The same principle also underpins the layman's 'hair of the dog' remedy in the treatment of hangover. Indeed this Law of Similars or correspondences, the idea of connection through a context of analogy, was established in ancient times by Hippocrates and was fundamental to medicine until the modern scientific era. Hahnemann revived this ancient doctrine but in so doing his thinking was well ahead of his time.

Underpinning this principle was the understanding that as all substances have an electromagnetic field there may be an effect on the electromagnetic field of the body caused by the corresponding electromagnetic field of a substance, provided the vibration levels are close enough for one to resonate with the other.[3] Accordingly, the sensitivity of a person to a given substance can be an expression of resonance between the person and the substance and this affinity can be used therapeutically.

The principle of resonance is also the basis for Hahnemann's insistence on taking into account the totality of presenting symptoms. In order to strengthen the entire electromagnetic field or dynamic plane of action it is necessary to find the resonant frequency of the entire organism. This involves taking into account both psychological and biological features. Hence in homeopathy the choice of medicine is always approached with respect to 'bio-emotional wholeness'.[4] Diagnostic indications for potentially beneficial medicines always have to include temperamental and emotional features as these have primacy over physical factors.

If only a partial image of the total symptom picture is acquired, the effect of the therapeutic substance on the organism will be limited only to that vibrational level. If a patient comes to a homeopath complaining of arthritis, for instance, and the only symptoms noted are those relating to the joints while ignoring the rest of the physical plane, the emotional plane, and the mental plane, the prescription can be expected only to act on the joints. Such a procedure is unlikely to produce a cure, and moreover may well result in degeneration in deeper levels.[5]

The aim of homeopathic treatment is to establish a total pattern of symptoms that mirrors the whole patient and is a reflection of his or her overall pattern of adjustment.

The apparency of anything can be annulled by the creation of a perfect duplicate. The homeopathic physician seeks to create a perfect duplicate of the patient's illness by selecting a medicine whose properties produce an artificial illness that exactly mimics the patient's illness.[6]

Hahnemann realised that in order to produce lasting curative results it is necessary to increase the intensity of the electrodynamic field of the therapeutic agent. 'In other words, we must liberate the energy contained within the substance in such a way as to make it more available to interaction with the dynamic plane of the organism.'[7] Hahnemann achieved this by the method of *potentisation*. This involves serial dilution and *succussion* or shaking up of the substance. His crucial observation was that the therapeutic potency of a substance increases the more it is diluted and succussed while simultaneously its toxic effects are nullified. In many homeopathic remedies the active ingredient is so diluted that it is unlikely to contain a single molecule of the original substance.

Once the original substance is no longer present, the remaining energy in the solvent can be continually enhanced *ad infinitum*. The solvent molecules have taken on the dynamic energy of the original substance. We know from clinical results that the therapeutic energy still retains the 'vibrational frequency' of the original substance, but the energy has been enhanced to such a degree that it is capable of stimulating the dynamic plane of the patient sufficiently to produce a cure.

Hahnemann's discoveries of the process of potentization and the Law of Similars have truly revolutionised the scientific potential of therapeutics. On the one hand, the principle of the Law of Similars provides us with a method of matching resonant vibrations of virtually any substance in the environment with that of the patient. As we have seen in instances of temporary relief, through administration of crude therapeutic agents, the crude form often possesses insufficient intensity to produce permanent cure. On the other hand, with Hahnemann's discovery of a technique to increased therapeutic intensity on the dynamic plane indefinitely, we now possess a way to stimulate the defence mechanism of the patient with whatever intensity is needed to overpower the force of the disease.[8]

However, within homeopathy the therapeutic relationship is also recognised as crucial to the effectiveness of any treatment It is by its nature intimate because the homeopath becomes involved in all aspects of the patient's life. Nevertheless, the relationship is non-intrusive and non-directive. The homeopath avoids leading questions and putting words in the patient's mouth and accurately records the patient's responses in exact quotes. These are not taken at face value but explored in depth. Each symptom is also attended to in great detail. Indeed, the level of attention given to the patient in homeopathy has led to the suggestion[9] that the therapeutic relationship is the crucial resonance and that the remedies are merely a crutch. This would be disputed by the vast numbers of people throughout the world who use homeopathic remedies in self-treatment most effectively without recourse to any homeopathic practitioner. Arguably the therapeutic relationship and the remedies in homeopath are mutually reinforcing.

Hahnemann's system of medicine differs from conventional Western medicine in a number of significant ways. His approach to medicine was fundamentally spiritual rather than material or physical.

Homeopathy demonstrates that non-material force fields —

'souls' as it were — of practically any and every existing substance are able to aid in psychosomatic transformation and effectively to influence health and counter disease.[10]

Like the spiritual traditions that underpin healing systems throughout history homeopathy emphasises the correspondence between the organism and the universe and reinforces the ancient idea of the sympathy of all things. It uses this principle as the basis of treatment.

> If all forms of human pathology correspond to a 'similar' dynamic inherent in some substance 'field' of a plant, mineral or animals substance 'out here', it is as though all of the human functional patterns of health and disease, somatic and psychic functioning, are reflected in some 'outer world' element, plant, animal or mineral. Through a matching of the dynamics within and without, a healing process is initiated. Hahnemann's deed was the demonstration of the effectiveness of an isomorphic or syntonic rather than oppositional approach, that is, of the effectiveness of going *with* rather than *against* the pattern one wishes to influence.[11]

Homeopathic treatment therefore consists not of opposing a problem, as in conventional allopathic medicine by introducing a condition different to the cause of the disease, but in using the problem as its solution. Hahnemann's approach was closely allied to that of Hippocrates and Paracelsus. He used the term 'vital force' to describe the balancing process within each living organism that promotes, or at least protects, health. He claimed that this vital force, comparable with Hippocrates' *vix medicatrix naturae*, is stimulated by internal and external factors to build up a counteractive reaction. The result of the interaction between the vital force and the conditions that set it in motion produces various symptoms in the body revealing that an imbalance has occurred. Disease is thus a product of stress and failure of the body's own attempt to heal itself, whereas health is the maintenance of the vital force or inner nature of the organism itself. Accordingly, homeopathy treats the person rather than the disease, and the cause of the disease rather than its symptoms.

In theory and practice homeopathy has parallels with ancient traditions of medicine. It also has marked similarities with twentieth-century psychotherapy, notably the person-centred therapy of Carl Rogers, who shared Hahnemann's view of the conditions in which the vital force flourishes and the idea that solutions to problems can be facilitated by accurate reflection of their symptoms.

This is not the only sense in which Hahnemann's thinking is contemporary.

> In ... discovering the effectiveness of highly attenuated, indeed really dematerialized 'substances' Hahnemann stumbled upon a phenomenon that is barely beginning to be understood in modern physics, a dynamic that might be likened to spirit, information or meaning in matter — a mapping for empirical experiential verification of that ... border area where material and nonmaterial, mind and matter, psyche and soma seem to overlap or even be one. All functions of humans, animals or even plants seem to interact in terms of such transmaterial fields, a sort of 'structured nothingness'.[12]

By directing treatment at this non-material level homeopathy is modifying information and thereby dealing indirectly with the chemistry and structure of the physical body. It treats energies on the psychological and emotional level that inform the body, giving it structure and form. As such Hahnemann's system of medicine is both ancient and modern, directed to what Plato referred to as the realm of perfect forms, or the soul, and to the dynamic fields of energy, information and intelligence of contemporary physics. It can also be classed as subjective medicine. 'In part because it deals with energy that can strongly be perturbed by the mental and emotional activity of individuals and in part because there has not been any diagnostic equipment to support the homeopathic physician.'[13] Quintessentially, however, homeopathy is psychological medicine, applying knowledge of the soul in the art of healing.

Homeopathy is widespread throughout Europe and has been available through the National Health Service in the United Kingdom since 1977. In addition to six homeopathic hospitals there are numerous homeopathic physicians within orthodox medical practice, whose most distinguished patrons include the Royal Family.

Homeopathy is also widely and is increasingly practised within the field of veterinary medicine. However, there remains a great deal of opposition to homeopathy within orthodox Western medicine. The effects of homeopathy, where acknowledged at all within orthodox medicine, are often dismissed as placebo effects because the dose of remedies used are considered too minute to have any pharmacological potency. The counter-argument is that the vibrational character of that substance — and hence the information it contains — is retained and potentised through succussion or vigorous shaking. The active component of the homeopathic remedy is thus physical rather than chemical and operates on similar principles to dissipative structures in that by shaking up existing patterns of energies within the body it enables the system to reorganise and a new form to emerge. Since, at a fundamental level, energy is information, it is hypothesised that this information can be transferred to water or other solvents, stored and passed to a biological system if it is in a sensitised state. An appropriate model for its action is the computer disk.

> If you had a homeopathic 'ultra-molecular' dilution chemically analysed, it would be found to contain nothing but water, ethanol (the dilution medium) and lactose (from the tablets onto which the dilutions are absorbed). However, if you had the same chemist analyse a computer disk, it would be found to consist only of vinyl and ferric oxide, yet for all the chemist knew it might contain the complete works of Shakespeare! The point is that the information is stored in physical, not chemical, form. This model also emphasises the importance of pre-sensitisation — you could only read the information on the disk if you had the right kind of computer with the right operating system and software.[14]

Despite its plausibility in physical terms, the concept of information medicine is not widely acknowledged within medicine and the effectiveness of homeopathic remedies still remains an issue. From the outset, homeopaths have conducted 'provings' of remedies on volunteers in order to determine their effects. Orthodox physicians often dismiss this proof, claiming that their efficacy has not been demonstrated in clinical trials. These are complicated in homeopathy by the highly individualised nature of the treatment. However, there is growing evidence from appropriately controlled studies reported in leasing medical journals that homeopathy is effective in the treatment of various conditions. A review of 107 clinical trials of homeopathy[15] found that 77 per cent gave positive results, though admittedly this is insufficient evidence from which to draw definite conclusions. Other controlled studies have found that in the treatment of some conditions homeopathy performs better than placebo. Support for the effectiveness of homeopathic remedies also comes from the growing number of studies in veterinary medicine, where placebo effect is controlled for in the very nature of the animal subjects.

Flower remedies

The principles of homeopathy put forward by Hahnemann greatly influenced the British physician Edward Bach. In 1919 Bach became a bacteriologist and pathologist at the London Homoeopathic Hospital where he developed various oral bacterial vaccines, or nosodes, that are still widely used in homeopathic practice. He shared Hahnemann's view that disease cannot be cured or eradicated by materialistic methods because it is immaterial in origin, the end product of deep and long-acting forces. He believed that apparently successful materialistic methods of treatment provide only temporary relief unless the real cause of disease is removed. For Bach the real cause of disease is a distortion in the body's energy field resulting from conflict between the essential self or soul and the mind or personality. His ideas, like those of Hahnemann, share much in common with the theories of Carl Rogers. This conflict produces negative states of mind that deplete the natural vitality of the body and render it susceptible to infection and illness. Like Hahnemann, Bach looked to natural remedies to restore healthy states of mind.

His clinical experience confirmed his belief that disease is 'the consolidation of mental attitude' — the coming into form of negative states of mind. Hence mental attitude should be used as a guide to necessary treatment because the mind shows the onset and cause of disease more definitely and much sooner that the body. In 1930, aged 43, he gave up his Harley Street practice to search for a method of treatment even more natural than homeopathy, which did not require 'anything to be destroyed or altered'.

Bach's research led him to conclude that positive, healthy states of mind could be restored by the energies found in flowering plants, trees and shrubs and special waters. Initially he discovered twelve healing herbs each with a natural affinity to certain mental traits. He believed these showed the same vibrational character as the quality concerned but without the distortion and at the natural rhythm, and so could be used to re-establish its harmonious vibration through the principle of resonance. Accordingly, by operating at subtle energy levels these flowers can act as a catalyst for reintegration and healing.

> They are able like beautiful music or any glorious thing that gives us inspiration to raise our very natures and bring us nearer to our souls, and by that very act bring us peace and relieve our sufferings. They cure not by attacking disease, but by flooding our bodies with the beautiful vibrations of our Higher Nature, in the presence of whom disease melts away as snow in sunshine.[16]

Bach subsequently identified 38 healing remedies that he believed could be used to remedy all the known states of mind that afflict humankind. He considered his flower remedies to be a complete system of healing requiring 'no extension or alteration'. Like Hahnemann, he believed that the patient should be treated rather than the disease, and the cause rather than its effects.

Bach tested the remedies on himself and also treated many patients successfully with them. His findings were verified by a medical colleague who used the remedies in his own practice. After his death his work was continued in his name. Bach believed his system to be complete but in recent years many other systems of treatment with flower essences have been developed. Some of these are considerably more extensive than Bach's system. However, they all utilise similar principles. Flower essences have been described as 'liquid pattern-infused solutions made from individual plant flowers, each containing a specific imprint that responds in a balancing, repairing and rebuilding manner to imbalances in humans on their physical, emotional, mental and spiritual or universal levels'.[17] This 'imprint' is the vibrational character of the flower — its soul — and the information it conveys.

> It's commonly understood that everything in the universe has a vibration to it. What makes something red is its vibration. Scientifically, you'd say red is its vibration. Flowers have a certain frequency too. If you process a flower into an essence and you take it into your body, it starts to vibrate at that frequency. It starts to create a synchronization of other cells and tissues in your body, causing them to vibrate at that level.[18]

This synchronisation can be likened to the way a tuning fork behaves. Striking a tuning fork causes others near to it to begin vibrating at the same frequency. As Bach noted, the effects of flower essences may also be likened to hearing a particularly moving piece of music whose sound vibrations indirectly affect physiological processes such as breathing, pulse rate, and other physical states. Certainly there is now abundant evidence that emotions produce hormonal changes that trigger biochemical responses, which in turn bring about changes in nerve function, digestion, respiration, circulation and the immune system.[19] However, the role of flower essences in these processes has still to be scientifically investigated and established. It needs to be shown first that infusions of flowers carry vibrations that trigger changes in the energy of the human body and that this particular energy change is related to emotions.

Nevertheless, flower remedies are now known and used world-wide in the treatment of humans, animals and plants. However, although tested in a manner similar to the provings of homeopathy, these flower essences have not been subjected to clinical trials and are not recognised within orthodox medicine.

Anthroposophical medicine

Anthroposophical medicine shares many principles in common with the systems of psychological medicine advocated by Hahnemann and Bach. It was developed by Rudolph Steiner (1861–1925) who put forward a 'fourfold picture of man'. He considered there to be three energy 'bodies' or levels of existence and consciousness beyond the physical:

- etheric

- astral

- spiritual.

Disease occurs when a person's four bodies malfunction in some way. As these four levels of being interrelate, psychosomatic processes work in both directions: the mind can produce malfunctions in the body and the body can produce mental disturbances. Therefore Steiner believed that any physical treatment should always be supported by treatment of the mind. Ultimately, however, in Steiner's system the root cause of all disease, mental or physical, is spiritual. The anthroposophical physician (only medically qualified doctors are allowed to train in and practice anthroposophical medicine) works to discover what underlies an illness and requires a spiritual awareness not demanded of orthodox doctors. The physician also administers remedies, mainly natural substances whose energies can be utilised to rectify energetic imbalance in the different energy bodies of man, notably homeopathic remedies which Steiner recognised as working on a spiritual level.

Radionics

Radionics also sees diseases and remedies as having their own frequency or vibration. Whereas treatment by homeopathy, flower essences and anthroposophical medicine involves prescriptions of natural sources of the correctional vibrational frequencies, radionics practitioners transmit vibrational energy of the needed frequency back to the patient using radionics devices. However the radionic rates of homeopathic, herbal, flower, gem and many other remedies can also be established in order to determine the most helpful treatments for any condition. Based on the work of George de la Warr, who developed radionics equipment which incorporated sound waves, practitioners have been able to transmit simulations of homeopathic remedies.

Psychological factors in illness

Emotions and their expression

The forms of healing described above are claimed by their exponents to exert their influence at the level of the energy field that controls the physical body. They are considered to achieve their effect by attunement to and amplification of the higher vibrations of the organism, resulting in the stimulation of the body's self-healing processes. Such healing can be likened to applying jump leads to a car battery, the depleted energies of which are boosted enabling the car to charge itself. Fundamentally the methods address the individual's psychological and emotional energies which are considered to be at a higher level than the physical energies of the body. The idea that these energies 'inform' the body, which is the fundamental principle of psychological medicine, is not new. Hippocrates viewed health as the balance of bodily humours that were affected by thoughts, feelings, emotions, behaviours and environmental factors. Accordingly, healing involved restoring equilibrium by regulation of psychological and environmental factors and lifestyle. Galen who, in the second century AD, systematised Hippocratic medicine, considered the emotional aspects of personality, notably depression, hostility, apathy and optimism, to be directly linked to health. He noted that cancer more commonly occurred in women of melancholic disposition than in those of more sanguine personality type. This view has found support among physicians throughout history and has been supported by modern research.[20–3]

Other psychological factors have been identified in cancer patients including the repression and denial of emotions, the inability to express hostile feelings, poor outlet for emotional discharge, a tendency towards self-sacrifice and blame, rigidity, impaired self-awareness and a predisposition to hopelessness and despair. Cancer has also been described as a disease following emotional resignation and loss of hope,[24] which is found in those who try to gain approval from others, suppress anger and experience other negative emotions,[25] and research evidence strongly suggests that cancer patients characteristically suppress emotion and seem to ignore negative feelings such as hostility, depression and guilt. Differences have been found between benign and malignant breast cancer patients in their expression of anger.[26] Long-term survivors of breast cancer express much higher levels of hostility, anxiety, alienation and other negative emotions than short-term survivors[27] and patients with malignant tumours have also been found to be more repressed in the expression of anxiety and to be more passive and appeasing.[28] Patients who express emotion freely and show active determination to fight their disease live longer than those who are meek, passive, complaining or defeatist.[29] Cancer patients have also been identified as being characterised by a greater tendency to hold resentment and not forgive, to be self-pitying, have a poor ability to develop and maintain meaningful long-term relationships and a poor self-image. Cancer patients report more subjectively experienced stress than controls.[30] Indeed the link between cancer and stress is well-established in the psychological literature.[31]

Recognition of the psychological characteristics of cancer patients has led to the notion of the cancer-prone or 'Type C' personality.[32] There is some evidence to support such a proposition but this is far from conclusive. It has also been argued[33] that cancer patients are no different from patients who develop other serious diseases and that there is a common group of causes for cancer, heart attack, stroke, and related thrombotic diseases which includes chronic stress, a predisposed personality type and chronic hyperactivation of neural, endocrine, immune, blood clotting and fibrinolytic systems. A number of studies have suggested a common pattern of psychological helplessness and hopelessness in various diseases. Women with rheumatoid arthritis have been found to be tense, moody, and depressed; concerned with rejection they perceived from their mothers and the strictness of their fathers; to show denial and inhibition of the expression of anger; and to reflect compliance, subserviance, conservatism, shyness, introversion and the need for security on standard tests of personality.[34] Emotional or affective factors have also been linked with respiratory and infectious diseases, and with multiple sclerosis (MS). There is a greater incidence of overt depressive disorders in MS populations, and a large proportion of MS patients exhibit depressive characteristics.[35]

Nevertheless there are numerous difficulties in studying possible psychological causes of illness, especially cancer. Although spoken of as one illness, cancer takes many forms that may have quite different causes. Factors that may be responsible for the initial onset of the disease may be different from those involved in its subsequent development. The onset of cancer may occur many years before any signs of disease are evident, so factors that are cited as antecedent conditions may in fact have occurred after the cancer became established. It is also possible that the presence of cancer, whether recognised by the patient or not, may have influenced the patient's psychological state by its physical effects on brain and body chemistry. Consequently the problems involved in designing research studies that will produce valid information about the psychological precursors of cancer or other diseases are formidable. Currently there is no generally accepted means of exactly defining and measuring many of the psychological variables investigated with the result that the findings of different studies vary with the different methods used. Nevertheless, there is abundant evidence supporting the influence of emotional factors on endocrine and immune functions.

Psychoneuroimmunology attempts to explain the mechanisms by which the mind works upon the body to influence illness, health and healing. Its central focus is to advance understanding of immunity. During the 1920s the Russian physiologist Ivan Pavlov established that guinea pigs could learn to produce specific antibodies in response to being handled by research workers in the laboratory. Some fifty years later it was found that rats can learn to enhance or suppress immune functions. The finding that cells in the immune system of rats could be trained initially attracted a good deal of scepticism but has now been conclusively demonstrated in numerous studies. Research findings from hundreds of studies relating to the influence of the mind on immunity have now been published. All of them point to the conclusion that the immune system is controlled by structures, particularly those involved in emotion, such as the hypothalamus and pituitary gland, and can be artificially stimulated to increase or decrease immune functioning. Moreover, thought and emotion produce molecules known as peptides that have receptors throughout the body. Intelligence and emotion are thus happening everywhere simultaneously, and as peptides are the place where learning occurs, memory is also located throughout the body. This has important implications for treatment.

Biofeedback

'A body that can "think" is far different from the one medicine now treats.'[36] It can learn to respond in various ways. This principle underpins biofeedback, which demonstrates that organisms can learn to control bodily processes and functions formerly considered involuntary or autonomic if feedback of information about that process or function is provided. There is nothing new in this principle. For over 5000 years Indian masters have taught their students to consciously self-regulate their psychological and physiological processes, and throughout the world many people have for centuries used various aspects of self-regulation in healing rituals. Modern biofeedback uses various devices such as the electrical skin resistance meter (ESRM) and the electroencephalograph (EEG) to provide information about bodily processes. EEG studies have revealed that every physiological state is accompanied by an apparent change in emotional and mental state, conscious and unconscious, and conversely that every conscious or unconscious emotional or mental state is accompanied by apparent change in physiology. By producing a pleasant sound that increases when *alpha* brain waves fall below a certain level, it was established that most subjects could learn to produce or suppress *alpha* waves at will and that *alpha* waves seemed to be associated with feelings of well-being. Gradually it emerged that any neurophysiological or other biological function that can be monitored or amplified and fed back can be regulated. Over a period of weeks subjects can acquire control of heartbeat, overcome rhythmic disabilities of atrial fibrillation and premature ventricular contraction, control high blood pressure without the use of drugs, vary the temperature of the hands, regulate stomach acidity and alter blood platelet formation. Research into these functions was greatly assisted by the development of the polygraph, an instrument for simultaneous electrical or mechanical recording of several involuntary physiological activities including blood pressure, pulse rate, respiration and perspiration. Using the information it provides, subjects are able to make links in their behaviour and make regulation possible. So self-regulation feats considered 'paranormal' only a few years ago, such as control over blood pressure or heart rate, can now be trained in half an hour.

Biofeedback has been used successfully in the treatment of numerous conditions. However, while many effects have been demonstrated in the laboratory or clinic, these are not necessarily or readily achieved outside these environments. This is because the bulky and expensive equipment capable of precisely monitoring subtle biological changes means that it is generally laboratory based. However, other methods of training subtle biological processes show more promise for use outside the laboratory or clinic.

Aromatherapy

In the same way that the immune systems of rats can be trained to associate the scent of camphor with immuno-enhancement or suppression, so different aromas may be used to condition the immune response, reduce heart rate, blood pressure or pain. These applications of aromatherapy and phytotherapy are currently being explored in both human and animal treatment.

The powerful effects of plant odours on emotions and mental processes have been recognised for centuries. The sacred scriptures of India, the Upanishads, describe the art of energising body, mind and soul through breathing, and aromatic plants have been used for this purposes in many traditional healing practices. The ancient Egyptians used perfumes to induce sleep, stimulate dreaming and reduce anxiety and in ancient Greece aromatic oils were variously used for their antidepressant, soporific, stimulant or aphrodisiac effects.

The chemistry of plant oils and the brain are now more widely understood and it is recognised that plant odours stimulate different parts of the brain. When inhaled they are transmuted into nerve messages that are initially translated by the amygdala and hippocampus, memory centres in the limbic system that have a major role in emotional response. Hence at this point an odour may trigger a recent or long-established memory. Some odours may then stimulate the thalamus to produce enkephalins, painkilling substances that also have an uplifting effect. Others may stimulate the pituitary gland to secrete endorphins that induce euphoria, or the raphe nucleus and locus ceruleus to produce the stimulants serotonin, and noredrenaline. Aromatic oils may therefore be used to produce these effects directly. They may also be used to produce certain effects indirectly by learned associations. By linking a certain learned response such as lowering blood pressure with a specific odour, a person or animal can be trained to produce that response every time they inhale the odour. In this way control of autonomic functions may be achieved.

However, a more recent approach to aromatherapy is concerned with plant oils not as chemical mixtures but as 'liquid vibrations', each having a certain resonance with a colour, sound and different bodily organs. By stimulating the organs and energies of the body these oils can bring about physical, mental, emotional or spiritual effects, whether simply by warming the body, stimulating circulation and relaxing muscle tension, enhancing positive emotions and feelings of well-being, or 'raising the spirits' in a more transcendent sense. Odours can thus be used to treat disease on a level that corresponds to the subtle energies of the person.

Colour therapy

Many of the effects produced by odours can be elicited by colour and light, which are merely different vibrational forms. In the ancient world each of the energies that make up sunlight was considered to reflect a different aspect of the divine and to influence different qualities of life. The origins of healing with colour in Western civilisation can be traced back to the mythology of ancient Egypt and Greece. Interest in the physical nature of colour developed in ancient Greece alongside the concept of elements. Each element was associated with a certain colour. Hence colour had an intrinsic role in healing, which involved restoring the balance of these elements. Coloured garments, oils, plasters, ointments and salves were used to treat disease and Pythagoras and Hippocrates referred to them in several treatises on medicine.

A disciple of Aristotle, the Arabic physician Avicenna (980–1037) indicated the importance of colour in both diagnosis and treatment in his *Canon of Medicine*. He noted that colour is an observable symptom of disease and developed a chart to relate colour to temperament and the physical condition of the body. He also used colour in treatment and wrote about its possible dangers, observing that a person with a nose-bleed should not gaze on things of a brilliant red colour or be exposed to red light as this would stimulate blood flow, whereas blue would reduce it.

During the Middle Ages, Paracelsus used colour and light extensively in treatment but, with the advent of physical medicine in the seventeenth century and its emphasis on surgery and antiseptics, interest in healing with colour declined and did not resurface until the nineteenth century.

Since then extensive research on colour has established many of its therapeutic properties. It has been used in orthodox medicine to prevent scar tissue forming, in the treatment of tuberculosis, neonatal jaundice, cancers, non-malignant tumours, arthritis, seasonal affective disorder, anorexia, insomnia, jet lag, drug dependency, impotence, depression, migraine, and headache.

Colour has also been successfully used in many non-medical settings. Studies have shown that viewing red light increases subjects' strength by 13.5 per cent and elicits 5.8 per cent more muscular activity in the arms and muscles. Hence it is often used in gymnasia. Red light is also used to improve the performance of athletes. It appears to help them achieve short, quick bursts of energy, whereas blue light assists in performances requiring a steady energy output.

Colour also affects emotion. Pink has been found to have a tranquillising and calming effect within minutes of exposure. It suppresses hostile, aggressive and anxious behaviour and reduces muscle strength within 2.7 seconds of exposure. It appears that in pink surroundings people cannot be aggressive because the colour saps their energy.[37] Hence pink holding cells are widely used in prisons and reformatories to reduce violent and aggressive behaviour.

Other studies have confirmed the effects of colour on emotions[38] as suggested in phrases like 'seeing red', 'feeling blue' and 'being in the pink'. However, research has also confirmed that colour need not be visually perceived for it to have definite psychological and physical effects. It can be distinguished by blind, colour-blind and blindfold subjects.

The connection between emotion and physiology

The connection between emotion and the autonomic nervous system was first indicated in the 1920s. By the 1950s it had been established that a close affinity exists between some neurotransmitters and some endocrines, and between the pituitary or master gland and one of the chief regulating systems of the brain, the hypothalamus. It thus became clear that hormones are a more important regulator of behaviour than had previously been recognised by psychologists. This new awareness gave rise to a new field of investigation, that of psychoneuroendocrinology, which was the precursor to psychoneuroimmunology.

The endocrine system was thought to be the sole mediator between the brain and the immune system until the 1980s. Then neural projections were identified from the spinal cord and medulla to the thymus gland (which stimulates the production of the T-cells of the immune system) in both rats and mice. This suggested a role for these functions in the regulation of thymic functions and established the role of the lower brain areas with regard to immunity, but not of the mind which is usually synonymous with the higher areas of the cortex of the brain. However, the hypothalamus, which has an important regulatory role in immune function, is intimately connected with the limbic system, part of the brain involved in emotion. The limbic system, in turn, forms a connecting network with the frontal lobes, which are the most evolved part of the cortex. The existence of connections between the brain and the immune system raised the question of whether behaviour or events modulated by various brain areas can be associated with changes in immune functions, and whether the findings of animal studies can be generalised to humans.

Research in the field of psychoneuroimmunology has shown that psychological distress can lead to adverse immunological changes providing one pathway through which major and minor life events might result in an increased incidence of infectious and malignant disease.[39] Consequently it is now widely accepted that both the neuroendocrine and immune systems can be influenced by external stress once it has been perceived by the central nervous system. Stress is characterised by activation of both the autonomic nervous system and the hypothalamo–pituitary–adrenal axis. The resulting neurochemical changes have been demonstrated to affect the immune system both directly and indirectly. While elucidation of the pathways of communication between the central nervous system and the immune system has advanced largely from animal studies, there is also a wealth of supporting evidence from human studies. Knowledge about the mechanisms of action is still limited but there is a growing literature describing such relationships, and their health-related consequences.

As a result the catalytic effect of stress on individuals with a predisposition to auto-immune diseases can now be explained. For over a century the relationship between stress and auto-immune disease has been recognised. In 1881 the association between MS and emotional disturbances was reported. There have since been many reports that support the claim that stress and psychosocial factors contribute to human auto-immune disease. A large body of evidence suggests that the onset of rheumatoid arthritis usually conforms to one of two patterns. It may occur after a single abrupt life event, such as the death of a spouse or close relative, separation from a loved one due to illness or divorce; loss of employment or sudden financial loss; or after a long series of unpleasant experiences. This may include long-term family discord, work stress or pressures associated with other responsibilities. The onset of auto-immune thyroid diseases and insulin dependent diabetes mellitus also show a link with stressful life events,[40] and patients with multiple sclerosis report a higher level of distress or stressful life events occurring just prior to the onset of MS symptoms. Other studies have revealed an association between MS and emotional disorders.

Emotional traits such as easily aroused hostility are also a feature of the personality type thought to be associated with coronary heart disease. Other characteristics of this 'Type A' personality include ambitiousness, acquisitiveness, competitiveness, preoccupation with deadlines, a continual sense of urgency, and fierce impatience. These traits, which are relatively enduring and consistent over the lifespan, translate into physical behaviours such as brisk body movements, fist-clenching during normal conversation, explosive and hurried speech, upper chest breathing, muscle tension. These are associated with physiological effects such as high blood pressure, raised levels of certain blood hormones such as adrenaline, norepinephrine, insulin, growth hormone and hydrocortisone, increased respiratory rate and activity of the sweat glands. These are all characteristic symptoms of stress and reflect the fact that the Type A person is constantly stressed. By contrast the 'Type B' personality is largely free of the sense of urgency that characterises Type A individuals. They are more leisurely and relaxed, though no less successful than Type A persons because they also tend to be generally well organised and efficient. They are also healthier, showing significantly fewer signs of coronary heart disease, but these findings are not as clear cut as was initially supposed.

The problem with research that tries to link personality with the onset and development of specific illnesses is that personality is a complex construct. It refers to the sum total of all the behavioural and psychological characteristics by means of which an individual is recognised as being unique. It comprises emotions, attitudes and disposition, beliefs, moods and coping styles. These factors are not discrete but interact in complex ways. This is evident in relation to stress.

Stress

There is now little doubt that stress contributes to a great deal of illness, both psychological and physical, and it became fashionable to think of stress itself as the major disease of the late twentieth century. Increasing concern about the stress of modern life led to various attempts during the 1960s, and subsequently, to score the stress impact of life events and produce 'stress' tables as a guide to the amount of stress a person can withstand. Typically events were rated on a scale between 0 and 100, with an event such as death of a spouse being assigned the maximum rating. Consequently the view of stress most widely promoted is that stress is caused by external factors beyond personal control and so must be avoided. Stress has therefore become a negative concept and stress avoidance the goal of many people pursuing health. However, by the late twentieth century it had been recognised that the interaction between life events and the individual is considerably more complex. An unhappy marriage or poor working conditions, while not events *per se* may nevertheless be highly stressful. Moreover, not only life events but ordinary everyday occurrences and irritations need to be taken into account; they frequently accompany major life events and in the short term they are better predictors of psychosomatic and physical symptoms than major life events.[41, 42]

While awareness of these factors appears to justify the growing concern with stress, the stress impact of an event, whether major or minor, when viewed objectively may be very different from the way it is experienced subjectively. Furthermore, the impact of the same event may vary, often dramatically, from person to person and in the same individual over time. Assigning a fixed numerical stress rating to an event can therefore be very misleading. Recently developed stress scales are more sensitive and score events on a ten-point scale. They also include items such as buying, selling and moving house, having a child commence school and pet-related problems. Nevertheless, their emphasis on stressful events implies that stress is 'out there' in the world, beyond the control of individuals, and obscures their role in determining stress. Ultimately, however, stress depends on the individual's attitude towards and interpretation of events and how he or she copes with them. As a result of research it is becoming increasingly evident that these factors are instrumental in determining the impact of stress on the autonomic nervous system, the immune system and susceptibility to disease.

Having the right attitude

The stress associated with an event depends to a great extent on whether a person appraises it as a threat or a challenge, as positive or negative. Those who view an event positively tend to see it as an opportunity to learn, grow and develop, whereas those who view it negatively tend to experience it aversively, as stressful and try to avoid it. The former not only cope with events that others find stressful, but may actually thrive as a result.[43] These differences in appraisal can result in enormous differences in how people respond to potentially stressful events and the amount of stress they experience. In a study[44] conducted in a US company during a prolonged and uncertain period of wide-sweeping and major reorganisation, psychologists found that half the executives experienced high levels of stress whereas the other half remained healthy. The latter were similar in terms of income, job status, educational levels, age, ethnic background and religious affiliation but their attitudes towards themselves, their jobs and fellow workers were totally different. Characteristically these executives had a strong commitment to themselves, their work and families; a sense of control over their lives; and an ability to see change in their lives as a challenge rather than a threat. They accepted that change, rather than stability, is the norm in life and welcomed it as an opportunity for growth and self-development. They sought novelty, tolerated ambiguity and showed mental flexibility and a strong sense of purpose in dealing with life's problems. Moreover, they looked to other people for support when they needed it.

By comparison, the executives who were less hardy experienced a sense of powerlessness, were threatened by change, anxious in the face of uncertainty and lacked social support. However, their most marked characteristic was alienation, not only from themselves but also from others. In other words, these non-hardy types experienced their world and others as unfriendly and hostile.

Subsequently the characteristics of psychological hardiness identified in this study — commitment, control and challenge — were confirmed in studies of managers, other professional groups and patients. However, a significant factor emerged in relation to army officers. While a sense of commitment and control appeared to protect officers from stress, those who were oriented towards challenge were in fact more prone to illness. This suggests that when a person's need for stimulation is not matched by opportunities for it, more illness can result. The results of the army study therefore highlighted the importance of finding the proper balance of stimulation and challenge in life.

The tendency to accentuate the negative outcomes of stress obscures the important stimulus value of change, challenge and novelty in spurring people on to achievements and satisfactions. If avoided entirely boredom would result, which ultimately might prove more stressful and hazardous because studies of sensory deprivation show that under-stimulation can cause the central nervous system to produce mental and physical disorders. Accordingly the concept of stress has been modified in recent years so as to distinguish between stress, that is, the subjectively experienced effects of an event, and stressors, the events *per se*. It also now takes into account, not only the nature of the stressor — its frequency, duration and intensity — and the individual's resources for dealing with it, but also other psychological variables, such as the need for stimulation and excitement, and the person's attitude towards, and interpretation of events. Hardiness induction groups, in which highly stressed hypertensive executives are helped to cope with stressors by appraising themselves and their stressors positively, have shown that after eight weekly sessions they score higher on tests of hardiness, report fewer symptoms of psychological stress and have lower blood pressure than executives in an untreated control group.[45] These results show that people can learn to avoid the negative consequences of stress by changing their attitude towards it.

Studies of cancer patients[46] have suggested that their attitude is vitally important in determining the outcome of the illness. Those with spontaneous remission of cancer are found to be positive in attitude. A clear correlation is also found between mental attitude and length of survival.[47] Cancer patients who outlive predicted life expectancies have been found to refuse to give up in the face of stress, to be more non-conformist, with greater psychological insight and flexibility.[48] Flexibility, or the willingness to make changes, seems to be a particularly crucial factor in recovery. Those who respond poorly to treatment are usually characterised by rigidity and holding on to self-image and the familiar.

Attitudinal healing

In contrast positive attitudes are widely considered life-enhancing and even life-giving. Therefore creating attitude change — sometimes known as attitudinal healing — focuses on trying to shift a person in a more positive direction. It works on the principle that if a person can change their outlook they can change themselves and the world around them. Rigidity is viewed as a response to fear, so the person is encouraged to confront the fear, let go of it and transform it into positive emotion and acceptance. This principle forms the basis of a good deal of psychotherapy and also various widely popularised self-healing approaches.[49] The requirements for such attitude change include the ability to accept criticism; self-acceptance and affirming self-worth; seeing the positive in all circumstances, and problems as situations to learn from; looking forward with joy rather backwards with sorrow, focusing on what one has rather than what one lacks; letting go of what is no longer needed and making the most of what one attracts. Essentially, attittudinal healing can be viewed as cultivating a relaxed approach to life.

Relaxation

It is now widely accepted that relaxation is an antidote to stress and as such is valuable in the prevention and treatment of illness and maintenance of health. By promoting heightened awareness of muscle tension within the body it increases physical self-awareness and attention to bodily cues and may reveal pain and other symptoms of illness ordinarily masked by high levels of tension. This is particularly important in persons with a tendency to repress painful and distressing conditions. However, relaxation is not concerned simply with the body and bodily tensions and associated physiological processes, but also with psychological factors. Indeed it can only be fully effective when mental attitudes, beliefs, negative emotions and expectancies are relaxed because physical tensions are the inevitable consequence of mental tensions and conflicts. Hence all forms of relaxation aim at suspension of ordinary mental activity which predominantly involves verbal thinking. Relaxation of verbal thinking enables access to ordinarily inaccessible regions of the self, which because they are beyond normal awareness, may be considered unconscious. These regions constitute non-ordinary reality and awareness of them amounts to an altered state of consciousness in which the person establishes contact with living energies conveying information and ideas. Relaxation therefore puts people more in touch with their souls, and by way of it a person can gain insight into his or her condition and influence it. Relaxation of verbal thinking is achieved by encouraging non-verbal mental images — traditionally considered the specific utterances of the soul. Imaginative methods are therefore common to many different forms of relaxation, and to certain forms of yoga, meditation, biofeedback, hypnosis and autogenic training, all of which are now recognised as promoting strikingly similar effects consistent with a physiological state of deep relaxation. These include: the quieting of the sympathetic nervous system, as manifested in altered skin resistance, brain wave and breathing patterns, and reduction in other measures of physiological arousal such as muscle activity, heart and pulse rate, blood pressure and blood hormone levels.

Music therapy

Many of these physiological effects can be elicited by music. Throughout the ancient world, music was widely acknowledged to be therapeutic and there is a long-standing tradition in both Eastern and Western cultures of healing with music. Now contemporary music therapy is applied within psychotherapy and psychiatry, principally to assist relaxation and to alleviate anxiety, but also in the treatment of schizophrenia, depression, Alzheimer's disease, learning difficulties and autism. Similarly it is used in some coronary care units and in hospices, in the treatment of cancer and some neurological problems, and also for pain relief, which, like its other benefits, can largely be attributed to its relaxing effects. Music is often used as an aid to relaxation through commercially produced and widely used relaxation audiotapes.

Pets as therapy

Petting animals also has relaxing, stress-relieving effects. It reduces anxiety and tension, blood pressure and heart rate,[50–55] and enables people to express affection. Animals can also act as a stress buffer by providing companionship, increasing social contacts, and promoting exercise. The benefits to health of the human–animal bond have been reported for a variety of specific illnesses[56, 57] and in a number of medical and psychotherapeutic interventions.[58–63] As a result animals are being used therapeutically in a wide variety of institutional contexts.

Laughter therapy

Humour and laughter can play an important role in relaxed living. A sense of humour enables people to see the funny side of situations that might otherwise be stressful and so take themselves less seriously. Not only can it help overcome negative attitudes and emotions but it may also assist in overcoming illness. While it is widely accepted that laughter may help a person feel better, it is only relatively recently that its physical effects have been investigated. Psychologically, laughter is inconsistent with anger, which is widely considered to be a factor in the onset of many cancers and other illnesses associated with suppression of the immune system. Claims regarding the benefits of laughter focus on neurotransmitters. The preliminary results of studies suggest that laughter reduces levels of neurotransmitters such as cortisol and adrenaline whose levels increase in response to stress and bring about immunosuppression. Evidence for immuno-enhancement has been demonstrated in response to humour, humorous films[64] and audiotapes.[65] Laughter also seems to stimulate the secretion of catecholamines, which in turn release endorphins, neurotransmitters that stimulate the pleasure centre in the brain and promote feelings of well-being and relaxation. In this way laughter may counteract the negative effects of stress and negative emotions that can trigger suppression of immune functions.

Laughter also has measurable physical effects on bodily processes.

A 'good' laugh exercises the muscles of the face, shoulders, diaphragm and abdomen and more robust laughter involves the arm and leg muscles. It has been claimed that laughing 100–200 times a day is equal to about ten minutes of rowing. 'Hearty' laughter speeds up heart rate, raises blood pressure, accelerates breathing and oxygen consumption. It produces huffing and puffing similar to that resulting from exercise, and so has been described as 'internal jogging'.[66] As laughter subsides it is followed by a brief period of relaxation during which respiration and heart rate slow down, often to below normal levels, blood pressure drops and muscles relax. 'Mirthful laughter' can also have a significant effect on immune functioning, producing significant reductions in the plasma levels of various stress hormones. It is as yet unclear whether the brief immunological changes associated with laughter can exert lasting health benefits. It is more likely that possessing an enduring sense of humour is more important.

Recognition of the therapeutic value of humour has led to 'laughter therapy' being promoted as part of health care and stress management programmes in both the USA and the UK. However, the ancient Greeks regarded laughter as highly therapeutic and for this reason Greek physicians recommended that patients watched comedy in the theatre.

The ability to see the lighter side of life is now being widely claimed to be advantageous in the cure of illness, pain control, increasing chances of survival and improving quality of life in the seriously ill. These claims are support by a number of studies.[67] They have established that showing elderly patients humorous movies has a significant effect in relieving pain and improving mood, and that listening to humorous audiotapes reduces stress levels.[68]

The suggestion that encouraging attitude change by teaching patients various psychological methods could increase their chances of survival has found support in various studies. Cancer patients using psychological methods have been found to survive two to three times longer than would have been predicted on the basis of national norms. After five years, 51 per cent of those who did so were living compared with only 16 per cent of patients who had not received the same treatment.[69] However, medical opinion on the issue remains divided. On the one hand doctors agree that patients' attitude is vitally important to their survival and that it is important to do everything possible to support those with serious illness. Yet on the other hand they tend not to agree on whether or not it is appropriate to offer specific psychological approaches because to do so could imply that they might cure or influence the course of the disease. Accordingly the medical establishment has been slow in implementing psychological approaches or carrying out controlled trials of their effectiveness. Attempts to establish a scientific basis for psychological approaches have been hampered because accounting for psychological factors complicates medical investigations with multiple variables that exceed the capacity of current research paradigms. Findings concerning psychological interventions are thus still limited, and both controlled clinical trials and carefully documented case studies are still needed. In practice, doctors often ignore psychological factors totally and programme patients with negative rather than positive expectancies and beliefs. Conventional medical approaches are therefore likely to increase the likelihood of stress rather than reduce it and to prompt some patients to seek other approaches that offer hope, and the prospect of recovery — that is, that give them something positive to believe in.

Faith healing

'A belief is a strong emotional state of certainty that you hold about specific people, things, ideas or experiences of life.'[70] Beliefs are pre-formed pre-organised approaches to perception that limit a person's view of what is possible. It is not therefore the case that 'seeing is believing', as is so often supposed, but that believing is seeing. What a person believes, what he or she thinks is possible or impossible, determines to a great extent what he or she can or cannot do. 'It is our belief that determines how much of our potential we'll be able to tap.'[71]

Studies on the placebo effect and hypnosis show that belief changes physiology. 'Whatever we're certain of in our hearts shows up in our bodies. Bodies are a print-out of our thinking.'[72] However, just as orthodox medicine has largely ignored the effects of the placebo, it has also blinded itself to the power behind them. In practice, medical practitioners often instil negative beliefs. The most common example is telling a person about to receive an injection 'this may hurt'. By setting up this expectancy — belief in a certain outcome — they are initiating what in many cases becomes a self-fulfilling prophecy. Other examples of this process in action are the tendency to encourage women giving birth to focus on the pain rather than the pleasure, and to deliver diagnoses and prognoses, which may act as powerful nocebos. Unsurprisingly, therefore, the belief systems of those patients who eventually succumb to cancer are characteristically negative, whereas those patients whose cancers show spontaneous remission tend to be positive.

The placebo effect clearly shows that people are able to convert a belief into a biological reality within the body. It therefore follows that by gaining control over inner certainty a person can change his or her biological reality. This may be at the level of the molecule, in the sense of producing from the body's 'exquisite pharmacy'[73] interleukin and interferon which make the crucial difference between life and death, or endorphin and enkephalin that could relieve pain. Or it may be at a more gross level.

It is now recognised that the body is a dynamic field of energy, intelligence and information that is constantly renewing itself in every moment of existence. It renews itself totally every year. Every molecule of DNA, the body's raw material, 'comes and goes like migratory birds'[74] every six weeks. The body is therefore always in-form-ation. This is also true of tumours and other tissue abnormalities of the body. Every molecule is constantly renewed so that a tumour that appears on a scan or X-ray is not actually the same tumour as six months previously although it may appear to be. It seems this way because the blueprint or matrix of the tumour remains unaltered. Deepak Chopra likens this process to rebuilding a house. If the same plan is followed as previously the building will, to all and intents and purposes, be the same as before. The meaning or interpretation that a person gives to his or her cancer — the beliefs he or she holds consistently about it — like the building plan, determines what is possible and the likely outcome.

> The same is true for everything in life. If we represent to ourselves that things aren't going to work, they won't. If we form a representation that things will work, then we create the internal resources we need to produce the state that will support us in producing positive results.[75]

In this way positive and negative beliefs produce different physiology and different outcomes. This is not a new insight. In 1904 Thomas Troward wrote 'the basis of all healing is a change in belief.'[76] Healing is, fundamentally, an attempt to replace negative beliefs with positive expectancies. In this sense all healing is ultimately faith healing.

Psychological medicine involves various technologies that have been developed to help individuals change their negative beliefs and create empowering new positive beliefs. These include cognitive behavioural therapies, such as rational-emotive therapy, cognitive therapy, neuro-linguistic programming (NLP) and neuro-associative conditioning. These identify and explore a person's belief systems, the mental syntax used by the person to code and consistently communicate these beliefs internally, and the way in which they manifest in physiology and behaviour. Having done so, they introduce strategies to model new and positive possibilities, basic to which is self-belief: faith in the self and its creative powers.

Meditation
In this respect these psychological approaches have much in common with the ancient healing tradition of Ayurveda, which encourages people to have faith in themselves first. Central to Ayurveda, and most other Eastern approaches to healing, is meditation. It can be regarded as a method of self-referral, of knowing the true self or soul.

> When you discover your essential nature and know who you really are, *in that knowing itself* is the ability to fulfil any dream you have, because you are the eternal possibility, the immeasurable potential of all that was, is and will be ... because underlying the infinite diversity of life is the unity of one all-pervasive spirit. There is no separation between you and this field of energy. The field of pure potentiality is your own Self. And the more you experience your true nature, the closer you are to the field of pure potentiality.[77]

Through meditation comes understanding of the physical laws of the universe and the way these can be applied in everyday life.

> All of creation, everything that exists in the physical world, is the result of the unmanifest transforming itself into the manifest.

Everything that we behold comes from the unknown. Our physical body, the physical universe — anything and everything that we can perceive through our senses — is the transformation of the unmanifest, unknown and invisible, into the manifest, known and visible.

The physical universe is nothing other than the Self curving back within Itself to experience Itself as spirit, mind and physical matter. In other words, all processes of creation are processes through which the Self or divinity expresses Itself. Consciousness in motion expresses itself as the objects of the universe in the eternal dance of life.

... The physical laws of the universe are actually the whole process of divinity in motion, or consciousness in motion. When we understand these laws and apply them in our lives, anything we want can be created, because the same laws that nature uses to create a forest, or a galaxy or a star or a human body can also bring about the fulfilment of our deepest desires.[78]

Irrespective of what method is used, the fundamentals of meditation are the same:

- relaxing the mind

- adopting a relaxed attitude of watchfulness and acceptance — a state of simply watching and accepting whatever is going on, of being rather than doing

- relaxing or letting go of beliefs about the self and its limitations.

There is little doubt that meditation promotes healing. It has many well-attested beneficial effects on the autonomic nervous system such as changes in brain wave activity, slowing of the heart rate and lowering of blood pressure, all consistent with a state of deep relaxation. In addition to these physiological effects it also has many psychological effects. It reduces anxiety and susceptibility to depression; increases the sense of being effective in the world rather than being a passive victim of circumstance; improves mood states; and reduces reliance on alcohol, cigarettes and coffee.

Transpsychic healing

While it is possible through meditation for individuals to change their beliefs about themselves and the universe and to use this knowledge for self-healing, change in belief is also the basis of healing in which the healer consciously and wilfully attempts to use knowledge of unity to influence another person. This has been termed 'mental'[79] or 'transpsychic'[80] healing to distinguish it from healing or the laying-on of hands which arouses and strengthens the patient's own healing resources through a partnership of harmony and cooperation.

> The sequence from which this results is as follows: — the subjective mind is the creative faculty within us, and creates whatever the objective mind impresses upon it; the objective mind, or intellect, impresses its thought upon it; and thought is the expression of belief; hence whatever the subjective mind creates is the reproduction externally of our beliefs. Accordingly our whole object is to change our beliefs ... the wrong belief which externalises as sickness is the belief that some secondary cause, which is really only a condition, is a primary cause ... There is only one primary cause, and this is the factor which in our own individuality we call subjective or sub-conscious mind.[81]

Troward indicates that when a healer has established rapport with a person and 'both are concentrated into a single entity'[82] the healer can through the principle of suggestion:

> ... make the mental affirmation that he shall build up outwardly the correspondence or that perfect vitality which he knows himself to be inwardly; and this suggestion being impressed by the healer's conscious thought while the patient's conscious thought is at the same time impressing the fact that he is receiving the active thought of the healer, the result is that the patient's sub- conscious mind becomes thoroughly imbued with the recognition of its own life-giving power, ... and proceeds to work out this suggestion into external manifestation, and thus health is substituted for sickness.[83]

LeShan indicates that the result of this mental action can be remarkable, even miraculous, producing physical change generally 'believed' to be beyond the body's ability for self-repair. He attributes to it the dramatic and well-documented cures of famous healers such as Harry Edwards and George Chapman.

However, as in meditation, these possibilities are within the belief system of the healer.

> Knowing for the moment that you are part of the total One of the cosmos, and that there are vast energies which maintain the universe on its course (so to speak, the cosmic 'homeostatic forces'), you attempt by total concentration and 'will' to bend these energies to increase the harmony of the healee, another part of the cosmos. Knowing yourself a part of an all-encompassing energy system, you will the total system to direct additional energies to the repair and harmonization of a part that needs it.[84]

In this sense mental or transpsychic healing can be considered faith healing as it proceeds from the beliefs of the healer, rather than the person being healed. Equally, however, faith healing can be achieved if a person believes in this possibility.

Changing belief is crucial to all healing, but many powerful beliefs are unconscious, that is, they are not represented in consciousness as thought. They are represented internally and structured through the five senses — sight, sound, touch, taste and smell. This means that people experience the world in the form of visual, auditory, kinaesthetic, gustatory and olfactory sensations and so their experiences are represented through these senses, though primarily through the three major modalities, the visual, auditory and kinaesthetic. These experiences are expressed in sensory images and therefore beliefs influencing health may be accessed and explored by way of the imagination — the means by which these images are produced. The power of the imagination is highlighted by placebos and hypnosis, which achieve their effects largely because the person imagines they will. Similarly most stress is caused by a person's 'worst imaginings'.

Imaginative medicine

Imaginative methods, which use spontaneous personal images to access, explore and make unconscious beliefs conscious, have been extensively and effectively used in psychotherapy, not only by Sigmund Freud and Carl Jung but by many other therapists. Guided imagery techniques have also been developed to provide a person with images that afford novel representations of issues that capture new and positive beliefs and unleash greater creative potentials.

These imaginative methods were used to good effect by the oncologist Carl Simonton and his co-workers who used the images produced by cancer patients in visualisation and artwork to identify negative beliefs about and attitudes towards their cancer and its treatment. By working with the patients they were able to introduce healthy images that captured positive expectancies. Similar techniques have been used in a variety of health care settings in recent years and have proved effective in the treatment of chronic pain and many other conditions.

Simonton and his colleagues considered that visualisation may also help cancer patients to confront their fears of hopelessness and helplessness, enabling them to gain a sense of control and change in attitude. This is particularly important in cancer patients in whom repression has been identified as a coping strategy. They typically deny the experience of stress, yet react to stress with high autonomic arousal.[85] Repressors who report low anxiety and high defensiveness actually show physiological responses to anxiety-provoking stimuli that equalled or surpassed those subjects who reported high anxiety. Repressors also report significantly lower levels of emotional pain than non-repressors, and it is suggested that since they fail to experience the emotional discomfort associated with anxiety and pain, they may lack the motivation to gain control over a stressful stimulus or event.[86] This is significant because animal studies have shown that variations in perceived control of a stressor affect arousal level and lymphocyte responses. Hence the controllability of stress factors appears to be critical in modulating immune function.

The psychiatrist Elisabeth Kubler-Ross[87] also used imagery and artwork to good effect in helping people express and confront their fears about death, dying and bereavement.

Imaginative methods, such as drawing, painting, sculpting,

modelling, mask-making, puppetry, dance, drama, poetry, storytelling and the creation of mandalas have been considered 'healing arts' throughout history. Art therapy *per se* was not used in Britain until the 1940s and until the 1980s there were no criteria for the professional training of art therapists. There is still no generally agreed consensus about its scope and applicability. Commonly it is viewed as a way of dealing with mental illness, because it has been developed and most widely used in the field of mental health, but it can be used by anyone as a medium for self-exploration and expression. Some proponents of art therapy view it purely as a diagnostic tool, and it has been applied effectively in this way in the field of physical medicine. Freud viewed art diagnostically, as evidence of a patient's pathology while Jung viewed the images of artwork, like those of dreams, therapeutically as a key to the artist's unconscious life and a means to healthy self-expression and transformation. These differing views are still evident within art therapy. Some therapists pay little attention to the production of art. They consider that the therapy lies in the discussion of the completed work, while others feel that the process of making art is intrinsically therapeutic and is the most important aspect of promoting change in a person. Nevertheless, they all recognise that everything a person makes or creates is an expression of imaginal experience and is therefore a portrait of psychic life.

Art therapist Shaun McNiff considers that the use of arts in therapy represents a return to the shamanic origins of art as medicine. 'Images and the artistic process are the shamans and familiar spirits who come to help people regain the lost soul'. Thus the creative art therapies are 'contemporary manifestations of ancient shamanic continuities'.[88] McNiff takes the view that loss of soul is a metaphor for detachment from feelings and the essential self. He believes that this estrangement from the essential self or soul results in mental and physical illness. While the soul cannot be lost in a literal sense because it is ever present, contact with or sight of it can be lost. People lose a sense of themselves and contact with their feelings because of the influence of the rational, logical, intellectual mind that always strives for control. This aspect of mind has to be relaxed in order for the essential self to be experienced. Salvation of the soul comes about when people engage with their environment and restore their relationship to it.

Art is one way in which this occurs, and theatre is another.

Engaging in the dramatic process, whether by acting or watching, brings about these kinds of insights and transformations when the fantasy is entered into wholly. It then becomes a reality, but can only do so if there is a suspension of disbelief, of rational thinking. This state can be regarded as being on automatic pilot, because the normal control mechanism — the reality factor, the thinking or conscious mind — and the beliefs it supports, is relaxed. The dramatic element comes about, as in Jungian therapy, by establishing dialogue with images. This gives expression to unconscious processes and emotions.

This was clearly understood by the ancient Greeks who recognised the ability of theatre to shake up or perturb. They believed that the evocation, through tragedy, of unsettling emotions such as fear and pity caused a profound change to take place, an emotional purging, which Aristotle termed 'catharsis'.

> The assumption is that the emotional stresses within us, often subconscious, and the moral contradictions too, likely to be equally deeply buried, need to be relieved and resolved. By losing our everyday awareness of ourselves and by identifying with the actors — themselves divested of self in the drama's heightened world — we expose ourselves to the full force of their sufferings and sins as we may never be able to own, and this effects relief ... Aristotle thought that to witness tragedy in the theatre is one of the ways in which human beings can be purged of stress and inner conflict. Our own pity and fear draws us towards a point of balance, and from this comes a sense of health and therefore pleasure.[89]

The Greeks also understood that laughter could purge an audience and used comedy as therapy several thousand years before its healing effects were pointed out in the twentieth century.

Emotional purging may also be effected by bioenergetic and bodywork approaches such as those of Wilhelm Reich, Ida Rolf, David Boadella and others, and by exercise.

These apparently very diverse approaches, by addressing psychological features such as emotions, thoughts, attitudes, beliefs and coping styles, all come under the umbrella of psychological medicine. They are all concerned with accessing and influencing processes of information so as to prevent or treat disease at the mental or emotional level. These approaches are necessary because:

> ... in order to influence effectively an upset or disturbed field, a healing approach must avail itself of and access the relevant dynamic systems in order to make the healing approach 'heard'. It is for this reason that good will and rational understanding are of so little use in emotionally determined conditions and organically encoded difficulties. Many tissue pathologies may have to be approached psychologically if (and whenever) their roots happen to be 'state bound' at that level. Often the approach will have to be directed to the unconscious mythological or even magical level rather than to rational understanding, while some emotional or mental disorders when encoded organically — such as psychotic or borderline conditions — may call for bodily approaches.[90]

What this highlights for us is that, as Hippocrates observed, a physician should have knowledge of the whole of things and be able and willing to draw on all the resources of the universe — human, animal, vegetable, mineral, material and immaterial — and to apply them in healing. He or she should be able to apply knowledge of the soul, in every sense, in the art of healing.

POSTSCRIPT

When I had completed the foregoing chapters, Janet and Dominic kindly agreed to be interviewed and generously gave their time for this purpose. I had met them only once previously, briefly in a social context. Apart from a brief telephone conversation to arrange the interviews, there had been no other contact between us.

Janet described having developed a severe headache one weekend. She and Dominic initially thought it might be an adverse reaction to the fumes of creosote with which Dominic had been painting the garden fence. However, over the next couple of days Janet 'felt something else taking over'... a slightly different personality'. While Janet appeared simply rather bemused by this, Dominic described it as 'really terrifying because Janet was no longer Janet'. It was as though she had 'absented herself' in some way. Much later, when Janet saw an inscription she had written at the time in a book she had bought for her daughter's birthday, she was shocked to see that the handwriting 'was like someone else's', not at all like hers own. She continued to drift in and out of this state for a couple of days, during which time she was seen by three doctors, who diagnosed her symptoms as those of 'flu.

Dominic was progressively alarmed by the changes in Janet's condition and later in the day after she had been seen by the third doctor, he summoned an ambulance. Janet remembers being highly amused as the ambulance men struggled to manoeuvre her downstairs to the waiting vehicle. By the time she reached hospital, her condition had deteriorated and shortly after admission it was decided that she should have a lumbar puncture. At this point Janet thought to herself 'I can't stand this. I'm off. I'm not hanging around for this' and instantly 'went off'. Looking back on this 'decision' she said, 'I knew I could control it — what an odd thing':

From then on — for the rest of it — I was in this other world I think. A most peculiar world of the left and the right, good and evil, in and out of various sorts of states which were horrible to very pleasant.

She found herself in New England, talking with people she didn't know — 'at no point did I meet anyone I knew'. She didn't feel that she had a body but people knew she was there. They could see her and they talked to her. The experience was very vivid — 'as real as being here'. These experiences occurred in a left-side sensory field. Simultaneously, on the right side, she was in Florence, apparently protecting an elderly Italian friend from seeing 'something horrible', 'nasty happenings' being projected onto her bedroom walls. She remembered being with my sister, realising how worried she was and telling her that she should go home as it was 2 am. Every now and then she had a sense of being in the clinic. She remembered a black nurse asking her, 'How are you, dear?' She also remembered hearing people say that she was in a persistent vegetative state and would never recover. These experiences all occurred in the same time frame, in the here and now.

Although not convinced she was in a clinic, Janet was aware she was in bed and in trying to rationalise why she was there, concluded 'rather stupidly' that she had undergone facial plastic surgery. She remembers hearing the registrar say to her. 'Do you know where you are? You're in the ... Hospital and you've been here for a while.' This annoyed her. She wanted him to stop saying things that weren't true and mentally she rudely dismissed him.

She felt very differently towards a healer from a local church, who had been summoned to the hospital by the family of a road traffic accident victim. Dominic had learned of his presence in the hospital and asked him if he would give healing to Janet. He agreed. Janet remembers him sitting beside her surrounded by a yellow light. 'It was there. It was concrete.' She realised he was a very special kind of person — a 'simple soul' — and that he didn't think she was dead. He told her when she met him after her recovery that there had been a yellow light around her that reflected the love of her family and God.

The healer attended to Janet twice, visiting her some time before it was planned to move her from the intensive care unit to a general ward. In the meantime, Janet's experience — 'the left and right, the good and bad split' — reached what she describes as a crescendo. She became aware of a menacing presence in her right field. She described him as like the devil, something she had never previously believed in. He was telling her that the idea of God was nonsense, that people were made in factories, that he would take her there and show her. She refused to listen to or accept what she was hearing and turned her back on him, saying repeatedly, 'I don't believe you.' In her mind there was no question about it, 'He was talking rubbish.' With hindsight, she was surprised by her uncharacteristic assertiveness. Simultaneously in the left field she sensed a presence with a fatherly quality, although it was not her father. He told her, 'You have had a horrible experience. You have made your judgement, and you are right.' As he did so she felt the 'bad' lifted from her. He then told her, 'It is not your time to come here. You're going to go back and it's going to be wonderful. Your daughter Catherine is going to have a baby. It's a girl. She needs you there.' Yet these words made Janet feel unhappy. 'Coming back instead of being where the father was felt like a consolation prize.' Janet thinks that she was conscious at this point.

Shortly afterwards she was aware of her daughters by her bedside. They were trying to remember the name of the actor who starred in the film *On the Waterfront*. One of them said, 'If mum were here she'd know.' And so it was that Janet's first words were 'Marlon Brando'. She then asked for tea and toast, thinking as she did so 'something awful has happened' because her family all looked so terrible. She realised her headache had gone.

Recalling the experience, Janet said, 'I don't see it in terms of being ill — I see it in terms of something being revealed in me — a revelation. A spiritual experience, not an illness. It feels like a precious thing to me. It feels like you've had a glimpse of something quite extraordinary. It feels like you've been shown something; something has been revealed.'

When asked what, she replied, 'A higher being, I think. The whole thing seems like a gift from God. I hesitate to say it because it seems presumptuous. Why me? I don't think I deserve it.' Janet added that just as she had previously never believed in the devil, she had not believed in God, having had a totally agnostic upbringing.

Asked to assess the impact of the experience on her life, Janet said,

'A big part of me will never be the same. A big part of me will be enhanced by the experience because I think it was a gift and I think I can use it and I have used it. I've changed because I don't have fears about dying. I know that dying won't be terrible because I think I've been there. I'm not a better person but different in the way I think about things. I know things, feel I'm *party* to things. I seem to have an instinct for things, a deeper intuition. I believe everyone in life is somehow joined. Life is not random. Things happen for a reason.'

Janet hopes that she may be able to use her experience to help other people to cope with illness and to raise awareness of the experiences of those in coma. This is why she had agreed to be interviewed.

At the end of the interview, Janet asked about the subject of my book. She knew only that it was about 'psychological medicine' and was interested in the relevance of her experience to this subject. Very briefly I explained that I was interested in the soul and its relevance to healing. She looked surprised and rather puzzled. I asked her whether it had ever occurred to her that when she was in coma her soul might have left her body. She was silent for some time, gazing at the floor as if in deep thought. She then looked up and straight at me and said with a sense of dawning awareness and conviction, 'That's it. That is exactly what it was.'

Larry Dossey[1] has talked of what he terms 'spiritual agoraphobia' in Western culture. He suggests that, like their counterparts who suffer from the *psychological* affliction of agoraphobia — fear of open spaces — *spiritual* agoraphobics have a deep-seated fear of vast expanses, the infiniteness in time and space suggested by non-local mind. They feel safer when things are closed in, finite and 'local' — such as a mind that is confined to the individual brain and body, and a mind that stays put in the here and now. 'A mind, in other words, that is soulless.'[2]

But

> Suppose for the moment that we *could* show that the human mind is nonlocal; that it is ultimately independent of the physical brain and body, and that, as a correlate it transcends time and space ... with one sweep, this discovery would redirect the imperatives of medicine. No longer would it be the ultimate

goal of the modern to forestall death and decay, for these would lose their absolute status if the mind were ultimately transcendent over the physical body. The mad, frenzied, life-at-any-cost dictum that prevails today could be modulated in its intensity, along with the despair that dying men feel. And once again we might recover something that has been notably absent in our experience of late: the human soul.[3]

NOTES

INTRODUCTION

1 Dossey, L. *Recovering the soul: a scientific and spiritual search*, New York: Bantam, 1989, p.1
2 *Ibid.* p.1
3 *Ibid.* p.2
4 Smart, N. *The world's religions*, Cambridge: University of Cambridge Press, 1992

CHAPTER ONE **Students of the soul**

1 Hearnshaw, L.S. *The shaping of modern psychology: an historical introduction*, London: Routledge, 1989
2 Hardy, J. *A psychology with a soul: psychosynthesis in evolutionary context*, London: Penguin, 1989, p.10
3 Butler, W.E. *Magic: its ritual, power and purpose*, Wellingborough, Northants: Aquarian Press, 1982
4 Happold, F.C. *Mysticism: a study and an anthology*, Harmondsworth: Penguin, 1970, p.19
5 Russell, B. *Mysticism and logic and other essays*, London: Allen and Unwin, 1959
6 Lévy-Bruhl, L. *The 'soul' of the primitive*, London: Allen and Unwin, 1928, quoted Hearnshaw *op. cit.* p.9
7 Johnson, E.L. 'Whatever happened to the human soul? A brief genealogy of a psychological term', *Journal of Psychology and Theology*, 26:1 (1998), 16–28, esp. p.17
8 Kalweit, H. *Dreamtime and inner space: the world of the shaman*, translated by W. Wunsche, Boston and London: Shambhala, 1988, pp.26–7
9 *Ibid.* pp.27–8
10 *Ibid.* p.24
11 Eliade, M. *From primitives to zen: a thematic sourcebook of the history of religions*, London: Collins, 1967
12 *Ibid.*
13 Jung, C.G. *The structure and dynamics of the psyche*, collected works of C.G. Jung, translated by R.F.C. Hull, London: Routledge and Kegan Paul, 1960, p.346

14   *Ibid.* p.347

15   Kalweit *op. cit.* pp.9–10

16   Huxley, A. *The perennial philosophy*, New York: Harper and Row, 1944, p.vii

17   Brett, G.S. *A history of psychology*, 3 vols, London: MacMillan, 1912–21

18   Hearnshaw *op. cit.* p.12

19   *Ibid.* p.13

20   *Ibid.* p.9

21   Eliade op. cit.

22   Chevalier, J. and A. Gheerbhant *A dictionary of symbols*, translated by J. Buchan-Brown, London: Blackwell, 1994, p.893

23   *Genesis* 2:7

24   Bloom, W. *Working with angels, fairies and nature spirits*, London: Book Club Associates, 1998, p.137

25   *Genesis* 9:4

26   *Leviticus* 17:11

27   *Deuteronomy* 12:23

28   *Genesis* 35:18

29   *Psalms* 119:28

30   *Lamentations* 3:20

31   Johnson *op. cit.* p.18

32   Guttman, J. *Philosophies of Judaism: the history of Jewish philosophy from biblical times to Franz Rosensweig*, London: Routledge and Kegan Paul, 1964

33   Kuperstok, N. 'Extended consciousness and Hasidic thought' in Bulka, R.P (ed.) *Mystics and medics: a comparison of mystical and psychotherapeutic encounters*, New York: Human Sciences Press, 1979, pp.87–97, esp. p.92

34   Goleman, D. *Varieties of Meditative experience*, London: Rider, 1977

35   Guttman *op. cit.* p.35

36   *Ibid.*

37   Chevalier and Gheerbhant *op. cit.* p.895

38   Claus, D.B. 'Toward the soul', *Yale Classical Monographs* 2, New Haven and London: Yale University Press, 1981

39   Jaynes, J. *The origin of consciousness in the breakdown of the bicameral mind*, Harmondsworth: Penguin, 1993, p.291

40   Claus *op. cit.*

41   Lovejoy. A. *The great chain of being*, Harvard University Press, 1978, p.29

42   Guthrie, W.K.C. *A history of Greek philosophy* 1, Cambridge: Cambridge University Press, 1962

43 *Ibid.* p.461
44 Koestler, A. *The sleepwalkers: a history of man's changing vision of the universe*, Harmondsworth: Penguin, 1984, p.27
45 *Ibid.* p.25
46 Guthrie *op. cit.* p.306
47 Hearnshaw *op. cit.* pp.16–17
48 Happold *op. cit.*
49 Russell *op. cit.*
50 Schlolem, G. (1961) quoted Hardy *op. cit.* pp.110–11
51 Robinson. T.M. *Plato's psychology*, Toronto: University of Toronto Press, 1970, p.3
52 *Ibid.* p.22
53 *Ibid.* p.8
54 Hearnshaw *op. cit.*
55 Aristotle quoted *ibid.*
56 Hardy *op cit.* pp.112–13
57 Plotinus *The essential Plotinus*, translated by E. O'Brien, London: Blackwell, 1964, p.25
58 Hardy *op. cit.* p.125
59 Plotinus quoted *ibid.*
60 *Ibid.*
61 *Ibid.*
62 Hearnshaw *op. cit.* p.17
63 *Ibid.* p. 17
64 *Mark* 8:36
65 Johnson *op. cit.* p.18
66 *Matthew* 10:28
67 *Revelations* 6:9
68 *Corinthians* 5:8
69 Duvall, N. S. 'From soul to self and back again', *Journal of Psychology and Theology*, 26:1 (1998), 6–15, esp. p.10
70 Hearnshaw *op. cit.*
71 Johnson *op. cit.*
72 quoted Hardy *op. cit.* p.102
73 Barrett, W. *Death of the soul: philosophical thought from Descartes to the computer*, Oxford: Oxford University Press, 1987, p.3
74 Hearnshaw *op. cit.* p.63
75 *Ibid.* p.67
76 Marchant, C. *The death of nature*, London: Wildwood House, 1982, p.111
77 Hearnshaw *op. cit.* p.67
78 Barrett *op. cit.* p.20

79   *Ibid.*

80   Van Peursen, C.A. *Body, soul, spirit: a survey of the body mind problem*, London: Oxford University Press, 1966, p.72

81   Ryle, G. *The concept of mind*, New York: Barnes and Noble, 1949

82   Van Peursen *op. cit.* p.20

83   *Ibid.* p.21

84   Hearnshaw *op. cit.* pp.68–9

85   Coren, S. *The intelligence of dogs: canine consciousness and capabilities*, UK: Headline Book Publishing, 1994, pp. 5–6

86   *Ibid.* p.60

87   Van Peursen *op. cit.* p.19

88   Hearnshaw *op. cit.* p. 73

89   *Ibid.* p.87

90   Duvall *op. cit.* p.10

91   Barrett *op. cit.* p.203

92   Van Peursen *op. cit.* p.4

93   Fromm, E. *Psychonanalysis and religion*, London: Gollancz, 1951

94   Zohar, D. The quantum self, London: Bloomsbury, 1990, p.2

95   Hearnshaw *op. cit.* p.77

96   Johnson *op cit.* p.20

97   Hearnshaw *op. cit.* p.98

98   *Ibid.* p.97

99   Johnson *op. cit.* p.21

100   Hardy *op. cit.* p.105

101   Darwin quoted *ibid.* p.105

102   Ornstein, R.E. *The psychology of consciousness*, Harmondsworth: Penguin, 1975

103   Johnson *op. cit.* p.21

104   Watson, J.B. *Behavior*, New York: Holt, 1914

105   Wigner, E.P. *Symmetries and reflections: scientific essays*, Cambridge MA: MIT Press, 1970, p.12

106   Capra, F. *The turning point: science, society and the rising culture*, London: Wildwood House, 1982, p.181

107   Heather, N. *Radical perspectives in psychology*, London: Methuen, 1976

108   Watson *op. cit.*

109   Skinner, B.F. *Beyond freedom and dignity*, Harmondsworth: Penguin, 1973

110   Eysenck, H.J. *The scientific study of personality*, London: Routledge and Kegan Paul, 1952

111   Fromm *op. cit.* pp.13–14

112   Burt, C. 'The concept of consciousness', *British Journal of Psychology*,

53:3 (1962), 229–42, esp. p.229

113 Jeans, J. *The mysterious universe*, London: Longmans, 1930

114 Naranjo, C. *The one quest*, London: Wildwood House, 1974

115 Jung *op. cit.* p.344

116 Moreland, J.P. 'Restoring the substance to the soul of psychology', *Journal of Psychology and Theology*, 2:1 (1998), 29–43, esp. p.43

117 Johnson *op. cit.* p.22

CHAPTER TWO **Saviours of the soul**

1 Butler, W.E. *Magic: its ritual, power and purpose*, Wellingborough: Aquarian Press, 1982

2 Kalweit, H. *Dreamtime and inner space: the world of the shaman*, translated by W. Wunsche, Boston and London: Shambhala, 1988, p.11

3 *Ibid.* p.16

4 *Ibid.* p.12

5 Harner, M. 'Shamanic counselling' in Doore, G. (ed.) *Shaman's path: healing, personal growth and empowerment*, Boston: Shambhala, 1988, pp.179–88

6 Kalweit *op. cit.* p.15

7 Metzner, R. 'States of consciousness and transpersonal psychology' in Valle, R.S. and S. Halling (eds), *Existential–phenomenological perspectives in psychology*, London: Plenum, 1989, pp.329–38, esp. p.333

8 Millenson, J.R. *Mind matters: psychological medicine in holistic practice*, Seattle: Eastland Press, 1995, p.210

9 McNiff, S. *Art as medicine: creating a therapy of the imagination*, London: Piatkus, 1992, p.21

10 Saint-Exupéry, A. de *The little prince*, London: Pan, 1974

11 Watson, L. *Supernature: the natural history of the supernatural*, London: Hodder and Stoughton, 1973

12 Kalweit *op cit.* pp. xii–xiii

13 *Ibid.* p.17

14 Eliade, M. *Shamanism: archaic techniques of ecstasy*, New York: Pantheon, Bollingen Foundation, 1964, pp. 216–17

15 Kalweit *op. cit.* p.30

16 *Ibid.* pp.29–30

17 Drury, N. *The elements of shamanism*, Shaftesbury: Element Books, 1991, p.5

18 Eliade *op. cit.*

19 *Ibid.*

20 Harner *op. cit.*

21   Strong, R. *The greatest benefit to mankind: a medical history of humanity from antiquity to the present*, London: Harper Collins Fontana, 1999, p.50

22   Hearnshaw, L.S. *The shaping of modern psychology: an historical introduction*, London: Routledge, 1989, p.152

23   *Ibid.* p.152

24   Strong *op. cit.* p.187

25   Achterberg. J. *Imagery and healing: shamanism in modern medicine*, New York and London: Science Library, Routledge and Kegan Paul, 1985

26   Cooter, R. 'Alternative medicine: alternative cosmology' in Cooter, R. (ed.) *Studies in the history of alternative medicine*, London MacMillan, 1988

27   Strong *op. cit.* p.169

28   *Ibid.* p.195

29   *Ibid.* p.218

30   Siegel, B.S. *Love, medicine and miracles*, London: Rider, 1986, p.65

31   Dossey, L. *Space, time and medicine*, Boulder and London: Shambhala, 1982, p.14

32   *Ibid.*

33   Engel, B.J. 'The need for a new medical model: a challenge to biomedical science', *Science*, 196 (8 April 1977), 129

34   Strong *op. cit.* 219

35   *Ibid.* p.215

36   *Ibid.* p.215–16

37   Hearnshaw *op. cit.* p.108

38   Strong *op. cit.* pp.249–50

39   *Ibid.*

40   Chopra, D. *Quantum healing workshop*, New York: Sound Horizons Audio-video Inc., 1990

41   Jung, C.G. *Modern man in search of a soul*, London: Routledge and Kegan Paul, 1966, p.203

42   Hearnshaw *op. cit.* p.121

43   Strong *op. cit.* pp.7–8

44   *Ibid.* p.8

45   Jung *op. cit.* pp.203–204

46   Brett, G.S. quoted Peters, R.S. *Brett's history of psychology*, London: Allen and Unwin, 1953, p.37

47   Pagels, H.R. *The cosmic code: quantum physics as the language of nature*, London: Michael Joseph, 1983, p.101

48   Heutzer. C.S. 'The power of meaning: from quantum mechanics to synchronicity', *Journal of Humanistic Psychology*, 24 (1984), 80–94, esp. pp.89–90

49 Bohm, D. *Wholeness and the implicate order*, London: Routledge and Kegan Paul, 1980
50 *Ibid.*
51 Pribram, K. *Consciousness and the brain*, New York: Plenum, 1976
52 Bohm *op. cit.*
53 Pribram *op. cit.*
54 Bohm *op. cit.*
55 Dossey *op. cit.* p.202
56 Jaynes, J. *The origin of consciousness in the breakdown of the bicameral mind*, Harmondsworth: Penguin, 1993
57 Dossey *op. cit.* p.86
58 Hearnshaw *op. cit.* p.86
59 Taggart, L.M. *What doctors don't tell you: the truth about the dangers of modern medicine*, London: Thorsons, 1996
60 Dossey *op. cit.* p.xii
61 Capra, F. *The turning point: science, society and the rising culture*, London: Wildwood House, 1982, p.118
62 Dossey *op. cit.*
63 *Ibid.* p.144
64 *Ibid.* p.190
65 *Ibid.* p.70
66 *Ibid.* p.111

CHAPTER THREE **Seers of the soul**

1 Kalweit, H. *Dreamtime and inner space: the world of the shaman*, translated by W. Wunsche, Boston and London: Shambhala, 1988, p.22
2 *Ibid.* p.21
3 Watts, A. *Psychotherapy east and west*, New York: Pantheon, 1961, p.19
4 Ornstein, R.E. *The psychology of consciousness*, Harmondsworth: Penguin, 1975
5 Tart, C.T. (ed.) *Transpersonal psychologies*, London: Routledge and Kegan Paul
6 Parrinder, G. *The indestructible soul: the nature of man and life after death in Indian thought*, London: George Allen and Unwin, 1973, p.9
7 Parrinder, G. *Upanishads, Gita and Bible: a comparative study of Hindu and Christian scriptures*, London: Faber, 1967
8 *Brihad-avaiyaka Upanishad*, 3 9:26
9 *Chandogya Upanishad*, 6 1:4–6
10 *Brikadaranvakopanishad* 1V iv 2022 quoted Besant, A. *The ancient wisdom*, Aberdeen University Press, 1899, p.16

11   Ramaswami, S. and A.A. Sheikh, 'Buddhist psychology: implications for healing' in Sheikh, A.A. and K.S Sheikh (eds) *Eastern and western approaches to healing: ancient wisdom and modern knowledge*, New York: Wiley, 1989, pp.91–123

12   Sandweiss, S.H. *Spirit and the mind*, Andhra Pradesh: Sri Sathya Sai Books and Publications Trust, 1985, p.287

13   Sai Baba quoted *ibid*. pp.287–8

14   Nikhilananda, S. *Hinduism: its meaning for the liberation of the spirit*, Myalore Madras: Sri Ramakrishna Math, 1968, p.42

15   Folkert, K.W. 'Jainism' in Hinnells, J.R. (ed.) *A handbook of living religions*, Harmondsworth, Penguin, 1985, pp.256–77, esp. p.262

16   Radhaskrishnan *Indian philosophy* 1, New York: MacMillan, 1951, p.369

17   Parrinder *op. cit.* 1967, p.34

18   *Ibid.* pp.35–6

19   Nakamura quoted Wilson-Ross, N. *Hinduism, Buddhism, Zen*, London: Faber, 1973

20   Chopra, D. 'Power talk', interview with Anthony Robbins, Robbins Foundation, 1991

21   Nyanatiloka cited Ramaswami and Sheikh *op. cit.* p.98

22   Parrinder *op. cit.* 1967, p.36

23   Wilson Ross, N. *Hunduism, Buddhism, Zen*, London: Faber, 1973, p115

24   Evans-Wentz, W.Y. Preface to the second edition of the *Tibetan Book of the Dead*, Oxford: Oxford University Press, 1976, p.xviv

25   *Ibid.* p.xxxix

26   Wilson Ross *op. cit.* p.115

27   Jung, C.G. Psychological commentary to the *Tibetan Book of the Dead*, (ed.) Evans-Wentz *op. cit.* pp.xxxix–xl

28   Evans-Wentz *op. cit.* p.2

29   Ring, K. *Life after death*, New York, 1981, quoted Kalweit *op. cit.*

30   Wilson Ross *op. cit.* p.139

31   Sasaki quoted *ibid.* p. 145

32   Watts, A. *Tao: the watercourse way*, London: Jonathan Cape, 1976, p.26

33   Chuang Yuan *Creativity and Taoism*, London: Wildwood House, 1975, p.31

34   Saso, M. 'Chinese religions' in Hinnells, J.R. (ed.) *A handbook of living religions*, Harmondsworth: Penguin, 1985, pp.344–64, esp. p.349

35   *Ibid.*

36   Wilson Ross *op. cit.* p.141

37 Frager, R. 'Transpersonal psychology: promise and prospects' in Valle, R.S. and S. Halling (eds.) *Existential–phenomenological perspectives in psychology*, New York and London: Plenum Press, 1989, pp.289–309, esp. p.307

38 Stoddart, W. *Sufism*, New York: Paragon House, 1985

39 Arasteh, A.R. and A.A. Sheikh *Sufism: the way to universal self* in Sheikh A.A. and K.S. Sheikh (eds) *Eastern and Western approaches to healing: ancient wisdom and modern knowledge*, New York: Wiley, 1989, pp. 91–123

40. *Ibid.*

41 Rumi (1952) quoted *ibid.* p.156

42 Buddhist scholar Nakamura cited Wilson Ross *op. cit.* p.121

43 Wilson Ross *op. cit.* pp.121–2

44 Von Franz. M.L. *Number and time: reflections leading towards a unification of psychology and physics*, London: Rider and Co, 1974, p.157

45 *Ibid.*

46 Sheikh, A.A. and K.S. Sheikh (eds) *Eastern and western approaches to healing: ancient wisdom and modern knowledge*, New York: Wiley, 1989, p.xiv

47 *Ibid.* p.xvii

48 Walsh, R. 'Towards a synthesis of Eastern and Western psychology' in *ibid.* pp.542–55, esp. p.543

49 *Ibid.* p.543

50 Dossey, L. *Recovering the soul: a scientific and spiritual search*, New York: Bantam, 1989, p.4

51 Walsh *op. cit.* p.549

52 Dossey *op. cit.*

53 Walsh *op. cit.*

54 Sims, A. 'The cure of souls: psychiatric dilemmas', *International Review of Psychiatry* 11:2–4 (1999), pp.97–102

55 Evans-Wentz *op. cit.* p.viii

56 Sheikh and Sheikh *op. cit.* p.xiv

57 Kenton, L. *Journey to freedom, 13 quantum leaps for the soul*, London: Harper Collins, 1998, p.34

58 Huxley, A. *The perennial philosophy*, New York: Harper and Row, 1944

59 Wilber, K. *The spectrum of consciousness*, Wheaton IL: Theosophical Publishing House, 1977

60 Ornstein, R.E. *The mind field*, Oxford: Pergamon, 1976

61 *Ibid.* p.31

CHAPTER FOUR   **Doctors of the soul**

1   Crawford, C. 'Ayurveda: the science of long life in contemporary perspective' in Sheikh, A.A. and K.S. Sheikh (eds) *Eastern and western approaches to healing: ancient wisdom and modern knowledge*, New York: Wiley, 1989, pp.3–32

2   Kakar, S. *Shamans, mystics and dctors: a psychological enquiry into India and its healing traditions*, London: George, Allen and Unwin, 1982, pp.227–8

3   Woocher, J.S. 'The Kabbalah, Hasidism and the life of unification' in Bulka, R.P. (ed.) *Mystics and medics: a comparison of mystical and psychotherapeutic encounters*, New York: Human Sciences Press, 1979, pp.27–52

4   Patel, C.H. 'Yoga and biofeedback in the management of hypertension', *Lancet*, 10 November 1973

5   Dostalek, C. 'The empirical and experimental foundation of yoga therapy' in Gharote, D. and M. Lockhart (eds) *The art of survival: a guide to yoga therapy*, London: Unwin Hyman, 1987

6   Ramaswami, S. and A.A. Sheikh 'Buddhist psychology: implications for healing' in Sheikh, A.A. and K.S. Sheikh, (eds), *Eastern and western approaches to healing: ancient wisdom and modern knowledge*, New York: Wiley, 1989, pp.91–123, esp. p.104

7   *Ibid.* p.120

8   Marahishi Mahesh Yogi *The science of creative intelligence*, Los Angeles: Maharishi International Press, 1969, p.287

9   Sugi, Y. and Akutsu, K. *Science of Zazen: energy metabolism*, Tokyo: Japan Publications Inc, 1964

10   Wallace, R.K. and M.B. Benson 'The physiology of meditation in altered states of awareness' in *Readings from Scientific American*, CA: W.H. Freeman, 1972, pp.125–31

11   Fenwick, P.B. 'Can we still recommend meditation?' *British Medical Journal*, 287, 12 November 1983, p.1401

12   Stoyva, J. and M. Budzynski 'Cultivated low arousal — an antistress response' in Decara, I.V. (ed.) *Recent advances in limbic and autonomic nervous system research*, New York: Plenum, 1973

13   Dhonden, Y. quoted Anderson, N. *Open secrets: a western guide to Tibetan Buddhism*, Harmondsworth: Penguin, 1982, p.219

14   Epstein, M. and L. Rapgay 'Mind, disease and health in Tibetan medicine' in Sheikh, A.A. and K.S. Sheikh (eds) *Eastern and western approaches to healing: ancient wisdom and modern knowledge*, New York: Wiley, 1989, pp.124–79, esp. p.125

15   Motoyama, H. 'Yoga and acupuncture' in Gharote, D. and M. Lockhart (eds) *The art of survival: a guide to yoga therapy*, London: Unwin Hyman, 1987

16 *Ibid.*

17 Pierrakos, J.C. *Core energetics*, Mendocino CA: Life Rhythm, 1990

18 Schwarz, J. *Human energy systems*, Hillsdale NJ: Erlbaum, 1980, p.21

19 Scott, W. (translator) *Hermetica* 4 vols, Oxford: Clarendon Press, 1923–36

20 Bruyere, R.L. *Wheels of light: chakras, auras and the healing energy of the body*, New York: Simon and Schuster, 1994

21 *Ibid.*

CHAPTER FIVE **Seekers of the soul**

1 Hearnshaw, L.S. 'The psychology of religion' in Hearnshaw, L.S. *A short history of British psychology 1840–1940* London: Methuen, 1964, pp.252–5, esp. p.252

2 *Ibid.*

3 Edwards, H. *A guide to spirit healing*, tenth impression, London: Psychic Press, 1987, p.4

4 *Ibid.*

5 Jung, C.G. *Psychology and religion*, New Haven, London and Oxford: Yale University Press, 1946, p.10

6 Sims, A. 'The cure of souls: psychiatric dilemmas', *International Review of Psychiatry* 11:2–3 (1999), 97–102

7 Frankl, V.E. *The doctor and the soul*, London: Souvenir Press, 1969

8 Jung, C.G. *Modern man in search of a soul*, London: Routledge and Kegan Paul, 1966, p.433

9 Gay, P. *A Godless Jew: atheism and the making of psychoanalysis*, New Haven CT: Yale University Press, 1987

10 Jacobs, M. *Freud*, London: Sage, 1992

11 Jung, C.G. *Memories, dreams and reflections*, London: Fontana/Collins, 1972, p.173

12 Hearnshaw, L.S. *The shaping of modern psychology: an historical introduction*, London: Routledge, 1989, p.157

13 Jackson, R. 'Psychotherapy: beyond a phoney love', *Leading Edge*, 6 (1992), 14–15

14 Jacobs *op. cit.*

15 Jung *op. cit.* 1972, p.84

16 Capra, F. *The turning point: science, society and the rising culture*, London: Wildwood House, 1982, p.186

17 Gay *op. cit.*

18 Millenson, J.R. *Mind matters: psychological medicine in holistic practice*, Seattle: Eastland Press, 1995, p.213

19 *Ibid.*

20   *Ibid.* p.211

21   Blazer, D. *Freud vs God: how psychiatry lost its soul and Christianity lost its mind*, Downers Grove, ILL: Inter Varsity Press, 1998, p.249

22   Jung *op. cit.* 1966, p.259

23   Sandweiss, S.H. *Spirit and the mind* Andhra Pradesh: Sri Sathya Sai Books and Publications Trust, 1985, p.14

24   Tart, C. Introduction to Tart, C. (ed.) *Transpersonal psychologies*, New York: Harper and Row, 1975, p.5

25   Jung *op cit.* 1946, p.11

26   Jacobi, J. *The psychology of Jung*, fifth edition, London: Routledge and Kegan Paul, 1962, p.5

27   *Ibid.* p.1

28   Jung *op. cit.* 1966, p.138

29   Jung, C.G. *The symbolic life*, Princeton NJ: Princeton University Press, 1976, p.122

30   Blair, L. *Rhythms of vision*, London: Croom Helm, 1975, p.106

31   Storr, A. *Jung*, Glasgow: William Collins, 1973, p.88

32   Von Franz, M.L. *C.G. Jung: his myth in our time*, London: Hodder and Stoughton, 1975, p.112

33   Vaughan-Lee, L. 'The light hidden in the darkness: alchemical symbolism in dreams', *Caduceus*, 19 (1992), 4–7

34   Butler, W.E. *Magic: its ritual, power and purpose*, Wellingborough: Aquarian Press, 1982

35   Jung *op. cit.* 1972

36   Drury, N. *Inner visions: explorations of magical consciousness*, London and Henley: Routledge and Kegan Paul, 1979, p.93

37   Jung *op. cit.* 1966, p.259

38   Jung, C.G. *Face to Face with C.G. Jung*, BBC television interview with John Freeman, first broadcast October 1959, repeated October 1988

39   Jung, C.G. *Synchronicity: an acausal connecting principle*, translated by R.F.C. Hull, London: Routledge, 1972

40   Watts, A. *Psychotherapy east and west*, New York: Pantheon, 1961, p.19

41   Totton, N. and E. Edmondson *Reichian bodywork: melting blocks to life and love*, Bridport, Dorset: Prism Press, 1988, p.36

42   Bugenthal, J. Foreword to Valle, R.S. and S. Halling (eds) *Existential–phenomenological perspectives in psychology*, New York: Plenum, 1989, p.xi

43   Heather, N. *Radical perspectives in psychology*, London: Methuen, 1976

44   Schatzman, M. *Soul Murder*, Harmondsworth: Penguin, 1976

45   Boyd, J.H. *Reclaiming the soul: the search for meaning in a self-centred culture*, Cleveland OH: Pilgrim Press, 1996

46   Bloom, A. *The closing of the American mind*, New York: Simon and Schuster, 1987

47   *Ibid.*

48   Duvall, N.S. 'From soul to self and back again', *Journal of Psychology and Theology*, 26:1 (1998), 6–15, esp. p.8

49   Davis, C. *Our modern identity*, 1990, pp.72–3 quoted *ibid.*

50   Lonergan, B.J.F. (1974) cited Duvall *op. cit.*

51   Duvall *op. cit.* p.13

52   Atwood, G.E. and R.D. Stolrov *Structures of subjectivity: explorations in psychoanalytic phenomenology*, Hillsdale NJ: Analytic Press, 1984, p.3

53   Szasz, T.S. *The myth of psychotherapy: mental healing as religion, rhetoric and repression*, Oxford: Oxford University Press, 1979

54   Daws, P.P. *Early days: a personal review of the beginnings of counselling in English education during the decade 1964–74* Cambridge: Hobson's Press, 1966

55   Lesh, T.V. 'Zen meditation and the development of empathy in counsellors' in Shapiro, D.H. and R.N. Walson *Meditation: classical and contemporary perspectives*, New York: Aldine, 1984, pp.152–87

56   Herrigel, E. *Zen in the art of archery*, New York: Pantheon, 1953, p.56

57   Gallup Poll, *Newsweek* 6 September 1976

58   Valle, R.S. 'The emergence of transpersonal psychology' in Valle, R.S. and S. Halling, *Existential–phenomenological perspectives in psychology*, New York: Plenum, 1989, pp.257–68, esp. p.257

59   Zohar, D. *The quantum self*, London: Bloomsbury, 1990, p.138

60   Duvall *op. cit.* p.7

61   Cushman, P. 'Why self is empty', *American Psychologist*, 45 (1990), 599–611, esp. p.599

62   Stephens, M. (1992) p.42 quoted Duvall *op. cit.*

63   Duvall *op.cit.* p.15

64   Maslow, A.H. *Towards a psychology of being*, New York: Van Nostrand, 1968, pp.iii–iv

65   Sandweiss *op. cit.* p.273

66   Lajoie, D.H. and S.I. Shapiro 'Definition of transpersonal psychology: the first twenty-five years', *Journal of Transpersonal Psychology*, 24 (1992), 79–98

67   Strohl, J.E. 'Transpersonalism: ego meets soul', *Journal of Counseling and Development*, 71 (Fall 1998), pp.397–403, esp. p.398

68   Valle *op. cit.* p.262

69   Hardy, J. *A psychology with a soul: psychosynthesis in evolutionary context*, Harmondsworth: Penguin, 1989, p.210

70   Wittine, B. 'Basic postulates for a transpersonal psychotherapy' in Valle and Halling *op. cit.* pp.269–87, esp. p.280

71   *Ibid.*

72   Grof, S. *Beyond the brain*, New York: State University of New York Press, 1985

73   Metzner, R. 'States of consciousness and transpersonal psychology' in Valle and Halling *op. cit.* pp.329–38

74   Myss, C. M. 'Intuition as a prerequisite for 21st century medicine', 'Energy and Medicine', first networking conference, London 30 November 1991

75   Wittine *op. cit.* p.282

76   Drob, S.L. 'The depth of the soul: James Hillman's vision of psychology', *Journal of Humanistic Psychology*, 39:3 (Summer 1999), Sage Publications, pp.56–72, esp. p.56

77   *Ibid.* p.56

78   Hillman, J. *Revisioning psychology*, New York: Harper, 1977, p.158

79   Wilber, K. *The spectrum of consciousness*, Wheaton ILL: Theosophical Publishing House, 1977

80   Sandweiss *op. cit.* p.14

81   Lasch, C. *The cult of narcissism: American life in an age of diminishing expectations*, New York: Norton, 1978

82   Duvall *op. cit.* p.8

83   Bugenthal *op. cit.* p.ix

CHAPTER SIX   **Scientists of the soul**

1   Besant, A. *The ancient wisdom* Aberdeen: Aberdeen University Press, 1899, pp.69–70

2   Moreland, J.P. 'Restoring substance to the soul of psychology', *Journal of Psychology and Theology*, 26:1 (1998), 29–43, esp. p.30

3   Davies, P. *God and the new physics*, Harmondsworth: Penguin, 1987, pp.79–80

4   *Ibid.*

5   *Ibid.* p.80

6   Moreland *op. cit.* p.29

7   *Ibid.*

8   Chopra, D. 'Power talk', interview with Anthony Robbins, Robbins Foundation, 1991

9   Bohm, D. *Wholeness and the implicate order*, London: Routledge, 1980

10   *Ibid.* p.209

11   *Ibid.*
12   Von Franz, M.L. *Number and time: reflections leading towards a unification of psychology and physics*, London: Rider, 1974, p.157
13   Chopra, D. *Quantum healing workshop*, New York: Sound Horizons Audio-Video Inc., 1990
14   Bohm *op. cit.* p.210
15   Zohar, D. *The quantum self*, London: Bloomsbury, 1990
16   Eddington, A. *The nature of the physical world*, Cambridge University Press, 1931, p.332
17   Finkelstein, D. 'A theory of the vacuum' in Sanders, S. (ed.) *Philosophy of the vacuum*, quoted Zohar *op. cit.* p.207
18   Wilson-Ross, N. *Hinduism, Buddhism, Zen*, London: Faber, 1973, p.121
19   Wilber, K. (ed.) *Defense of mysticism: quantum questions. Mystical writings of the world's greatest physicists*, Boston: New Science Library, 1984, p.206
20   Schrödinger, E. *What is life? and mind and matter*, London: Cambridge University Press, 1969, p.145
21   Dossey, L. *Recovering the soul: a scientific and spiritual search*, New York: Bantam, 1989, p. 176
22   *Ibid.* pp.176–7
23   Sperry, R. 'Annual review of neurosciences' quoted in R.Targ and K. Harary *The Mind Race* New York: Villard Books, 1984, p.xv
24   Pert, C. 'Molecules of emotion', interview by Martin Redfern, *Network*, 68 (1998), 9–11, esp. p.10
25   Pert, C. 'Interview with Candace Pert', *Omni* February 1982, p.64, quoted Sandweiss, S.H. *Spirit and the mind*, Andhra Pradesh: Sri Sathya Sai Books and Publications Trust, 1985, p.274
26   Pert *op. cit.* 1998, p.9
27   *Ibid.* p.10
28   Pert *op. cit.* 1985, p.274
29   Dossey *op. cit.* p.162
30   Markowitz, H. quoted *ibid.*
31   Davies *op. cit.* p.82
32   Sheldrake, R. *A new science of life: the hypothesis of formative causation*, London: Blond and Briggs, 1981
33   Eden, J. *Energetic healing; the merging of ancient and modern medical practices*, New York: Plenum, 1993, p.98
34   Sheldrake, R. The rebirth of nature, *Caduceus*, Winter 1991, 20–22, esp. p.22
35   Watson, L. *Lifetide: a biology of the unconscious*, London: Hodder and Stoughton, 1979, pp.156–60

36   *Ibid.* p.156
37   *Ibid.* p.157
38   Sheldrake *op. cit.* p.22
39   Eden *op. cit.* p.99
40   Chopra, D. *Creating affluence*, London: Transworld Press, 1999
41   Sheldrake *op. cit.* p.20
42   *Ibid.*
43   *Ibid.* pp.20–21
44   Schrodinger, E. *Science theory and man*, New York: Dover, 1957
45   Chopra *op. cit.* p.26
46   *Ibid.* p.79
47   Bloom, W. *Working with angels, fairies and nature spirits*, London: Book Club Associates, 1998
48   *Ibid.* p.137
49   *Ibid.* p.117
50   *Luke* 9:29
51   Day, L. with G. de la Warr *New worlds beyond the atom*, London: Vincent Stuart, 1956
52   Edelstein, E.J. and Ł. Edelstein *Asclepius: a collection and interpretation of his testimonies*, Baltimore, MD: Johns Hopkins University Press, 1945
53   Webster, C. 'The nineteenth century after-life of Paracelsus' in Cooter, R. (ed.) *Studies in the history of alternative medicine*, London: MacMillan, 1988, pp.79–88
54   Inglis, B. *Trance: a natural history of altered states of mind*, London: Paladin, 1990
55   Hearnshaw, L.S. *The shaping of modern psychology: an historical introduction*, London: Routledge, 1989
56   Day *op. cit.* p.13
57   Kenyon, J.J. 'Human energy fields: a doctor's view from science and medicine Part III' *Caduceus*, 21 (1993), 14–15, esp. p.14
58   Kilner, W.J. *The aura*, New York: Samuel Weiser, 1974
59   Adamenko, V. G. Kirlian photography, *Caduceus*, 12 (1990), 18–21
60   Inyushin, V.M. *On the biological essence of the Kirlian effect*, Kazach State University: Alma-Ata, 1968
61   Tomkins, C. and C. Bird *The secret life of plants*, London: Penguin, 1973
62   Adamenko *op. cit.*
63   Adamenko, V.G. 'Kirlian photography: a tool in the diagnosing of psychopathy', *Journal of Biological Photography*, 56 (1988), 385–8
64   Adamenko *op. cit.*

65 Maragoni, V., Evangelopolou, T. and J. Yfantapoulos 'Kirlian photograpy: a tool in the diagnosis of psychopathology', *Journal of Biological Photography*, 56 (1988), 3

66 Adamenko *op. cit.* 1990

67 Adamenko *ibid.* p.21

68 Quickenden, T.I. and S.S. Que Hee 'On the existence of mitogenetic radiation', *Speculative Scientific Technology*, 4 (1981), 453–64

69 Niggli, H.J. 'Biophotons: our body produces light! A review of work over the past seventy years on the emission of ultraweak electromagnetic radiation by human cells', *Network*, 68 (1998), 16–17

70 Colli, L., Facchini, U., Guidotti, G. Dugnami, A., Lonali, R. Arsengo, M. and O. Sommariva 'Further measurements on the bioluminescence of seedlings', *Experientia*, II (1955), 479–81

71 Popov, G.A. and B.N. Tarusova 'Nature of spontaneous luminescence of animal tissues', *Biophysics*, 8 (1963), 372

72 Quickenden, T.I. and Que Hee, S.S. 'The spectral distribution of the luminescence emitted during growth of the yeast *saccaromyces cervisiae* and its relationship to mitogenetic radiation', *Photochemical Photobiology*, 23 (1976), 201–204

73 Popp, F.A. and Ruth, B, 'Untersuchungen zur ultraschwachen Lumineszenz aus biologischen Systemen unter Berücksichtigung der Bedeutung fur die Arzneimittelforschung' ['Investigations into ultraweak bioluminescence in consideration of its value in medical research'], *Drug Research*, 27 (1977), 933–40

74 Inaba, H., Shimizu, Y., Tsuji, Y. and A. Yamagishi 'A photon-counting spectral analysing system of extra-weak chemi- and bioluminescence for biochemical applications, *Biochemical Photobiology*, 30 (1979), 169–75

75 Deveraj, B, Scott, R.Q., Roschger, P. and H. Inaba 'Ultraweak light emission from rat liver nuclei', *Photochemical Biology*, 154 (1991), 289–93

76 Popp, F.A., Li, K.H. and Q. Gu, *Recent advances in biophoton research and its applications*, Singapore World Scientific, 1992

77 Nagl, N.W. and F.A. Popp (1987) in Barrett, T.W. and H.A. Pohl (eds) *Energy transfer dynamics*, pp.248–56 quoted Ho, M.W. and F.A. Popp 'On the inherent lightness of being', *Caduceus*, 13 (1991), 28–31, esp. p.28

78 Ho, M.W. and F.A. Popp 'On the inherent lightness of being', *Caduceus*, 13 (1991), p.28

79 *Ibid.*

80   Konikiewicz, L.W. 'Kirlian photopgraphy in theory and clinical application', *Journal of Biological Photography Association*, 45:3 (1977), 115–37

81   Chouhan, P.S. 'Bioelectrographic images in normals and patients with cervical cancer', thesis submitted to the International Institute of Integral Human Sciences, 1989, cited Kenyon *op. cit.*

82   Adamenko *op. cit.* 1990, p.20

83   Becker, R.O. *Cross currents: the promise of electro-medicine*, Los Angeles: J.P. Tarcher, 1990

84   Becker, R.O. and G. Selden *The body electric: electromagnetism and the foundation of life*, New York: William Morrow and Co, 1985

85   Bruyere, R.L. *Wheels of light: chakras, auras and the healing energy of the body*, New York: Simon and Schuster, 1994

86   Motoyama, H. 'Prepolarization resistance of the skin as determined by the single square voltage pulse method', *Psychophysics*, 21 (1985), 5

87   Motoyama, H. 'Before polarization current and the acupuncture meridians', *Journal of Holistic Medicine*, 8 (1986), 1–12

88   Bruyere *op. cit.*

89   Reported Brennan, B.A. *Light emerging: the journey of personal healing*, New York: Bantam, 1993, p.18

90   Bloom *op. cit.*

91   Extract from Project report: a study of structural integration from neuromuscular, energyfield and emotional approaches, Chapter IV Energy field studies, Electronic aura study by V.V. Hunt, Appendix 1, pp.219–33 in Bruyere *op. cit.*

92   Reported Brennan *op. cit.*

93   *Ibid.* p.18

94   Bensoussan, A. 'Acupuncture meridians — myth or reality?' Part 2, *Complementary Therapies in Medicine*, 2 (1994), 80–85, esp. p.81

95   *Ibid.*

96   Zhang, C.L. and F.A. Popp 'Standing wave superposition hypothesis of acupuncture', unpublished manuscript, 1992, cited Rubik, B. 'Can western science provide a foundation for acupuncture?' *Alternative therapies*, 1:4 (September 1995), 41–7

97   Rubik, B. 'Can western science provide a foundation for acupuncture?' *Alternative therapies*, 1:4 (September 1995), p.44

98   Ho and Popp *op. cit.* p.28

99   Rubik *op. cit.* p.44

100 Kenyon *op. cit.* p.15

101 Zohar *op. cit.* p.68

102 *Ibid.* pp.68–70

103 Brennan, B. *Hands of light: a guide to healing through the human energy field*, New York: Bantam, 1988, p.89

104 Davies *op. cit.* pp.vii–ix

105 Kalweit, H. *Dreamtime and inner space: the world of the shaman*, translated by W. Wunsche, Boston and London: Shambhala, 1988, p.xii

106 Eliade, M. *Yoga, immortality and freedom*, Princeton University Press, 1958

107 Kalweit *op. cit.*

108 Bruyere *op. cit.* p.232

109 Kalweit *op. cit.* p.xiii

110 Dossey *op. cit.* p.32

111 Gauld, A. *Mediumship and survival: a century of investigations*, London: Granada Paladin, 1983

112 Reported Norton, C. 'Near-death experiences triggered by stress not delusion or mental illness', *Independent* 4 February 2000

113 Mindell, A. *Coma: key to awakening*, Boston and Shaftesbury: Shambhala, 1989

114 *Ibid.* p.53

115 *Ibid.* p.70

116 *Ibid.* p.77

117 *Ibid.* p.79

118 Kalweit *op. cit.* p.67

119 *Ibid.* p.58

120 Carpenter, E. *The drama of love and death*, 1912, quoted *ibid.* p.235

121 Gauld *op. cit.* p.222

122 Reported *Mysteries* BBC1 4 November 1999

123 Dossey *op. cit.* pp17–18

124 Sandweiss, S.H. *Spirit and the mind* Andhra Pradesh: Sri Sathya Sai Books and Publications Trust, 1985, p.276

125 Bloom *op. cit.*

126 Huxley, A. *The doors of perception*, London: Chatto and Windus, 1954

127 James, W. quoted Sandweiss *op. cit.*

128 Zohar *op. cit.* p.123

129 Dossey *op. cit.* pp.290–91

CHAPTER SEVEN **The therapeutic relationship: being a soul-mate**

1 Tredgold, A, *Psychological medicine*, Baltimore: Williams and Wilkins, 1945

2 Millenson, J.R.E. *Mind matters: psychological medicine in holistic practice*, Seattle: Eastland Press, 1995, p.5

3   Millenson *op. cit.* p.6

4   Stanway, A. *Alternative medicine: a guide to natural therapies*, Harmondsworth: Penguin, 1982, p.23

5   Chopra, D. *Quantum healing workshop*, New York: Sound Horizons Audio-Video Inc., 1990

6   Dossey, L. *Space, time and medicine*, Boulder and London: Shambhala, 1982, p.11

7   Ornstein, R.E. and D. Sobel *The healing brain: a radical new approach to health care*, London: MacMillan, 1988, p.24

8   Fulder, S. *How to survive medical treatment: an holistic approach to the risks and side effects of orthodox medicine*, London: Hodder and Stoughton, 1987

9   McTaggart, L. *What doctors don't tell you: the truth about the dangers of modern medicine*, London: Thorsons, 1996, pp.95–6

10   Coleman, V. 'The betrayal of trust', *European Medical Journal*, 4 (1994)

11   Illich, I. *Medical nemesis: the expropriation of health*, London: Marian Boyars, 1975

12   LeShan, L. *Holistic health: how to understand and use the revolution in medicine*, Wellingborough: Turnstone Press, 1984, p.1

13   Stanway *op. cit.*

14   Lindop, E. 'Factors associated with student and pupil wastage', *Journal of Advanced Nursing*, 1987, 751–8

15   Illiffe, S. *Strong medicine*, London: Lawrence and Wishart, 1988, p.5

16   Burg, M.A. 'Women's use of complementary medicine: combining mainstream medicine with alternative practices', 1966, reported in *Positive Health*, 18 (1997), p.49

17   Copper, R.A. and S.J. Stoflert 'Trends in the education and practice of alternative medical clinicians', *Health*, 15:3 (1996), 226–38

18   Sharma, U. *Complementary medicine today: practitioners and patients*, London: Tavistock, 1992, p.26

19   Mason, K. 'A new biomedical model', *Energy and Medicine*, *Networking Journal*, London: Turning Points, 1 (1992), 16–18

20   Chopra, D. *Creating affluence*, London: Transworld, 1999, pp.79–80

21   Laing, R.D *Did you used to be R.D. Laing?* Channel 4 interview 27 April 1991

22   Vincent, C. and A. Furnham 'Why do patients turn to complementary medicine?: an empirical study', *British Journal of Clinical Psychology*, 35:1 (1996), 37–48

23   Jung, C.G. *Modern man in search of a soul*, London: Routledge and Kegan Paul, 1966, p.56

24 Vithoulkas, G. *The science of homoeopathy,* New York: Grove, 1980, p.140

25 Jung, C.G. *Memories, dreams and reflections,* London: Fontana, 1972, p.155

26 Anderson, N. *Open secrets: a western guide to Tibetan Buddhism,* Harmondsworth: Penguin, 1982, p.88

27 Jourard, S.M. *The transparent self,* London: Van Nostrand, 1971

28 Lesh, T.V. 'Zen meditation and the development of empathy in counsellors' in Shapiro, D.H. and R.N. Walson *Meditation: classical and contemporary perspectives,* New York: Aldine, 1984, pp.152–87

29 Chopra *op. cit.* pp.89–90

30 Rogers, C.R. quoted Jourard *op. cit.* pp.144–5

31 Robbins, A. *Unlimited power,* New York: Simon and Schuster, 1997, p.230

32 *Ibid.*

33 Mindell, A. *Coma: key to awakening,* Boston and Shaftesbury: Shambhala, 1989, p.235

34 *Ibid.* p.61

35 Benor, D.J. 'Psychic healing: research evidence and potential for improving medical care' in Salmon, S.W. (ed.) *Alternative medicines: popular and policy perspectives,* London: Tavistock, 1984

36 Benor, D.J. 'Survey of spiritual healing research', *Complementary Medicine Research,* 4:3 (1990), 9–33

37 Weatherhead, L.D. *Psychology, religion and healing,* London: Hodder and Stoughton, 1951, p.50

38 *Acts of the Apostles* 8:7, 3:10, 9:32–4, 9:17, 14:8, 28:7–8

39 Edwards, H. *A guide to spirit healing,* tenth impression, London: Psychic Press, 1987

40 LeShan, L. *Clairvoyant reality: towards a general theory of the paranormal,* Wellingborough: Turnstone Press, 1982, p.102

41 Grad, B., Cadoret, R.J. and G.J. Paul 'The influence of an unorthodox method of treatment on wound healing in mice', *International Journal of Parapsychology,* 3 (1961), 5

42 Grad, B. 'A telekinetic effect on plant growth', *International Journal of Paranormal Psychology,* 5 (1963), 117–34

43 Barry, J. 'General and comparative study of the psychokinetic effect on a fungus culture', *Journal of Parapsychology,* 32 (1968), 237–43

44 Grad, B. 'Some biological effects of the "laying on of hands": a review of experiments with animals and plants', *Journal of the American Society for Psychical Research,* 59 (1965), 95–129

45 Grad, B. 'The "laying on of hands": implications for psychotherapy, gentling and the placebo effect', *International Journal of the Society for Psychical Research,* 61 (1967), 286–305

46   Miller, R.N. 'The positive effect of prayer on plants', *Psychic*, 22 April 1972

47   Holmes, E. 'Thought as energy', *Science of Mind Annual 1975*, cited Benor *op. cit.* 1990

48   Krieger, D. 'The imprimatur of nursing', *American Journal of Nursing*, 5 (1975), 484–7

49   Krieger, D. *The renaissance nurse*, Philadelphia: J.B. Winnicott, 1981

50   Krieger, D. 'Therapeutic Touch', *Mediscope*, Manchester Medical Gazette, Manchester University 611 (1982), 10–12

51   Benor *op. cit.* 1990

52   Krippner, S. *Galaxies of life: human aura in acupuncture and Kirlian photography*, New York: Gordon and Breach, 1973

53   Adamenko, V.G. Kirlian photography, *Caduceus*, 12 (1990), 18–21

54   Cade, C.M. and Coxhead, N. *The awakened mind: biofeedback and the development of higher states of awareness*, Shaftesbury: Wildwood House, 1979

55   Gerber, R. *Vibrational medicine: new choices for healing ourselves*, Santa Fe NM: Bear and Co., 1988, p.306

56   LeShan *op. cit.*

57   Ouseley, S.G.J. *The power of the rays: the science of colour healing*, eleventh impression, London: L.N. Fowler and Co. Ltd, 1981, p.84

58   Chopra *op. cit.* 1999, p.91

59   LeShan *op. cit.* p.148

60   Troward, T. *The Edinburgh lectures on mental science*, London: L.N. Fowler and Co., 1904, p.77

61   *Ibid.* p.80

62   Jupp, A.C. 'Parapsychology and the counsellor', unpublished dissertation (Diploma of Advanced Study in Education), Keele University, 1976

63   Jourard *op. cit.*

64   *Ibid.*

65   Cousins, N. *Human Options*, New York: W.W. Norton, 1981

66   Rossi, E.L. *The psychobiology of mind–body healing: new concepts in therapeutic hypnosis*, New York: W.W. Norton, 1986

67   Cousins *op. cit.*

68   Chopra, D. 'Power talk', interview with Anthony Robbins, Robbins Foundation, 1991

69   *Ibid.*

70   Siegel, B.S. *Peace, love and healing: bodymind communicaton and the path to self-healing*, London: Rider, 1990, p, 96

71   Reported Dossey *op. cit.*

72   Rossi *op. cit.*

73   Mindell *op. cit.* p.20
74   Chopra *op. cit.* 1991
75   Bowers, K.S. *Hypnosis for the seriously curious*, Monterey CA: Brooks/Cole, 1976, p.152
76   Bresnitz, S. (ed.) *The denial of stress*, New York: International Universities Press, 1983
77   Glaser, R. and J. Kiecolt-Glaser (eds) *Handbook of human stress and immunity*, San Diego: Academic Press, 1994
78   Clare, A. quoted Zifr, N. and M. Slerin *Challenging cancer*, New York: Routledge, 1992
79   Harrison, J. *Love your disease: its keeping you healthy*, London: Angus and Robertson, 1984, p.172
80   Robbins, A. 'Power talk', interview with Deepak Chopra, Robbins Foundation, 1991
81   Achterberg, J., Simonton, O.C. and S.M. Simonton 'Psychology of the exceptional cancer patient: a description of patients who outlive predicted life expectatncies', *Psychotherapy: Theory, Research and Practice*, 14 (1977), 416–22
82   Greer, S., Morris, T. and K.W. Pettingdale 'Psychological response to breast cancer: a controlled study', *Lancet*, 2 (1979), 785–7
83   Nicholas, R.S. *et al.* 'Stress and immunity in humans: modifying variables' in Glaser and Kiecolt-Glaser *op. cit.*
84   Cousins *op. cit.* pp.56–7
85   Cousins, N. Intangibles in medicine: an attempt at a balancing perspective, *Journal of the American Medical Association*, 260:16 (11 September 1988), 1610–12, esp. p.1612
86   LeShan *op. cit.* p.2
87   Gillie, O. 'Treatment of pain', *Health Independent*, 3 January 1989
88   Ornstein and Sobel *op. cit.* p.30
89   *Ibid.*
90   Stuttaford, T. 'A doctor writes', *The Times* 1 February 2000, p.17

CHAPTER EIGHT   **Divining the soul: diagnosis**

1   Chopra, D. *The seven spiritual laws of success*, London: Transworld, 1999, p.87
2   Dossey, L. *Space, time and medicine*, Boulder and London: Shambhala, 1982, p.vii
3   Chopra, D. *Perfect health: a complete mindbody guide*, New York: Bantam, 1992, p.47
4   Shealy, C.N. in Shealy, C.N. and C.M. Myss *The creation of health: merging traditional medicine with intuitive diagnosis*, Walpole NH: Stillpoint Publishing, 1988

5   Page, I. quoted *ibid.* p.47
6   Shealy *op. cit.* p.67
7   *Ibid.*
8   McGarey, W. *The Edgar Cayce Remedies*, London: Bantam, 1983
9   Benor, D.J. Science looks at healing, *Caduceus*, 6 (1989), 18–20
10 Extracted from Leichtman, R. 'The Way of Health', quoted Shealy *op. cit.* p.69
11 Myss, C.M. in Shealy, C.N. and C.M. Myss *The creation of health: merging traditional medicine with intuitive diagnosis*, Walpole NH: Stillpoint Publishing, 1988
12 *Ibid.* p.90
13 Oppenheimer, R. quoted Whitmont, E.C. *The alchemy of healing: psyche and soma*, Berkeley CA: North Atlantic Books, 1993, p.42
14 Whitmont, E.C. *The alchemy of healing: psyche and soma*, Berkeley CA: North Atlantic Books, 1993, p.58
15 *Ibid.*
16 *Ibid.* p.62
17 Chopra *op. cit.* 1999, pp.68–9
18 Myss *op. cit.* p.88
19 Pierrakos, J. *Core energetics*, Mendocino CA: Life Rhythm, 1990
20 Damasio, A. *The feeling of what happens: body, emotion and the making of consciousness*, London: Heinemann, 1999
21 Karagulla, S. *Breakthrough to creativity*, Santa Monica CA: C.A. de Vorss, 1967
22 Davidson, J. *Subtle energy*, Saffron Walden:, C.W. Daniels and Co., 1987
23 Bell, A.H. (ed.) *Practical dowsing: a symposium*, London: G. Bell and Sons, 1965
24 Tansley, D.V. 'Radionics' in A. Hill (ed.) *Unconventional medicine*, London: New English Library, 1979
25 *Ibid.* p.161
26 Westlake, A.T. *A history of psionic medicine*, London: Psionic Medicine Society, 1977
27 Brennan, B. *Hands of light: a guide to healing through the human energy field*, New York: Bantam, 1988
28 Gerber, R. *Vibrational medicine: new choices for healing ourselves*, Santa Fe NM: Bear and Co., 1988
29 *Ibid.* p.227
30 Von Sratten, M. 'Iris diagnosis' in A. Hill (ed.) *Unconventional medicine*, London: New English Library, 1979, p.39
31 Mototyama, H. 'Yoga and acupuncture' in Gharote, D. and M.

Lockhart (eds) *The art of survival: a guide to yoga therapy*, London: Unwin Hyman, 1987

32   Achterberg, J. *Imagery in healing: shamanism and modern medicine*, London: Routledge, 1985, p.56

33   *Ibid.* pp.65–6

34   Oaklander, V. *Windows to our children: a gestalt therapy approach to children and adolescents*, Utah: Real People's Press, 1978

35   Simonton, O.C., Matthews-Simonton, S.M. and J. Creighton *Getting well again*, New York: Bantam, 1978

36   Myss *op. cit.*

37   *Ibid.* p.92

38   Achterberg *op. cit.* pp.101–102

39   Whitmont *op. cit.* p.62

40   *Ibid.* p.62

CHAPTER NINE   **Treating the soul**

1   British Medical Association Report of the Boards of Science and Education on Alternative Therapy, London, 1986, pp.61–75 in Saks, M. (ed.) *Alternative Medicine in Britain*, Oxford: Clarendon Press, 1992, pp.211–31

2   Graham, H. *Complementary therapies in context: the psychology of healing*, London: Jessica Kingsley, 1999

3   Vithoulkas, G. *The science of homoeopathy*, Wellingborough: Thorsons, 1986, p.99

4   Whitmont, E.C. *The alchemy of healing: psyche and soma*, Berkeley CA: North Atlantic Books, 1993

5   Vithoulkas *op. cit.* p.93

6   Hamlyn, E. *The healing art of homoeopathy: the Organon of Samuel Hahnemann*, Beaconsfield: Beaconsfield Publishing, 1979

7   Vithoulkas *op. cit.* p.101

8   *Ibid.* p.104

9   Capra, F. *The turning point: science, society and the rising culture*, London: Wildwood House, 1982, p.377

10   Whitmont *op. cit.* p.46

11   *Ibid.* p.7

12   *Ibid.*

13   Tiller, W. Foreword to Vithoulkas *op. cit.* p.xii

14   Fisher, P. 'The development of research methodology in homoeopathy', *Complementary Therapies in Nursing and Midwifery*, 1 (1995), 168–74, esp. p.170

15   Kliejnem, J., Knipschild, P. and G. ter Riet 'Clinical trials of homeopathy', *British Medical Journal*, 302 (1991), 316–23

16   Bach, E. quoted Ramsall, J. and N. Murray *Questions and answers: clarifying the basic principles of Bach Flower Remedies*, Mount Vernon: Mount Vernon Bach Centre, 1987, p.12

17   Wright, M.S. *Flower Essences*, Warrenton VA: Perelandra Ltd, 1988, p.3

18   Leonardi quoted Morrison, H. 'Nature's Prozac', *Natural Health*, May/June (1995), pp.80–128, esp. p.85

19   Pelletier, K.S. and D.L. Herzing 'Psychoneuroimmunology: towards a mind–body model' in Sheikh, A.A. and K.S. Sheikh *Eastern and Western approaches to healing: ancient wisdom and modern knowledge*, New York: Wiley, 1989, pp.344–94

20   Kissen, D.M. and H.J. Eysenck 'Personality in male lung cancer patients', *British Medical Journal*, 36 (1962), 123–7

21   LeShan, L. 'An emotional life-history pattern associated with neoplastic disease', *Annals of the New York Academy of Sciences*, 125 (1966), 780–93

22   Solomon, G.F. 'Emotions, stress, the CNS and immunity', second Conference on Psychophysiological Aspects of Cancer, *Annals of the New York Academy of Sciences*, (1969) 335–42

23   Abse, D.W. *et al.* 'Personality and behavior characteristics of lung cancer patients', *Journal of Psychosomatic Research*, (1974), 1001–13

24   Reich, W. *Reich speaks of Freud*, Harmondsworth: Penguin, 1975

25   Manning, M. 'Self healing', holistic health workshop, Farnham Holistic Health Centre, 30 April 1988

26   Greer, S., Morris, T. and K.W. Pettingdale 'Psychological responses to breast cancer: effect and outcome', *Lancet*, 2 (1979), 785–9

27   Derogatis, L., Abeloff, M. and N. Melisaratos 'Psychological coping mechanisms and survival time in metastatic breast cancer', *Journal of American Medical Association*, 242 (1979), 1504–1508

28   Temoshok, L. and B.W. Heller 'Biopsychosocial studies of cutaneous malignant melonomas: psychosocial factors associated with prognostic indicators, progression, psychophysiology and tumor-host response', *Social Science and Medicine*, 20:8 (1985), 833–40

29   Meares, A. 'Meditation: a psychological approach to cancer treatment', *Practitioner*, 222 (1979), 119–22

30   Hughes, J. *Cancer and emotion: psychological preludes and reactions to cancer*, Chichester: Wiley, 1987

31   Rosch, P.J. 'Stress and cancer' in C.L. Cooper (ed.) *Stress and cancer*, Chichester: Wiley, 1984

32   Temoshok, L. and B.W. Heller 'Stress and Type C versus epidemiological risk factors in melonoma', paper presented at the

89th Annual Convention of the American Psychological Association, Los Angeles, 1981, reported Temoskok and Heller *op. cit.*

33 Dattore, P.J., Schontz, F.C. and L. Coyne 'Premorbid personality differentiation of cancer and non-cancer groups: a test of the hypothesis of cancer proneness', *Journal of Consulting and Clinical Hypnosis*, 48 (1980), 388–94

34 Moos, R.H. 'Personality factors associated with rheumatoid arthritis: review', *Journal of Chronic Disorders*, (1969), 1741

35 Whitacre, C.C., Cummings, S.O. and A.C. Griffin 'The effects of stress on autoimmune disease' in Glaser, R. and J. Kiecolt-Glaser (eds) *Handbook of human stress and immunity*, San Diego: Academic Press, 1994, p.80

36 Chopra, D. *Quantum healing*, New York: Bantam, 1989, p.71

37 Schauss, A.G. 'Tranquilising effect of color reduces aggressive behaviour and potential violence', *Journal of Orthomolecular Psychiatry*, 84 (1974), 218 221

38 Aaranson, B.S. 'Color perception and affect', *American Journal of Clinical Hypnosis*, (1971), 1438–41

39 Glaser, R. and J. Kiecolt-Glaser (eds) *Handbook of human stress and immunity*, San Diego: Academic Press, 1994

40 Whitacre *et al. op. cit.* p.79–80

41 Kanner, A.D. *et al.* 'Comparison of two modes of stress measurement, daily hassles and upsets versus major life events', *Journal of Behavioral Medicine*, (1981), 1–39

42 Lazarus, K.S. 'Little hassles can be hazardous to health', *Psychology Today*, 15 (1981), 58–68

43 Ecker, R. *The stress myth*, Tring: Lion Publishing, 1989

44 Kobasa. S.C., Maddi, S. and S. Kahn Hardiness and health: a prospective study, *Journal of Personality and Social Science*, 42 (1982), 168–77

45 *Ibid.*

46 Achterberg, J., Simonton, S.M. and O.C. Simonton 'Psychology of the exceptional cancer patient: a description of patients who outlive predicted life expectancies', *Psychotherapy: Theory, Research and Practice*, 14:4 (1977), 416–22

47 Greer *et al. op. cit.*

48 Achterberg *et al. op. cit.*

49 Jampolsky, G.C. *Love is letting go of fear*, Berkeley CA: Celestial Arts, 1979

50 Muschel, I.J. 'Pet therapy with terminal cancer patients', *Journal of Contemporary Social Work*, (1984), 451–8

51 Baun M.M. *et al.* 'Effects of bonding vs. non-bonding on the physiological effects of petting', Proceedings of the Conferences on the Human–Animal Bond, University of Minnesota, 13–14 June 1983 and University of California 17–18 June 1983

52 Friedman, E. *et al.* Social interaction and blood pressure: influence of animal companions, *Journal of Nervous and Mental Disease*, 171:8 (1983), 461–5

53 Jenkins, J. 'Physiological effects of petting a companion animal, unpublished Masters thesis', San Francisco State University, 1984, cited Pelletier and Herzing *op. cit.*

54 Katcher, A. 'Interactions between people and their pets' in Fogle, B. (ed.) *Interrelations between people and pets*, Springfield ILL: Thomas, 1981

55 Arehart-Treichel, J. 'Pets: the health benefits', *Science News*, 121 (1982), 220–24

56 Holden, R.C. 'Human–animal relationship under scrutiny', *Science*, 214 (1981), 418–20

57 Smith, B. 'Project inreach: a program to explore the ability of Atlantic bottlenose dolphins to elicit communication responses from autistic children' in Katcher, A. and A. Beck (eds) *New perspectives on our life with companion animals*, Philadelphia: University of Philadelphia Press, 1982

58 Arkow, P. *Dynamic relationships in practice: animals in the helping professions*, Alameda CA: The Latham Foundation, 1984

59 McCulloch, M.I. 'Animal facilitated therapy: an overview', *California Veterinarian*, 8 (1982), 13–24

60 Corson, S.A. and E. O'Leary Corson 'Pet animals as nonverbal communication mediators in psychotherapy in institutional settings' in *Ethology and nonverbal communication in mental health: an interdisciplinary biopsychosocial exploration*, Oxford: Pergamon, 1979, pp.83–110

61 Corson, S.A. *et al.* 'Pet-facilitated psychotherapy in a hospital setting' in Masserman, J.H. (ed.) *Current Psychiatric Therapies*, 15 (1975)

62 Corson, S.A. *et al.* 'Pet dogs as non-verbal communication links in hospital psychiatry', *Comprehensive Psychiatry*, 18 (1977), pp.61–72

63 Mugford, R.A. and J.G. McComisky 'Some recent work on the psychotherapeutic value of caged birds with old people' in Anderson, R.S. (ed.) *Pet animals and Society*, London: Bailliere Tindall, 1975

64 Cousins, N. *Anatomy of an illness as perceived by a patient: reflections on healing and regeneration*, London: Bantam, 1981

65 Minchoff, K.M., Baker, B. and K.H. Dillon 'Positive emotional states and enhancement of the immune system', *International Journal of Psychiatric Medicine*, 15 (1985), 13–17

66 Cousins *op. cit.* p.138

67 Adams, E.R. and F.A. McGuire 'Is laughter the best medicine?' *Activities, Adaptation, Aging*, 8 (1986)

68 Minchoff, K.M., Baker, B. and K.H. Dillon *op. cit.*

69 Newbon, B.W. 'The use of hypnosis in the treatment of cancer patients: a 5-year report', presented at the Annual Scientific Progress of the American Association of Clinical Hypnosis, Minneapolis, 1980

70 Robbins, A. *Unlimited power*, New York: Simon and Schuster, 1997, p.107

71 *Ibid.* p.57

72 Robbins, A. 'Power talk', interview with Deepak Chopra, Robbins Foundation, 1991

73 Chopra, D. 'Power talk', interview with Anthony Robbins, Robbins Foundation, 1991

74 *Ibid.*

75 Robbins *op. cit.* p.44

76 Troward, T. *The Edinburgh lectures on mental health*, London: L.N. Fowler and Co. Ltd, 1904, p.74

77 Chopra, D. *The seven spiritual laws of success*, New York: Bantam, 1999, p.10

78 *Ibid.* pp.4–5

79 Troward *op. cit.*

80 LeShan, L. *Clairvoyant reality: towards a general theory of the paranormal*, Wellingborough: Turnstone Press, 1982

81 Troward *op. cit.* p.73–4

82 *Ibid.* p.78

83 *Ibid.* p.79

84 LeShan op.cit. p.150

85 Nicholas, R.S. *et al.* 'Stress and immunity in humans: modifying variables' in Glaser, R. and J. Kiecolt-Glaser (eds) *Handbook of human stress and immunity*, San Diego: Academic Press, 1994

86 *Ibid.*

87 Kubler-Ross, E. *On death and dying*, London: Tavistock, 1977

88 McNiff, S. *Art as medicine*, London: Piatkus, 1992, p.18

89 Harwood, R. *All the world's a stage*, London: Secker and Warburg, 1984, pp.53–4

90 Whitmont *op. cit.* p.63

POSTSCRIPT

1   Dossey, L. *Recovering the soul: a scientific and spiritual search,* New York: Bantam, 1989

2   *Ibid.* p.9

3   *Ibid.* p.8

INDEX